Early-life Environmental Exposure and Disease

Yankai Xia
Editor

Early-life Environmental Exposure and Disease

Facts and Perspectives

Springer

Editor
Yankai Xia
School of Public Health
Nanjing Medical University
Nanjing, Jiangsu, China

ISBN 978-981-15-3796-7 ISBN 978-981-15-3797-4 (eBook)
https://doi.org/10.1007/978-981-15-3797-4

This Springer imprint is published by the registered company Springer Nature Singapore Pte Ltd.
The registered company address is: 152 Beach Road, #21-01/04 Gateway East, Singapore 189721, Singapore

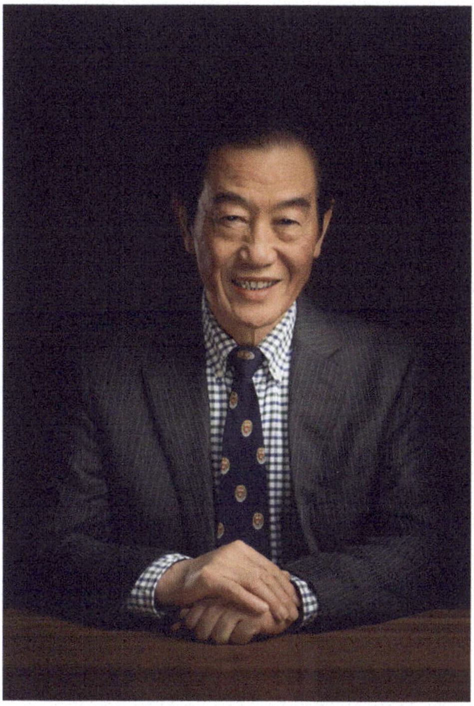

I dedicate this book to Professor Xinru Wang, for his great contributions in the field of environment and health.

Preface

Man and nature have always coexisted in harmony. Nature produces resources necessary for humankind's survival and development. In the long history of the Earth, various substances in the environment have cultivated living organisms ranging from prokaryotes to humans, who have constantly taken advantage of nature's great capacity for self-regulation to modify the environment to suit their needs. Regrettably, the rapid development of human activities has broken this balance, leading to resource shortages and severe environmental contamination, among other irreversible damages. Environmental pollutants spread and circulate in nature and eventually enter the human body, potentially causing changes in hormones, proteins, metabolites, and so on, ultimately resulting in various adverse health effects. Particularly, it should be noted that people are particularly vulnerable to these environmental risks in early life and pollutant exposure during this crucial period could result in intergenerational effects.

Nowadays, as life expectancy has risen to an unprecedented level, more attention has been paid to environmental chemical exposure, which is ubiquitous yet largely invisible. Environmental exposures include all the chemicals and compounds with which we come into contact. Evidence suggests that the elementary composition of the human body is identical with that of the Earth's crust, mainly as a result of the exchange of substances through metabolism, evidencing the intimate connection that the human body has with its surroundings. Toxins discharged as a result of industrial production or daily living activities enter the human body directly through polluted air, water, and soil or indirectly through food intake, due to the biomagnification properties of plants and animals.

Environmental chemical pollutants can enter the human body via inhalation, ingestion, or dermal contact, with inhalation being the most rapid route of uptake. Inhalation is the major route of polluted air and tobacco smoke exposure, which consists mostly of particulate matter (PM), heavy metals like lead and cadmium, polycyclic aromatic hydrocarbons (PAHs), volatile organic compounds (VOCs), and carbonyls. Ingestion exposure mainly occurs via consumption of contaminated food and drink or via the intentional or inadvertent non-dietary ingestion of soil, dust, or chemical residues on surfaces or objects containing complex chemical contaminants, which include pesticides, polybrominated diphenyl ethers (PBDEs), phenols, perfluorinated alkyl substances (PFAS), and heavy metals like lead and mercury. Especially for young children, ingestion exposure through hand-to-mouth or object-to-mouth activity must not be overlooked. Dermal exposure can result from skin contact with contaminated environmental media, including water, sediment, outdoor soil or dust, surfaces, and personal care products containing triclosan, oxybenzone, parabens, and heavy metals like lead and cadmium.

Humans encounter hundreds or even thousands of different environmental pollutants daily. Many substances appear almost harmless, others may be potentially harmful but are uneasily absorbed by the human body, and others may be incredibly harmful, even in very small quantities. Generally, environmental chemicals such as those listed in the above paragraph have the following characteristics. First, they affect a wide area and a large population. Second, there is a long term of exposure between the pollutant and the affected humans. Third, the environmental chemicals are commonly transformed and metabolized in nature and in humans. Fourth, a variety of substances can act on the human body at the same time, resulting in a joint effect. Fifth, humans are affected by environmental chemicals to a greater degree due to biomagnification. Considering the level and variety of contaminants in all environmental media, the chronic exposure that people face eventually leads to a high risk of adverse health effects.

Comprehensive assessment of exposure is particularly important. In addition to substances necessary for human survival, many known and potential toxins can be detected in blood, urine, hair, fingernails, and other tissues, acting as biomarkers of exposure. Different poisons can damage different systems of the human body, with special attention being paid to the nervous system, immune system, and reproductive system, as well as childhood growth and development. For example, the accumulation of lead in the body may cause syndromes affecting the nervous system, digestive system, and circulatory system, such as sensory and motor disorders, lead colic, and anemia. Due to the individual and combined effects of various toxins, the human body can experience damage at the system, organ, tissue, and cellular levels.

While such damage can occur in both males and females of all ages, women during pregnancy and lactation periods, infants and children are more sensitive to toxins, such that the same dosage of exposure may lead to more severe outcomes. For instance, studies indicate that prenatal exposure to organophosphate pesticides may not only cause health damage to the mother's neural system but also result in preterm birth and attention deficit hyperactivity disorder (ADHD) in the offspring. Given the potential for health damage to two or more generations, more studies ought to focus on the effects of toxins at these special stages, with further discussion on appropriate production limits to be enforced for the sake of prevention.

The issue of early-life environmental exposure and resulting diseases is one of the hottest topics in life sciences. Exposure to adverse environmental conditions during early life, a period critical for tissue organogenesis and functional development, can lead to lifelong negative health effects. The Developmental Origins of Health and Disease (DOHaD) theory posits that exposure to various substances during early life is an important potential contributor to long-term disease. From this theory, it can be inferred that the increased incidence of chronic noncommunicable diseases, such as allergic diseases, neurobehavioral developmental disorders, and metabolic disorders, can be attributed in part to harmful environmental exposure.

Adverse environmental conditions before conception, in utero, and during infancy can lead to negative health effects during the subsequent lifetime of the exposed individuals. Concerning the central topic of early-life environmental exposure and disease, our book is divided into five parts, starting with an overview of environmental exposure measurement and evaluation, followed by a review of the effects of various exposures like tobacco smoke, pesticides, metals, and stress on offspring's health. Next is a discussion of the developmental origins of various childhood diseases that affect growth, neural development, and reproductive health, as well as allergic diseases, highlighting the importance of longitudinal studies that measure exposure at potentially sensitive time points during childhood. The book then provides up-to-date evidence of early-life environmental exposure's intergenerational/transgenerational effects, especially through genetic and epigenetic pathways, underlining a crucial point in the book's discussion of pollutants' far-reaching potential for harm (Fig. 1).

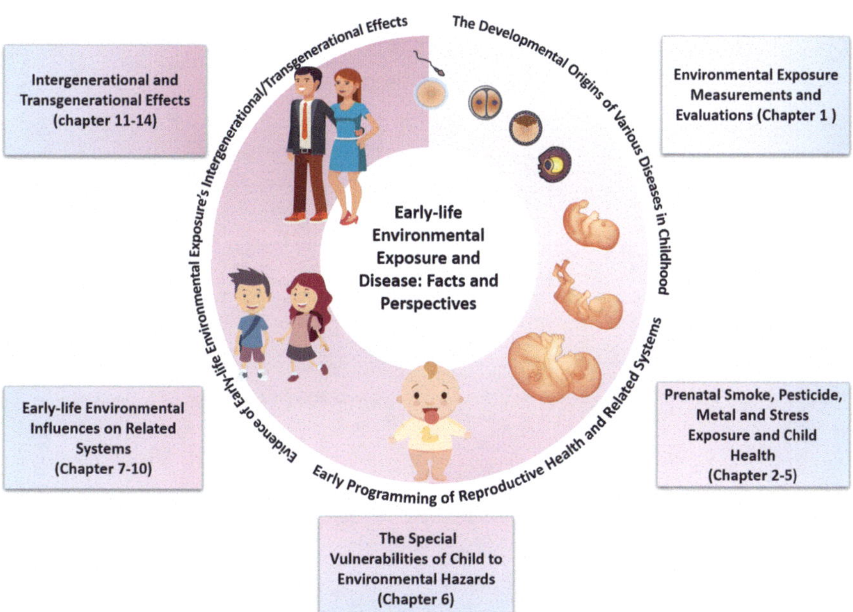

Fig. 1 The structure diagram of this book

The book provides readers a thorough understanding of the predominating perspectives of epidemiologic, clinical, and basic science studies in the burgeoning area of early-life environmental exposure and diseases. Importantly, the book also includes a comprehensive discussion of possible preventive measures. Unlike in any other book, we synthesize the existing knowledge of environmental exposure's impact on children's health in early life, systematically expounding different sources of environmental exposure and their impact on childhood development and disease and adding new discoveries and insights into their intergenerational/transgenerational effects.

With great pleasure, we extend our sincere thanks to all our well-qualified and internationally renowned contributors from various countries for providing the important, authoritative, and scientific information and technology to make this book a reality. Our contributors have enriched the book with cutting-edge knowledge and informative illustrations, tables, and figures. We are extremely thankful to Springer Nature for completing the review process expeditiously for publication. Finally, we express heartfelt thanks to our family members and friends for all the support they have provided in the preparation of this book.

In short, we hope for harmony between man and nature!

Nanjing, China Yankai Xia

Cover Page

Ministry of Education and Shanghai Key Laboratory of Children's Environmental Health, Institute of Early Life Health, Xinhua Hospital, Shanghai Jiao Tong University School of Medicine. junjimzhang@sina.com

It has been over 30 years since Dr. David Barker, an epidemiologist in U.K., published his milestone paper on a simple observation of the inverse association between birthweight and the risk of death due to coronary heart disease later in life. The theory of "fetal programming" or "Developmental Origin of Health and Disease (DOHaD)" has been confirmed both in human epidemiologic investigations and animal studies, and is now widely accepted. It has also become clear that the critical window of fetal programming and developmental elasticity is in early life, commonly defined as from conception to 2 years of age (approximately 1,000 days). Insults from external and internal sources on embryo, fetus and infant may leave a permanent mark with important health implications in future life. The underlying biological mechanisms are not totally clear but epigenetic changes caused by the insults have been proposed. In this emerging area, environmental exposure to pollutants and psychosocial factors during pregnancy and infancy are the prominent examples of such insults that have drawn keen interest worldwide.

The editor of this book, Professor Yankai Xia, Dean of School of Public Health, the Nanjing Medical University, China, led a team of esteemed international experts in the field of early-life environmental health, and produced this informative and timely book. It covers comprehensive yet closely related topics, ranging from common environmental exposures to health outcomes in children and adults. What makes this book more valuable and refreshing is that it addresses some practical issues such as cautions on contamination and other potential pitfalls in biosample collection, and includes topics such as paternal environmental exposure, impact of e-cigarettes, transgenerational effects, and molecular mechanisms.

The contents of this book are well organized, systematic and easy to read. The gathered evidence is up-to-date. This book is truly an objective review of rich scientific evidence, making it a “must-have” by researchers and graduate students in this field. Clinicians engaging in maternal and child health who often encounter patients with suspected environmental exposures may also find it a useful reference. More importantly, as two-thirds of the early-life window is at postpartum, this precious time may offer an opportunity to initiate clinical interventions for fetal reprogramming and avoid health consequences later in life. Furthermore, the evidence collected by this book may serve as a scientific basis for policy-makers to set up environment and health policies that could have wide and long-term impacts on human health.

Jun Jim Zhang
junjimzhang@sina.com

Acknowledgments

This book was supported by NSFC-NIH Biomedical collaborative research program (No. 81961128022) and the Priority Academic Program for the Development of Jiangsu Higher Education Institutions (Public Health and Preventive Medicine)

Contents

Environmental Exposure Measurements and Evaluations

Yankai Xia, Xu Wang, and Minjian Chen

1 Introduction

Environmental exposure is defined as the exposure of individuals to environmental factors in a specific period. The environmental factors include biological, chemical, physical, and sociopsychological factors [1].

Exposure assessment is a quantitative process for the measurement and following evaluation of exposure burden. Exposure assessment is an important part of environmental health risk assessment [2], and we need to identify the potential exposure population. Therefore, the understanding of environmental exposure measurements and evaluations is important for the assessment and prediction of the health risk caused by environmental factors in early life. Among the environmental factors, the studies on the assessment of chemical factor exposure in early life were widely reported.

This chapter focused on the topic of chemical exposure assessment. The chemical exposure assessment includes internal and external exposure assessment [3], and the future of a more comprehensive environmental exposure assessment was discussed, and the outline of the chapter is shown in Fig. 1.

2 Internal Exposure Assessment

Internal exposure assessment is to recruit a certain number of representative populations after exposure, collect and analyze the biomarkers in the human biomaterials, and estimate the exposure of environmental pollutants in biomaterials through the concentration of biomarkers [4].

Y. Xia · X. Wang · M. Chen (✉)
School of Public Health, Nanjing Medical University, Nanjing, China
e-mail: minjianchen@njmu.edu.cn

Y. Xia (ed.), *Early-life Environmental Exposure and Disease*,
https://doi.org/10.1007/978-981-15-3797-4_1

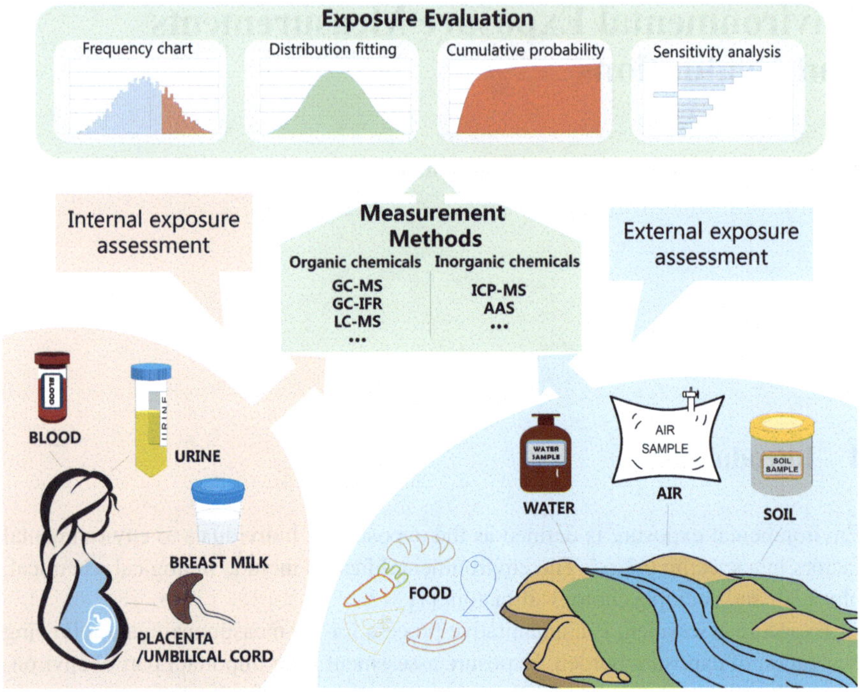

Fig. 1 Outline of the chapter

2.1 *Biomarkers*

Biomarkers might be specific to chemicals, so that the content of biomarkers is related to the degree of chemical exposure. For the biomarker of exposure, the process of chemical absorption, distribution, metabolism, and excretion (ADME) must be understood. This is important for choosing the appropriate biomaterials [5].

2.2 *Biomaterials*

In the selection of biomaterials, the ADME process of chemicals should be studied [6]. After the chemicals are absorbed into the blood, they are distributed to the whole body, so the blood is an important biomaterial for the detection of chemical exposures. The body's storage depot includes plasma proteins, the liver, the kidney, adipose tissue, and bone. Therefore, adipose tissue is also commonly used as a biomaterial for the detection of chemical exposures. One of the main ways of excretion is the kidney, so urine is also a main biomaterial. Chemicals can also be excreted through hair and nails, so these two are also major biomaterials. It should be noted that the placenta and umbilical cord (blood) are the main media of chemical transfer between mother and infant, and they are important biomaterials for chemical detection in early life.

Blood

After the chemicals are absorbed into the blood, they are distributed and metabolized, and the chemicals may also be released into the blood from the storage depot, so the blood is important for chemical internal exposure detection. Blood samples are easy to be obtained and can be divided into serum and plasma. Plasma samples are anticoagulated. Serum samples often encounter the problem of hemolysis, but the use of anticoagulants in plasma samples may cause the risk of pollution in the detection of some chemicals [7]. Therefore, for plasma samples, the blank samples should be tested to estimate the experiment contamination. Many unstable chemicals in blood may be oxidized, polymerized, or degraded after collection. And we need to ensure the reproducibility of the experiment and prevent the obvious dynamic changes of chemicals in blood after collection. Thus, standardized procedure should be conducted during and after blood sample collection. Attention should also be paid to fasting status, blood collection time and method, anticoagulant usage, blood collection volume, sample storage condition, hemolysis, etc. For example, if chemicals have a short half-life in the human body and are abundant in the food, the fasting status may have an obvious impact on these chemicals' levels in the blood [8].

Dry blood spots on paper are the standard clinical sample types for neonatal screening programs around the world [9]. The sample is collected by puncturing the infant's heel with the vent tube and dropping each drop of blood onto the standard paper, so that each blood spot in the collected blood sample contains about 50 μ l of blood. This kind of sample is easy to be obtained because of its clinical use, and can be used in exposure science [10]. However, the sample of this method has been dried with the risk of loss of some chemicals, and the chemicals on the paper can be contaminated by some chemicals. And the concentration of analyte in the center and periphery of the spot is often different.

Urine

Urine reflects the excretion of chemicals exposed to humans. Therefore, to select biomarkers in urine, we need to fully understand the ADME process of chemicals. Generally, morning urine is the commonly used sample [11]. Due to the large content of polar chemicals in urine, the specific polar chemical is the common detection target. The adequate separation of polar chemicals should be considered when using a chromatography-based method to avoid the detection interference/matrix effects. The advantages of urine samples are noninvasive, easy to be obtained, and large volume. Therefore, it is suitable for infant sample collection. Diapers are also used for urine collection [12], but attention should be paid to chemical loss and contamination. Urine samples are affected by the drinking and sweating of the subjects, and there is a phenomenon of urine concentration and dilution. Generally, urine creatinine and specific gravity are used for concentration detection correction [13].

Placenta

The placenta is a special endocrine organ during pregnancy. It is the place of chemical and metabolic waste exchange between mother and fetus [14]. The placenta is easy to be obtained in childbirth. It should be noted that the placenta has a barrier function [15], so it is necessary to distinguish its maternal side and fetal side. The blood supply of the mother penetrates from the maternal side of the placenta to the fetal side. There may be inhomogeneity in the concentration of chemicals on the maternal and fetal sides of the placenta [16]. Therefore, the analysis of the concentration of chemicals should not be randomly selected in any part of the placenta; otherwise, it may produce inaccurate estimation.

Umbilical Cord (Blood)

The umbilical cord is the only channel connecting the mother and the fetus. Its collection is simple and noninvasive. The determination of the chemicals in the umbilical cord or cord blood can provide a direct evaluation for the chemical exposure of the fetus in the mother [17]. Compared with the determination of the maternal blood, it can more directly link to the exposure of the fetus [18]. Notably, some researchers have pointed out that the umbilical cord is the best sample to evaluate the fetal exposure status of persistent organic pollutants (POPs) [19]. The umbilical cord (blood) has been used to determine trace metals (such as mercury and cadmium), polychlorinated biphenyls (PCBs), and organochlorine pesticides for early life exposure [20].

Breast Milk

Breastfeeding has always been considered as the safest and best way for healthy mothers to feed their babies. However, due to environmental pollution, it cannot be ignored that breast milk is also a way of excretion of chemicals, reflecting the internal exposure of the mother and indirectly revealing the exposure of the baby [21]. The pollutants that have been reported to be detected in human milk include pesticides, herbicides, drugs, industrial chemicals, toxic metals, and radionuclides. Among them, fat-soluble pollutants are the most important [22]. Breast milk contains milk fat. In addition, due to the concentration of milk tube, the concentration of pollutants in milk sometimes is several times higher than that in the blood of lactating mothers.

Saliva

Saliva has an excretory function, so it can reflect the internal exposure of chemicals [23]. Saliva sample collection is simple and noninvasive. Especially for the detection of chemicals in children, the collection of saliva has a higher acceptance. Attention should be paid to the standardization of methods when collecting saliva samples. Food and drink residues in the mouth can cause experiment contamination, which can be avoided by collecting saliva without eating for a period of at least 2–3 h [24]. In addition, the volume of saliva is small, so the error caused by evaporation should be avoided.

Hair

Hair sampling is simple and painless, which is easy to be stored. In addition, hair chemicals may reflect the dynamic changes of human chemical exposure in a certain period of time [25], so it has been used as an ideal biomaterial. Hair is mainly used for the detection of trace elements and drugs, such as arsenic and mercury [26]. The disadvantage of hair is that it is easy to be polluted by the environment, such as the substances passed by hand, the chemicals used in hair routine, and the deposition of atmospheric particles or aerosols in the environment. The use of washing to remove contamination may introduce new contamination [27]. Therefore, when using hair for internal exposure detection, we should fully consider the possible contamination of target chemicals.

Nails
Nail is a way of excretion of chemicals. The advantage is that nails are easy to be collected and stored. When the population is recruited, the sampling of children's nails can be simple, rapid, and easily accepted. The growth of foot nails can accurately record the metabolism of trace elements (such as arsenic, lead, cadmium, copper, and zinc) during this period [28]. Some studies have pointed out that nails can reflect chemical intake 6–12 months ago [28]. In addition, nails can also reflect drug exposure [29].

Teeth
Because deciduous teeth fall off naturally, they can be called noninvasive biomaterials, and they are easy to be stored. Another advantage of teeth is that they can record the exposure of chemicals for a long time (from birth to falling off) [30]. Teeth are mainly used to reflect the exposure of elements, such as calcium, lead, fluorine, and manganese [31, 32].

3 External Exposure Assessment

External exposure assessment measures the content of chemicals in the media (such as atmosphere, soil, water, personal care products, food, etc.) and calculates the level of individual exposure by combining the information of exposure source, route, and time [33]. External exposure assessment method is widely used in the science of exposure assessment, especially for large-sample-size human population study because of its easy collection and calculation [34]. The disadvantage of the external exposure method is that it ignores the bioavailability of chemicals in the human body [35]. In addition, if the external exposure information collection is not comprehensive, it may also cause incomplete evaluation [35]. These may lead to some deviation in the evaluation. The materials of external exposure analysis including air, water, and soil are disscussed.

Air
Air samples mainly reflect the chemicals entering the human body through the respiratory tract, and some chemicals can also enter the human body through the air due to swallowing into the digestive tract. The existing forms of air pollutants include gas, vapor, and aerosol. In general, direct collection method and enrichment

collection method can be used to collect air samples [36]. The direct collection method is suitable for the situation of high concentration of chemicals in the atmosphere. Generally, syringes, plastic bags, collection tubes, and vacuum bottles can be used to collect samples. The collection time is generally short, reflecting the situation of pollutants in the air in a short time. Therefore, it is necessary to increase the number of samples to achieve longer coverage or to use in the case of a stable pollution state. Enrichment collection method is a method of preconcentration of chemicals during collection by using liquid and solid absorbent. It is applicable to the situation of low concentration of chemicals [36]. The sampling time is generally long, which can represent the average concentration of the sampling time period and reflect the real situation of air pollution. Personal and area sampling can be used for air sample collection. Personal exposure assessment is more accurate, which can directly reflect individual exposure level [37]. Area sampling can reflect the exposure of a certain region. According to the spatial distance between the individual and each sampling point and other pollution-related information, individual exposure burden can be evaluated by calculation, which is suitable for epidemiological research of a large sample size.

Water

Pollutants in the water mainly enter the human body through the digestive tract, and can also volatilize into the air and enter the human body through the respiratory tract. The contact between human skin and polluted water can also make some chemicals enter the human body. Water sampling can be divided into natural water body, industrial wastewater, domestic sewage, and water supply pipe network sampling [38]. The setting of water sampling sites should be representative. The sampling should consider the frequency and time, consider the changes in the wet and dry periods, and consider the pollution information. For the detection of different chemical categories, different water collection and storage containers should be selected. For example, if the substance to be tested is a trace metal or glass component, glass bottle cannot be used. On the contrary, if plastic-related chemicals are to be assessed, plastic containers should be avoided. The amount of sampling should be enough to meet the needs of analysis. If the concentration of the tested chemical is very low and it needs to be preconcentrated [39], the sampling amount should be increased. In addition, attention should be paid to the storage method. According to the characteristics of the target chemical, freezing or cold storage should be considered or preservatives should be added [40].

Soil

The chemicals in the soil mainly enter the human body through air, water, and the food chain [41]. Therefore, the detection of soil chemical content can be used as an external exposure evaluation, reflecting the potential exposure route and burden in the human body. Soil can be used for the detection of organic and inorganic exposure. First of all, it should be noted that the containers in the experiment may cause contamination. For example, plastic containers can cause phthalate contamination. Volatile organic compound (VOC) detection may be contaminated by other organic solvents used in the analytical process. For heavy metal analysis, tree branches and other non-soil debris should be removed from soil samples before drying. The digestion method is used to make the metal in soil measurable. For the organic chemicals, the proper pretreatment method should be selected according to the physicochemical characters. For VOCs, the pretreatment may cause loss and contamination. The headspace injection method can be used for substances with low water solubility. For substances with high water solubility, vacuum distillation can be used [42]. For semi-volatile organic compounds, Soxhlet extraction and purification can be used to concentrate the target chemicals and remove the interferences.

4 Analytical Instruments for Environmental Exposure

4.1 Gas Chromatography

Gas chromatography (GC) is a chromatographic separation method using gas as a mobile phase. The vaporized chemicals are carried into the chromatographic column by carrier gas [43]. The stationary phase in the column has different molecular forces with the chemicals in the sample, so the chemicals can be separated. The retention time and chromatogram of each chemical can be recorded by the subsequent detection system. According to the retention time and order, the chemicals can be qualitatively analyzed; according to the peak height and area size, the compounds can be quantitatively analyzed. It can be used in combination with a flame ionization detector (FID), mass spectrometer (MS), etc. Generally, GC can be used for organic chemicals with heat stability and a boiling point of no more than 500 °C, such as volatile organic compounds, organic chlorine, organic phosphorus, polycyclic aromatic hydrocarbons, phthalates, etc. Nonvolatile liquid and solid substances can be analyzed by pyrolysis and gasification.

4.2 Liquid Chromatography

Liquid chromatography (LC) is a chromatographic separation method using liquid as a mobile phase. The chemicals are brought into the column by the liquid mobile phase, and the stationary phase in the column has different forces to the chemicals in the sample, so the chemicals can be separated. Similar to GC, LC can also provide information of the retention time and order, peak height, and area size of each chemical to the detector for qualitative and quantitative analysis. It can also be used in combination with mass spectrometry, etc. Modern LC consists of a high-pressure pump, injection system, temperature control system, chromatographic column, detector, signal recording system, etc. Compared with the classical liquid chromatography, it has the characteristics of high efficiency, rapidity, and sensitivity [44].

4.3 Capillary Electrophoresis

The capillary electrophoresis (CE) instrument uses the elastic quartz capillary as the separation channel and the high-voltage direct current electric field as the driving force to separate the components according to the difference of the mobility and distribution behavior of the chemicals in the sample. CE is particularly suitable for the separation of polar chemicals [45].

4.4 Ultraviolet–Visible Spectroscopy

Ultraviolet–visible (UV-Vis) spectrophotometer is a kind of analytical instrument which uses the radiation absorption of the UV-Vis spectral region (190–400 nm) of chemical substances [46]. It is mainly composed of a light source, monochromator, absorption cell, detector, and signal processor. The absorption spectrum of the chemical has characteristics related to its structure, so the UV-Vis spectrophotometer has a certain qualitative ability. When it is used for quantitative analysis, the absorbance of a certain concentration of sample solution is measured at the maximum absorption wavelength and compared with that of a certain concentration of reference solution to calculate the concentration of sample solution. It can be used for the determination of transition metal ions and highly conjugated organic compounds [47].

4.5 Fluorescence Spectroscopy

Fluorescence analysis is a method that can be used for qualitative or quantitative analysis, because some chemical substances are in excited state after being irradiated by ultraviolet (UV) light, and the fluorescence of excited state molecules can reflect the characteristics of the substance [48]. The advantage of fluorescence analysis is that there is a molecular excitation process, which greatly improves the sensitivity of fluorescence spectrum-based detection. Ultralow-concentration organic chemicals with UV excitation characteristics can be detected by fluorescence analysis [49].

4.6 Atomic Absorption Spectroscopy

Atomic absorption spectroscopy (AAS), also known as atomic spectrophotometry, is an analysis method for chemical element detection based on the absorption of optical radiation (light) by free atoms in the gaseous state. The limits of detection (LODs) can be reached to the 10^{-9} g/ml level by flame AAS (FAAS) and 10^{-13} g/ml by graphite furnace AAS (GFAAS). More than 70 kinds of inorganic elements can be detected by AAS [50].

4.7 Atomic Fluorescence Spectroscopy

Atomic fluorescence spectroscopy (AFS) is a method of element quantitative analysis by measuring the fluorescence emission intensity from atoms in the gaseous state that have been excited to higher energy levels by absorption of electromagnetic radiation. Atomic fluorescence photometer is suitable for the detection of inorganic elements [51]. Compared with the atomic absorption spectrometer, the atomic fluorescence photometer has a significantly improved sensitivity due to lower interferences [52].

4.8 Mass Spectrometry

Mass spectrometer (MS) has the structure of ion source, mass analyzer, and ion detector. The ion source is to ionize the chemical molecules under high vacuum. The ionized molecules will be further changed into many kinds of fragment ions and neutral particles with smaller mass due to receiving too much energy. The mass analyzer is a device to separate the ions of different masses into it at the same time according to the mass-to-charge ratio m/z. The separated ions enter the ion detector which collects and amplifies the ion signals, and then the computer draws a mass spectrogram. Mass spectrometer is divided into high resolution, medium resolution, and low resolution mass spectrometer. It can be connected with LC, GC, and CE [53]. It is widely used in the detection of organic and inorganic substances [54].

4.9 Nuclear Magnetic Resonance Spectroscopy

Nuclear magnetic resonance (NMR) spectrometer is one of the most powerful tools for the qualitative analysis of the composition and structure of substances [55], and sometimes it can also be used for quantitative analysis. NMR is mainly used for organic chemical analysis, and compared with a mass spectrometer, it has a nondestructive advantage for chemical analysis, but the detection sensitivity is often lower than that of a mass spectrometer [56].

4.10 *Direct-Reading Instruments*

Direct-reading gas detector, using the sensor principle, can quantitatively analyze a variety of toxic and harmful gases by replacing the corresponding sensor module. The precision of the instrument depends on the sensor. The result is directly readable, and the sensor does not need to be calibrated every time. The instrument can be used in field investigation [57]. In addition, there are also direct-reading water detectors. Attention should be paid to the differences between the detection principle of direct-reading detectors and that of the standard methods, so as to clarify the potential problems that need to be paid attention to when interpreting the detection results by direct-reading detectors [57, 58].

4.11 *Chromatography Tandem Mass Spectrometry*

It mainly includes GC tandem MS and LC tandem MS [59]. The combination of chromatography and MS occupies the primary position in the detection of organic compounds. GC is suitable for the detection of volatile and heat-stable substances. The derivatization method was used to expand the detection range of GC-MS [60]. LC-MS has a wide range of organic compound detection using columns of different retention characteristics [61]. Compared with LC-MS, GC-MS usually uses standard 70 eV high-energy electrons to interact with atoms or molecules in the gas phase to produce ions, which has high ionization efficiency and abundant fragments, so there is a relatively complete database that can be used for the qualitative analysis of chemicals for GC-MS [62].

4.12 *Inductively Coupled Plasma Tandem Mass Spectrometry*

Inductively coupled plasma tandem mass spectrometry (ICP-MS) is a mass spectrometry method that uses inductively coupled plasma to ionize samples. It atomizes the sample and produces atoms and small polyatomic ions, which are then detected by mass spectrometry. ICP-MS is more sensitive than GFAAS in the determination of many trace and ultra trace elements. ICP-MS can measure almost all kinds of samples, achieve simultaneous multielement determination at one time, and provide the information of isotopes [63]. The combination of chromatography and ICP-MS, in which ICP-MS is used as a detector, can determine the elements with different chemical valences in samples [64]. These properties establish the primary position of ICP-MS in trace element detection technology.

4.13 Capillary Electrophoresis Tandem Mass Spectrometry

Similar to CG-MS and LC-MS, capillary electrophoresis tandem mass spectrometry (CE-MS) combines the advantages of CE and MS, taking both the separation and molecular mass information into account. Ions are usually formed by electrospray [65]. It has a good detection performance for polar substances [45].

5 Analytical Methods for Environmental Exposure

Analytical methods for environmental exposure include the determination of organic/inorganic chemicals in environmental and biological samples (Table 1) [64–88].

5.1 Analytical Methods for Organic Chemicals

The stability, volatility, and other characteristics of chemicals should be considered in the collection and storage of samples for the detection of organic chemicals, and it should be noted that the containers used should not introduce new contamination. For example, phthalate determination is easily contaminated by plastic containers [91].

The sample preparation step for the measurement method of organic chemicals in a biological and environmental matrix is to separate or preconcentrate the target compounds from the matrix. For gas chromatography, because the detection substance sometimes does not have the characteristics for gas chromatography detection, it often needs derivative treatment [60]. For the pretreatment of liquid chromatography, the particulates in the sample should be removed to prevent the column from being blocked. At the same time, the proteins in the biological matrix should be also removed to prevent the column from being blocked due to the denaturation of proteins in the mobile phase. It should be noted that the more complex the sample preparation steps are, the greater the experimental error will be introduced [92].

The most common detection techniques for organic compounds include GC, LC, and CE, which are usually connected with a mass spectrometer. In the detection system, the specificity provided by a mass spectrometer is the strongest, while that provided by an ultraviolet spectrophotometer commonly is the lowest. LOD of most MS-based methods is in the range of pico- to nanogram per gram of matrix, which usually meets the sensitivity requirements of detecting the level of chemicals in the general population when the matrix is 1–10 g. The analysis deviation is usually between 10% and 20%.

Table 1 Analytical methods for environmental chemical exposure assessment in early life

Exposure family	Biomaterials (matrix)	Instrument (methodology)	No. of chemicals measured	No. of subjects	Volume/weight for analysis	References
Organic chemical						
Pesticides	Meconium of infants	GC-MS	8	200	0.5 g	[66]
	Urine of pregnant women and their infants	GC–MS/MS	6	273 maternal urine samples and 107 neonatal urine samples		[67]
	Urine of pregnant women	GC-MS	6	413		[68]
Antibiotics	Urine of pregnant women	UPLC–Q/TOF MS	21	536	1.0 mL	[69]
Phthalates	Urine of pregnant women	HPLC-MS/MS	18	642		[70]
	Urine of pregnant women	UPLC-MS/MS	7	1002	0.5 ml	[71]
	Urine of pregnant women	HPLC-MS	15	446	1 μl	[72]
Phenols	Urine of pregnant women	HPLC-MS	11	446		[72]
Parabens	Urine of pregnant women	LC-MS/MS	4	439		[73]
Polybrominated diphenyl ethers	Serum of pregnant women	GC/MS	8	185	0.5 ml	[74]
	Placenta, breast milk, fetal cord blood, and neonatal urine samples	GC/MS	17	30 paired placenta, breast milk, fetal cord blood, and neonatal urine samples		[75]
Perfluorinated alkyl acids	Blood of pregnant women and cord blood	LC-MS/MS	2	50	2 ml	[76]

	Serum of pregnant women	LC-MS/MS	7	1533		[77]
Polycyclic aromatic hydrocarbons	Placenta	GC–FID	16	84	10 g	[78]
	Urine of pregnant women	UPLC-MS/MS	1	627	1 ml	[79]
Cotinine	Saliva of pregnant women and their infants	LC-MS	1	147 maternal saliva samples and 120 infant saliva samples		[80]
	Urine of infants	GC-MS	1	265 maternal urine samples and 93 infant urine samples		[81]
Volatile organic compounds	Urine of pregnant women	UPLC-MS/MS and IC-ESI/MSMS	28	488		[82]
	Urine of pregnant women	UPLC-MS	3	29	5 ml	[83]
Polychlorinated biphenyls	Serum of pregnant women	GC-MS	7	281		[84]
Inorganic chemical						
Elements	Urine of pregnant women	ICP-MS	5	762		[85]
	Amniotic fluid	ICP-MS	22	65		[86]
	Breast milk	ICP-MS	7	35 of colostrum, 59 of transitional milk, and 92 of mature milk	0.2–0.3 g lyophilized breast milk sample	[87]
	Tooth of infants	ICP-MS	3	156		[88]
	Nail of pregnant women and their infants	ICP-MS	6	694	Approximately 1 cm in depth and 1–2 cm in diameter	[89]
	Hair of infants	ICP-MS	3	112	3 g	[90]

Other analytical methods that can be used for organic chemical determination also include immunoassay and bioassay [93]. These techniques are usually used for analysis by ultraviolet, fluorescence, or radioactivity detection. The sensitivity of some of these methods is suitable for human sample detection. It should be noted that, because these techniques do not use separation techniques, the problem about specificity may be encountered.

5.2 Analytical Methods for Inorganic Chemicals

The containers used for the detection of inorganic chemicals should not introduce new contamination into samples when samples are collected and stored. Sometimes, glass containers may introduce metal contamination [94].

The sample preparation of inorganic chemicals is often simple. In some cases, only dilution is needed for sample preparation [20]. However, we still need to pay attention to the detection process to avoid the introduction of contamination. For example, all the experimental equipment should be cleaned with acid.

The detection of inorganic elements mainly uses AAS or ICP-MS.

6 From Exposure Measurements to Evaluations: The Use of Models

The goal of chemical measurement is to be used in the research and the assessment of environmental exposure risk. Environmental exposure evaluation is one of the key contents of risk assessment, which needs to be implemented by using specific models and algorisms. The acquisition of exposure route, exposure frequency, exposure dose, and other data in different exposure events is necessary for exposure evaluation. Chemical measurement provides information of the internal and external exposure of chemicals for exposure evaluation. The exposure of the human body to chemicals can be divided into two forms: one is single exposure, i.e., a single kind of pollutant enters the human body through a single way; the other is mixed exposure, i.e., a variety of pollutants from multiple sources (diet, drinking water, and living environment) enter the human body through multiple routes (skin, mouth, and inhalation). The second one is more common. Through several links of exposure event loop, individual loop, time loop, and uncertainty loop, the models including data and the methods of demography, geostatistics, and biostatistics are used to simulate exposure events and conduct exposure evaluations [95]. The first step of exposure evaluation is to determine individual characteristic values, which are used to determine parameters of exposure events. After determining the individual characteristic values, exposure event loop should be established, which covers multi-source and multi-route exposures. For multi-route exposure, the amount of exposure should be calculated based on the consideration of exposure route information. Some routes may not occur in an exposure event, such as some chemicals only through dietary intake, some only through air inhalation, and some only through skin contact. When the calculation of the first individual's multi-source and multi-route exposure is completed, the exposure of the individual should be calculated with emphasis on describing the variability of individual exposure to chemicals. The exposure evaluation next describes the characteristics of exposure variability in different periods and calculates uncertainty factors, including the selection of sampling points, analysis methods, calculation methods, the use of alternative data, etc. There are several software that have been designed to conduct environmental exposure evaluation including Crystal Ball, LifeLine, Calendex, etc. [96].

7 Future Perspective

People in early life are exposed to a variety of environmental factors. Therefore, the future direction of environmental exposure assessment is from single exposure to comprehensive exposure assessment.

In recent years, "exposome" has become a hot topic in the environmental research area. Exposome is defined as the sum of human environmental exposure from early life to death [97]. The combination of exposome and genome can greatly improve our understanding of the cause of disease and various health outcomes.

The assessment of exposome includes a series of indicators of internal and external exposure, which need to cover all stages of life. Exposome also includes physical, biological, and sociopsychological factors, which need to be assessed by various detection technologies and investigation methods [98]. Indeed, exposome study remains challenging. In terms of chemical exposure assessment, the existing high-throughput methods encounter the problems of huge differences in chemical properties and concentrations in samples, which makes high-throughput methods often compromise the detection performance of some chemicals in the sample pretreatment and instrument analysis. Otherwise, the analysis can be conducted by a highly optimized method for the detection of special chemicals. Because the amount of information obtained from this kind of detection is relatively small, a variety of methods and several rounds of analysis are required, increasing the investment of time and cost for exposome analysis. And this kind of strategy is not suitable for samples with small volume. Therefore, the realization of the assessment of exposome depends on the development of high-throughput and high-sensitivity detection technology and requires a high degree of technology integration and teamwork. Fortunately, the concept of exposome has been introduced into several birth cohort studies related to early life exposure, and exposome is now moving from theory into practice [99]. These birth cohort studies are accumulating a large volume of information about pregnancy exposure and following children's outcomes, which holds a great promise for the study of environmental factors affecting children's growth and future health outcomes related to early life exposure.

Acknowledgments This work was supported by grants from the National Natural Science Foundation of China (81871210, MC) and the Key Natural Science Foundation of the Jiangsu Higher Education Institutions of China (18KJA320003, MC).

References

1. House JS (2002) Understanding social factors and inequalities in health: 20th century progress and 21st century prospects. J Health Soc Behav 43(2):125–142
2. Nieuwenhuijsen M, Paustenbach D, Duarte-Davidson R (2006) New developments in exposure assessment: The impact on the practice of health risk assessment and epidemiological studies. Environ Int 32(8):996–1009
3. Jiang Y, Yuan L, Lin Q, Ma S, Yu Y (2019) Polybrominated diphenyl ethers in the environment and human external and internal exposure in China: a review. Sci Total Environ 696:133902
4. Paustenbach D, Galbraith D (2006) Biomonitoring and biomarkers: exposure assessment will never be the same. J Environ Health Perspect 114(8):1143–1149
5. Ladeira C, Viegas SJB (2016) Human biomonitoring–an overview on biomarkers and their application in occupational and environmental health. J Biomonit 3(1)
6. Barr DB, Thomas K, Curwin B, Landsittel D, Raymer J, Lu C, Donnelly KC, Acquavella J (2006) Biomonitoring of exposure in farmworker studies. Environ Health Perspect 114 (6):936–942
7. Bowen RA, Remaley AT (2014) Interferences from blood collection tube components on clinical chemistry assays. Biochem Med (Zagreb) 24(1):31–44
8. Koch HM, Lorber M, Christensen KLY, Palmke C, Koslitz S, Bruning T (2013) Identifying sources of phthalate exposure with human biomonitoring: results of a 48 h fasting study with urine collection and personal activity patterns. Int J Hyg Environ Health 216(6):672–681
9. Therrell BL, Padilla CD, Loeber JG, Kneisser I, Saadallah A, Borrajo GJ, Adams J (2015) In current status of newborn screening worldwide: 2015, Seminars in perinatology. Elsevier, pp 171–187
10. Chaudhuri SN, Butala SJ, Ball RW, Braniff CT (2009) Rocky Mountain biomonitoring, C., pilot study for utilization of dried blood spots for screening of lead, mercury and cadmium in newborns. J Expo Sci Environ Epidemiol 19(3):298–316
11. Perez R, Domenech E, Coscolla C, Yusa V (2017) Human biomonitoring of food contaminants in Spanish children: design, sampling and lessons learned. Int J Hyg Environ Health 220 (8):1242–1251
12. Oya N, Ito Y, Hioki K, Asai Y, Aoi A, Sugiura Y, Ueyama J, Oguri T, Kato S, Ebara T, Kamijima M (2017) Quantitative analysis of organophosphate insecticide metabolites in urine extracted from disposable diapers of toddlers in Japan. Int J Hyg Environ Health 220(2 Pt A):209–216
13. MacPherson S, Arbuckle TE, Fisher M (2018) Adjusting urinary chemical biomarkers for hydration status during pregnancy. J Expo Sci Environ Epidemiol 28(5):481–493
14. Griffiths SK, Campbell JP (2014) Placental structure, function and drug transfer. Contin Educ Anaesthesia Crit Care Pain 15(2):84–89
15. Hameed ERA, Shehata MA, Waheed H, Samie OMA, Ahmed HH, Sherif LS, Ahmed A (2019) Heavy metals can either aid or oppose the protective function of the placental barrier. Open Access Macedonian J Med Sci 7(17):2814
16. Eaton B, Yudilevich D (1981) Uptake and asymmetric efflux of amino acids at maternal and fetal sides of placenta. Am J Phys Cell Phys 241(3):C106–C112

17. Remy S, Govarts E, Wens B, De Boever P, Den Hond E, Croes K, Sioen I, Baeyens W, van Larebeke N, Koppe J (2016) Metabolic targets of endocrine disrupting chemicals assessed by cord blood transcriptome profiling. Reprod Toxicol 65:307–320
18. Xu C, Tang M, Zhu S, Naranmandura H, Liu W (2016) Assessment of arsenic in colostrum and cord serum and risk exposure to neonates from an island population in China. Environ Sci Pollut Res Int 23(22):22467–22476
19. Leung M, Nøst TH, Wania F, Papp E, Herzke D, Al Mahmud A, Roth DE (2018) Maternal-child exposures to persistent organic pollutants in Dhaka, Bangladesh. J Expo Health:1–9
20. Silver MK, Arain AL, Shao J, Chen M, Xia Y, Lozoff B, Meeker JD (2018) Distribution and predictors of 20 toxic and essential metals in the umbilical cord blood of Chinese newborns. Chemosphere 210:1167–1175
21. Kunter I, Hurer N, Gulcan HO, Ozturk B, Dogan I, Sahin G (2017) Assessment of Aflatoxin M1 and heavy metal levels in mothers breast Milk in Famagusta, Cyprus. Biol Trace Elem Res 175 (1):42–49
22. Anadón A, Martínez-Larrañaga MR, Ares I, Castellano V, Martínez MA (2017) Drugs and chemical contaminants in human breast milk. In: Reproductive and developmental toxicology. Elsevier, pp 67–98
23. Hutchinson L, Sinclair M, Reid B, Burnett K, Callan B (2018) A descriptive systematic review of salivary therapeutic drug monitoring in neonates and infants. Br J Clin Pharmacol 84 (6):1089–1108
24. Elmongy H, Abdel-Rehim M (2016) Saliva as an alternative specimen to plasma for drug bioanalysis: A review. Trac-Trends Anal Chem 83:70–79
25. Liu LY, He K, Hites RA, Salamova A (2016) Hair and nails as noninvasive biomarkers of human exposure to brominated and organophosphate flame retardants. Environ Sci Technol 50 (6):3065–3073
26. Manceau A, Enescu M, Simionovici A, Lanson M, Gonzalez-Rey M, Rovezzi M, Tucoulou R, Glatzel P, Nagy KL, Bourdineaud JP (2016) Chemical forms of mercury in human hair reveal sources of exposure. Environ Sci Technol 50(19):10721–10729
27. Pozebon D, Scheffler GL, Dressler VL (2017) Elemental hair analysis: a review of procedures and applications. Anal Chim Acta 992:1–23
28. Gutierrez-Gonzalez E, Garcia-Esquinas E, de Larrea-Baz NF, Salcedo-Bellido I, Navas-Acien-A, Lope V, Gomez-Ariza JL, Pastor R, Pollan M, Perez-Gomez B (2019) Toenails as biomarker of exposure to essential trace metals: a review. Environ Res 179:108787
29. Concheiro M, Huestis MA (2018) Drug exposure during pregnancy: analytical methods and toxicological findings. Bioanalysis 10(8):587–606
30. Andra SS, Austin C, Arora M (2016) The tooth exposome in children's health research. J Curr Opin Pediatrics 28(2):221
31. Arora M, Bradman A, Austin C, Vedar M, Holland N, Eskenazi B, Smith DR (2012) Determining fetal manganese exposure from mantle dentine of deciduous teeth. Environ Sci Technol 46(9):5118–5125
32. Arora M, Kennedy BJ, Elhlou S, Pearson NJ, Walker DM, Bayl P, Chan SWY (2006) Spatial distribution of lead in human primary teeth as a biomarker of pre- and neonatal lead exposure. Sci Total Environ 371(1–3):55–62
33. Turner MC, Nieuwenhuijsen M, Anderson K, Balshaw D, Cui Y, Dunton G, Hoppin JA, Koutrakis P, Jerrett M (2017) Assessing the Exposome with external measures: commentary on the state of the science and research recommendations. Annu Rev Public Health 38:215–239
34. Chen H, Burnett RT, Kwong JC, Villeneuve PJ, Goldberg MS, Brook RD, van Donkelaar A, Jerrett M, Martin RV, Brook JR, Copes R (2013) Risk of incident diabetes in relation to long-term exposure to fine particulate matter in Ontario, Canada. Environ Health Perspect 121 (7):804–810
35. Zhu YY, Duan XL, Qin N, Li JH, Tian J, Zhong Y, Chen LG, Fan RF, Yu Y, Wu GP, Wei FS (2019) Internal biomarkers and external estimation of exposure to polycyclic aromatic

hydrocarbons and their relationships with cancer mortality in a high cancer incidence area. Sci Total Environ 688:742–750
36. Raza N, Hashemi B, Kim KH, Lee SH, Deep A (2018) Aromatic hydrocarbons in air, water, and soil: sampling and pretreatment techniques. Trac-Trends Anal Chem 103:56–73
37. Asbach C, Alexander C, Clavaguera S, Dahmann D, Dozol H, Faure B, Fierz M, Fontana L, Iavicoli I, Kaminski H, MacCalman L, Meyer-Plath A, Simonow B, van Tongeren M, Todea AM (2017) Review of measurement techniques and methods for assessing personal exposure to airborne nanomaterials in workplaces. Sci Total Environ 603–604:793–806
38. Zainudin FM, Hasan HA, Abdullah SRS (2016) Characterization of trihalomethanes (THMs) levels in surface water, domestic and industrial wastewater. J Environ Sci Technol 9 (3):268–276
39. Sohrabi R, Bahramifar N, Javadian H, Agarwal S, Gupta VK (2016) Pre-concentration of trace amount of bisphenol A in water samples by palm leaf ash and determination with high-performance liquid chromatography. J Biomed Chromatogr 30(8):1256–1262
40. Peacock M, Freeman C, Gauci V, Lebron I, Evans CD (2015) Investigations of freezing and cold storage for the analysis of peatland dissolved organic carbon (DOC) and absorbance properties. Environ Sci Process Impacts 17(7):1290–1301
41. Zhuang P, Huiling Z, Wensheng S (2009) Biotransfer of heavy metals along a soil-plant-insect-chicken food chain: field study. J Environ Sci 21(6):849–853
42. Hiatt MH, Youngman DR, Donnelly JR (1994) Separation and isolation of volatile organic compounds using vacuum distillation with GC/MS determination. J Anal Chem 66(6):905–908
43. Coskun O (2016) Separation techniques: chromatography. North Clin Istanb 3(2):156–160
44. Hamilton RJ, Sewell PA (1982) Introduction to high performance liquid chromatography. In: Introduction to high performance liquid chromatography. Springer, pp 1–12
45. Takahashi K, Kohno H (2016) Different polar metabolites and protein profiles between high- and low-quality Japanese Ginjo sake. PLoS One 11(3):e0150524
46. Kabir I, Hossain M, Al-Amin M, Shupta JA (2017) Portable UV-spectrophotometer to determine the concentration of potassium. BRAC Univeristy
47. Yang CM, Chen CY (2005) Synthesis, characterisation and properties of polyanilines containing transition metal ions. Synth Met 153(1–3):133–136
48. Parker C, Rees W (1962) Fluorescence spectrometry. A review. J Anal 87(1031):83–111
49. Bridgeman J, Bieroza M, Baker A (2011) The application of fluorescence spectroscopy to organic matter characterisation in drinking water treatment. Rev Environ Sci Biotechnol 10 (3):277–290
50. Helaluddin ABM, Khalid RS, Alaama M, Abbas SA (2016) Main analytical techniques used for elemental analysis in various matrices. Trop J Pharm Res 15(2):427–434
51. Wang Y, Lin L, Liu J, Mao X, Wang J, Qin D (2016) Ferric ion induced enhancement of ultraviolet vapour generation coupled with atomic fluorescence spectrometry for the determination of ultratrace inorganic arsenic in surface water. Analyst 141(4):1530–1536
52. Cabon JY, Giamarchi P, Le Bihan A (2010) Determination of iron in seawater by electrothermal atomic absorption spectrometry and atomic fluorescence spectrometry: a comparative study. Anal Chim Acta 664(2):114–120
53. Ramautar R, Somsen GW, de Jong GJ (2017) CE–MS for metabolomics: developments and applications in the period 2014–2016. J Electrophor 38(1):190–202
54. Kaufmann A, Widmer M, Maden K, Butcher P, Walker S (2018) Analysis of a variety of inorganic and organic additives in food products by ion-pairing liquid chromatography coupled to high-resolution mass spectrometry. Anal Bioanal Chem 410(22):5629–5640
55. Bhatia A, Sarma SJ, Lei Z, Sumner LW (2019) UHPLC-QTOF-MS/MS-SPE-NMR: a solution to the metabolomics grand challenge of higher-throughput, confident metabolite identifications. In: NMR-based metabolomics. Springer, pp 113–133
56. Jahangir M, Nuringtyas T, Ali K, Wilson E, Choi Y, Verpoorte R (2018) NMR-based metabolomics: Understanding plant chemistry and identification of biologically active compounds. In: NMR-based metabolomics, pp 246–263

57. Shi J, Chen F, Cai Y, Fan S, Cai J, Chen R, Kan H, Lu Y, Zhao Z (2017) Validation of a light-scattering PM2.5 sensor monitor based on the long-term gravimetric measurements in field tests. PLoS One 12(11):e0185700
58. Kim JY, Magari SR, Herrick RF, Smith TJ, Christiani DC (2004) Comparison of fine particle measurements from a direct-reading instrument and a gravimetric sampling method. J Occup Environ Hyg 1(11):707–715
59. Vestal ML (1984) High-performance liquid chromatography-mass spectrometry. Science 226 (4672):275–281
60. Snyder LR, Kirkland JJ, Dolan JW (2011) Introduction to modern liquid chromatography. Wiley, Hoboken
61. Xu RN, Fan L, Rieser MJ, El-Shourbagy TA (2007) Recent advances in high-throughput quantitative bioanalysis by LC–MS/MS. J Pharm Biomed Anal 44(2):342–355
62. Vijayabaskar G, Elango V (2018) Characterization of bioactive compounds in alcoholic extract of Hemidimus indicus and Alpenia officinarum using GC-MS technique. J World J Sci Res 3 (2):16–22
63. Balcaen L, Bolea-Fernandez E, Resano M, Vanhaecke F (2015) Inductively coupled plasma–tandem mass spectrometry (ICP-MS/MS): a powerful and universal tool for the interference-free determination of (ultra) trace elements–a tutorial review. J Anal Chim Acta 894:7–19
64. Nagaoka MH, Yamazaki T, Maitani T (2002) Binding patterns of vanadium ions with different valence states to human serum transferrin studied by HPLC/high-resolution ICP-MS. Biochem Biophys Res Commun 296(5):1207–1214
65. Soga T, Kakazu Y, Robert M, Tomita M, Nishioka T (2004) Qualitative and quantitative analysis of amino acids by capillary electrophoresis-electrospray ionization-tandem mass spectrometry. J Electrophor 25(13):1964–1972
66. Ostrea EM Jr, Morales V, Ngoumgna E, Prescilla R, Tan E, Hernandez E, Ramirez GB, Cifra HL, Manlapaz ML (2002) Prevalence of fetal exposure to environmental toxins as determined by meconium analysis. J Neuro-Oncol 23(3):329–339
67. Ein-Mor E, Ergaz-Shaltiel Z, Berman T, Göen T, Natsheh J, Ben-Chetrit A, Haimov-Kochman-R, Calderon-Margalit R (2018) Decreasing urinary organophosphate pesticide metabolites among pregnant women and their offspring in Jerusalem: Impact of regulatory restrictions on agricultural organophosphate pesticides use? Int J Hyg Environ Health 221(5):775–781
68. Wang YW, Chen LM, Wang CF, Hum Y, Gao Y, Zhou YJ, Shi R, Zhang Y, Kamijima M, Ueyama J, Tian Y (2017) Association between organophosphate pesticide exposure and thyroid hormones in pregnant women. Epidemiology 28:S35–S40
69. Wang H, Wang N, Qian J, Hu L, Huang P, Su M, Yu X, Fu C, Jiang F, Zhao Q, Zhou Y, Lin H, He G, Chen Y, Jiang Q (2017) Urinary antibiotics of pregnant women in eastern China and cumulative health risk assessment. Environ Sci Technol 51(6):3518–3525
70. Philips EM, Jaddoe VW, Asimakopoulos AG, Kannan K, Steegers EA, Santos S, Trasande L (2018) Bisphenol and phthalate concentrations and its determinants among pregnant women in a population-based cohort in the Netherlands, 2004–5. J Environ Res 161:562–572
71. Zhu YS, Wan YJ, Zhang B, Zhou AF, Huo WQ, Wu CS, Liu HX, Jiang YQ, Chen Z, Jiang MM, Peng Y, Xu SQ, Xia W, Li YY (2018) Relationship between maternal phthalate exposure and offspring size at birth. Sci Total Environ 612:1072–1078
72. Polinski KJ, Dabelea D, Hamman RF, Adgate JL, Calafat AM, Ye XY, Starling AP (2018) Distribution and predictors of urinary concentrations of phthalate metabolites and phenols among pregnant women in the healthy start study. Environ Res 162:308–317
73. Aker AM, Johns L, McElrath TF, Cantonwine DE, Mukherjee B, Meeker JD (2018) Associations between maternal phenol and paraben urinary biomarkers and maternal hormones during pregnancy: a repeated measures study. Environ Int 113:341–349
74. Eslami B, Hossein-Rashidi B, Naddafi K, Rastkari N, Djazayeri A, Malekafzali H (2016) Dietary and socio-demographic determinants of serum persistent organic pollutants (POPs) levels in pregnant women in Tehran. J Family Reprod Health 10(3):129–138

75. Chen Z-J, Liu H-Y, Cheng Z, Man Y-B, Zhang K-S, Wei W, Du J, Wong M-H, Wang H-S (2014) Polybrominated diphenyl ethers (PBDEs) in human samples of mother–newborn pairs in South China and their placental transfer characteristics. J Environ Int 73:77–84
76. Rovira J, Martinez MA, Sharma RP, Espuis T, Nadal M, Kumar V, Costopoulou D, Vassiliadou I, Leondiadis L, Domingo JL, Schuhmacher M (2019) Prenatal exposure to PFOS and PFOA in a pregnant women cohort of Catalonia, Spain. Environ Res 175:384–392
77. Bjerregaard-Olesen C, Bach CC, Long M, Ghisari M, Bossi R, Bech BH, Nohr EA, Henriksen TB, Olsen J, Bonefeld-Jørgensen EC (2016) Time trends of perfluorinated alkyl acids in serum from Danish pregnant women 2008–2013. J Environ Int 91:14–21
78. Agarwal P, Singh L, Anand M, Taneja A (2018) Association between placental polycyclic aromatic hydrocarbons (PAHS), oxidative stress, and preterm delivery: a case–control study. J Arch Environ Contam Toxicol 74(2):218–227
79. Li NN, Mu Y, Liu Z, Deng Y, Guo YX, Zhang XJ, Li XH, Yu P, Wang YP, Zhu J (2018) Assessment of interaction between maternal polycyclic aromatic hydrocarbons exposure and genetic polymorphisms on the risk of congenital heart diseases. Sci Rep 8(1):3075
80. Gavarkovs AG, Risica PM, Parker DR, Jennings E, Mello J, Phipps M (2018) Self-reported environmental tobacco smoke exposure and avoidance compared with cotinine confirmed tobacco smoke exposure among pregnant women and their infants. Int J Environ Res Public Health 15(5):871
81. Ein-Mor E, Berman T, Barnett-Itzhaki Z, Goen T, Ergaz-Shaltiel Z, Natsheh J, Ben-Chetrit A, Haimov-Kochman R, Calderon-Margalit R (2019) Newborn infant urinary cotinine and birth outcomes in the Jerusalem environment mother and child cohort study. Int J Hyg Environ Health 222(7):1054–1058
82. Boyle E, Viet S, Wright D, Merrill L, Alwis K, Blount B, Mortensen M, Moye J, Dellarco M (2016) Assessment of exposure to VOCs among pregnant women in the National Children's Study. Int J Environ Res Public Health 13(4):376
83. Caron-Beaudoin E, Valter N, Chevrier J, Ayotte P, Frohlich K, Verner MA (2018) Gestational exposure to volatile organic compounds (VOCs) in Northeastern British Columbia, Canada: a pilot study. Environ Int 110:131–138
84. Lignell S, Aune M, Darnerud PO, Stridsberg M, Hanberg A, Larsson SC, Glynn A (2016) Maternal body burdens of PCDD/Fs and PBDEs are associated with maternal serum levels of thyroid hormones in early pregnancy: a cross-sectional study. Environ Health 15(1):55
85. Song L, Liu B, Wang L, Wu M, Zhang L, Liu Y, Bi J, Yang S, Zhang B, Xia W (2020) Exposure to arsenic during pregnancy and newborn mitochondrial DNA copy number: a birth cohort study in Wuhan. Chin J Chem 243:125335
86. Henriquez-Hernandez LA, Luzardo OP, Boada LD, Gonzalez-Antuna A, Dominguez-Bencomo AI, Zumbado M, Burillo-Putze G (2019) Assessment of 22 inorganic elements in human amniotic fluid: a cross-sectional study conducted in Canary Islands (Spain). Int J Environ Health Res 29(2):130–139
87. LetiniĿ JG, SariĿ MM, Piasek M, JurasoviĿ J, Varnai VM, Grgec AS, Orct T (2016) Use of human milk in the assessment of toxic metal exposure and essential element status in breastfeeding women and their infants in coastal Croatia. J Trace Elem Med Biol 38:117–125
88. Cassidy-Bushrow AE, Wu KH, Sitarik AR, Park SK, Bielak LF, Austin C, Gennings C, Curtin P, Johnson CC, Arora M (2019) In utero metal exposures measured in deciduous teeth and birth outcomes in a racially-diverse urban cohort. Environ Res 171:444–451
89. Punshon T, Li ZG, Marsit CJ, Jackson BP, Baker ER, Karagas MR (2016) Placental metal concentrations in relation to maternal and infant toenails in a US cohort. Environ Sci Technol 50 (3):1587–1594
90. Dursun A, Yurdakok K, Yalcin SS, Tekinalp G, Aykut O, Orhan G, Morgil GK (2016) Maternal risk factors associated with lead, mercury and cadmium levels in umbilical cord blood, breast milk and newborn hair. J Matern Fetal Neonatal Med 29(6):954–961
91. Heffernan AL, Gomez-Ramos MJ, Symeonides C, Hare DJ, Vijayasarathy S, Thompson K, Mueller JF, Ponsonby AL, Sly PD, Group BISI (2020) Harmonizing analytical chemistry and

clinical epidemiology for human biomonitoring studies. A case-study of plastic product chemicals in urine. Chemosphere 238:124631

92. Fiehn O (2016) Metabolomics by gas chromatography–mass spectrometry: combined targeted and untargeted profiling. J Curr Protoc Mol Biol 114(1):30.4. 1–30.4. 32
93. Lang Y, Li K, Meng W, Liu R (2018) Development of a chemiluminescent enzyme immunoassay for the detection of bisphenol A in milk. Wei Sheng Yan Jiu 47(2):296–300
94. Shotyk W, Krachler M (2007) Lead in bottled waters: contamination from glass and comparison with pristine groundwater. Environ Sci Technol 41(10):3508–3513
95. Zartarian VG, Ozkaynak H, Burke JM, Zufall MJ, Rigas ML, Furtaw EJ Jr (2000) A modeling framework for estimating children's residential exposure and dose to chlorpyrifos via dermal residue contact and nondietary ingestion. J Environ Health Perspect 108(6):505–514
96. Cao H, Qiao L, Zhang H, Chen J (2010) Exposure and risk assessment for aluminium and heavy metals in Puerh tea. J Sci Total Environ 408(14):2777–2784
97. Dennis KK, Marder E, Balshaw DM, Cui Y, Lynes MA, Patti GJ, Rappaport SM, Shaughnessy DT, Vrijheid M, Barr DB (2017) Biomonitoring in the era of the exposome. Environ Health Perspect 125(4):502–510
98. Dennis KK, Auerbach SS, Balshaw DM, Cui Y, Fallin MD, Smith MT, Spira A, Sumner S, Miller GW (2016) The importance of the biological impact of exposure to the concept of the exposome. Environ Health Perspect 124(10):1504–1510
99. Vrijheid M, Slama R, Robinson O, Chatzi L, Coen M, van den Hazel P, Thomsen C, Wright J, Athersuch TJ, Avellana N, Basagana X, Brochot C, Bucchini L, Bustamante M, Carracedo A, Casas M, Estivill X, Fairley L, van Gent D, Gonzalez JR, Granum B, Grazuleviciene R, Gutzkow KB, Julvez J, Keun HC, Kogevinas M, McEachan RR, Meltzer HM, Sabido E, Schwarze PE, Siroux V, Sunyer J, Want EJ, Zeman F, Nieuwenhuijsen MJ (2014) The human early-life exposome (HELIX): project rationale and design. Environ Health Perspect 122(6):535–544

Early-life Tobacco Smoke/Nicotine Exposure and Offspring Health

Katherine M. Kuniyoshi, Bo Hang, and Virender K. Rehan

1 Introduction

The impact of environmental exposures on children's health is of worldwide concern. The World Health Organization (WHO) has declared that the deaths of 1.7 million children under the age of 5 in 2012 were attributed to the environment and that reducing these risks can potentially prevent 1 in 4 deaths [1]. Environmental exposures such as air pollution, hazardous chemicals, and smoke/tobacco pose significant risk to the health and well-being of children. The WHO has identified that despite numerous organizations reporting on the dangers of tobacco smoke, there are more than a billion smokers globally, which contributes to 5 million deaths yearly [2, 3]. Specifically in the United States, there were about 36.5 million smokers; nearly half of their deaths are related to smoking in 2015 [2, 4]. Despite awareness of the adverse effects to themselves as well as to their fetuses, approximately 10% of pregnant women smoke, leading to ~400,000 smoke-exposed infants born annually [4, 5]. These numbers are likely to be an underestimate since studies have shown that at least 20% of pregnant smokers lie about their habit [6]. Therefore, smoking during pregnancy continues to be a major public health crisis [4, 5]. In fact, smoking during pregnancy is the largest preventable cause of prematurity, low birth weight (LBW), intrauterine growth restriction, and perinatal mortality [7, 8]. The reason for its prevalence is multifactorial, including the highly addictive nature of

K. M. Kuniyoshi · V. K. Rehan (✉)
Department of Pediatrics, Lundquist Institute for Biomedical Innovation at Harbor-UCLA Medical Center, David Geffen School of Medicine, Los Angeles, CA, USA
e-mail: vrehan@lundquist.org

B. Hang
Biological Systems and Engineering Division, Lawrence Berkeley National Laboratory, Berkeley, CA, USA

Y. Xia (ed.), *Early-life Environmental Exposure and Disease*,
https://doi.org/10.1007/978-981-15-3797-4_2

nicotine, the negative reinforcement of withdrawal symptoms, and aggressive advertising strategies targeting the adolescent population [9, 10].

Here we first highlight the extent of the problem and review the various forms of tobacco smoke and nicotine exposures, including the marked increase in the usage of electronic cigarettes (e-cigs). We then review nicotine's transfer method and other potential short- and long-term outcomes of early-life exposure. We then discuss the transgenerational pulmonary effects following perinatal smoke/nicotine exposure and lastly discuss issues related to secondhand and thirdhand smoke (SHS and THS, respectively) exposures.

2 Early-Life Tobacco Smoke/Nicotine Exposure and Respiratory Morbidity

2.1 Types of Exposures

Directly attributed to maternal smoking, cigarette smoke exposure is the foremost preventable factor for childhood respiratory diseases, accounting for an approximately 20% of all healthcare expenses [11]. Remarkably, an even larger number of women and children are exposed to SHS and THS [12–14]. Secondhand smoke, or passive smoking, is the inhalation of smoke by persons other than the intended "active" smoker. In contrast, THS consists of residual tobacco smoke pollutants that remain on surfaces and in dust after tobacco has been smoked and includes secondary pollutants that result from chemical reactions of primary pollutants with each other and with oxidants in the environment [15]. The timescale for THS exposure is much longer than SHS, ranging from days to weeks and months.

E-cigs (vape pens) [16] were originally promoted as a safer alternative to reduce harm compared to traditional cigarettes [17]. On these presumptions, the use of e-cigs has grown exponentially, and based on projections of past sales, the consumption of e-cigs is predicted to surpass that of conventional cigarettes within the next decade, resulting in an estimated $50 billion global market by 2025 [18]. E-cig use has been particularly increasing among women of childbearing age [19–24], and women who already use these products are less likely than tobacco users to quit during pregnancy [25]. This is resulting in an unprecedented amount of developing embryos as well as fetuses exposed to e-cigs with unawareness of the hazard effects on their health. This is particularly concerning since nicotine concentrations in some e-cigs can be even higher in comparison to those found in traditional cigarettes [26, 27].

2.2 *General Overview of Respiratory Morbidity Following Early-Life Tobacco Smoke/Nicotine Exposure*

Early-life, in particular, prenatal environmental exposure (both active and passive) generates a lifelong decrease in pulmonary function of progeny, resulting in an ascending risk of asthma, pulmonary infections, and chronic lung disease (CLD), even though the offspring do not smoke [28–30]. Even more concerns are the potential effects on the developing fetus which are not confined to the exposed offspring but can be transmitted to subsequent generations' progeny as well, regardless of exposure [31, 32].

Extensive epidemiological and experimental data supports that perinatal exposure to cigarette smoke results in a decrease in forced expiratory flow volumes, functional residual capacity, alveolarization, and a higher risk for allergic asthma, and the effects are similar if either parent smoked [33–37]. Several studies have associated prenatal cigarette exposure, as opposed to postnatal exposure, to abnormal infant lung function [38–40], such as decreased passive respiratory compliance, decreases in forced expiratory flows, and altered tidal volume patterns [35, 41]. Moreover, infants who are exposed to smoke in utero are less likely to respond to bronchodilators as a treatment for peripheral airflow obstruction [42].

Evidence is also emerging to suggest that some specific attributes might render e-cigs potentially even doing more harm to developing organs. For instance, the use of higher temperatures in these devices can produce toxins such as formaldehyde hemi-acetyls [43]. Compounds used in e-liquids as aerosolizing agents (such as vegetable glycerin and propylene glycol) can produce toxic carbonyl compounds (acrolein, aldehyde, and formaldehyde) through oxidation [44, 45]. Metal coils used as heating agents can produce heavy metals, which can be inhaled or ingested through e-cig vapors [46–48]. Even the artificial flavoring could be converted into carcinogenic and/or toxic by-products when heated [49].

3 Nicotine Is the Primary Determinant of Early-Life Tobacco Smoke Exposure-Mediated Respiratory Morbidity

In addition to nicotine, many other components in cigarette smoke, such as polycyclic ammonia, aromatic hydrocarbons, hydrogen cyanide, and carbon monoxide, are considered harmful [50, 51]. However, evidence supports that nicotine mediates the effects of perinatal smoke and asthma [31, 32, 52]. Multiple animal models, including a nonhuman primate model [52–56], have demonstrated the same pulmonary phenotype seen following perinatal nicotine exposure as that seen in human infants exposed to prenatal smoke.

3.1 Animal Models Used to Study Early-Life Tobacco Smoke/Nicotine's Effects on the Developing Lung

In vitro studies have evidentially shown that the cells directly affected by nicotine are the pulmonary alveolar type II (ATII) cells as well as lung fibroblasts [57–59]. Airflow restriction due to modifications in pulmonary function and structure, such as thicker alveolar walls, increase in collagen, and airway smooth muscle deposition has been noted in primate, sheep, rat, and mice models [60–62]. Decreased expiratory flows along with dysanaptic lung growth and lung branching were noted in embryonic murine lung explants with dose-dependent nicotine exposure [63].

3.2 Critical Window for Tobacco Smoke/Nicotine's Effects on the Developing Lung

The development of the lung begins prenatally during the fourth week of gestation, with the majority of postnatal lung growth completed by 2 years of age, although it can persist into mid-adolescence [64–66]. The lungs are especially pregnable to the effects of nicotine in this entire process. The perinatal period is defined as starting at 22 completed weeks of gestation and lasting 7 days after birth [67]. In humans, this period has also been recognized as a time window from 20 completed weeks of gestation to the 28th postnatal day in general. This is the period during which lung growth and cellular differentiation occur rapidly and is the time period prior to widespread alveolarization, but after the completion of most lung branching [68]. It is suggested that nicotine significantly affects the cellular differentiation and conducting airways instead of alveolarization [63]. Recent studies have also suggested that lung function in children is more likely to be compromised if the fetus was exposed to tobacco smoke during gestation, particularly during the third trimester [69, 70].

3.3 Perinatal Nicotine Metabolism and Pharmacokinetics

Upon maternal nicotine exposure via any route, the lungs are the main storage area for the body [71]. It is then absorbed into maternal circulation, reaching peak concentrations in approximately 15–30 min [72]. Minimal biotransformation occurs from transition of nicotine into the placenta [73, 74]. The nicotine is then re-cycled from the placenta back into maternal circulation, but a fraction is excreted into the amniotic fluid via fetal urine. The nicotine can then be absorbed through the fetus's skin [75]. Compared to maternal levels, the fetal serum levels can be higher by 15% and amniotic fluid levels by more than 88% [76, 77]. Nicotine metabolizes in the fetal liver very slowly, explaining the prolonged fetal half-life of nicotine and higher fetal levels of nicotine compared to the maternal levels [78, 79], and the reason why the cells of the developing lung and other organs are exposed to higher concentrations of nicotine for longer periods. Cotinine is the main metabolite of nicotine, which can reach levels tenfold higher than nicotine itself [78].

The nicotine concentrations in breastmilk can be 2–3 times higher than that in the maternal plasma, primarily due to its high lipid content [80] and higher acidity [81]. Multiple experimental studies have demonstrated that even if the offspring was only exposed to nicotine/smoke postnatally, i.e., through breastmilk, a blunting of alveolarization occurs. For example, suppressed alveolarization and bigger alveoli in rat pups exposed to nicotine independently via breastmilk from postnatal day 2 to postnatal day 21 have been reported [82].

3.4 Early-Life Tobacco Smoke/Nicotine Exposure and Potential Long-Term Outcomes on Respiratory Health

In addition to the predisposition to childhood asthma following perinatal smoke exposure, increasing evidence is observed for an altered developmental programming that predisposes to CLD later in life, even with no subsequent smoke/nicotine exposure [28, 54, 83, 84]. The decreased lung function in children with prenatal smoke exposure persists later in life, attesting that the effects of smoke exposure on small airways are permanent [85]. Hypoplasia and arrested lung growth have been shown in animal models [55–57, 86–90]. The hypoplastic fetal lungs of the in utero smoke-exposed rat fetuses showed reduced parenchymal tissue and septal crests, decreased surface area for gas exchange, and larger and fewer saccules [87]. Again, as alluded to above, the risk of altered lung structure and function following perinatal smoke exposure extends beyond the exposed offspring to the progeny of subsequent non-exposed pregnancies as well [31, 32, 91–93].

3.5 Early-Life Tobacco Smoke/Nicotine Exposure and Offspring Predisposition to Respiratory Infections and Allergic Asthma

Due to changes in offspring immune responses and lung structure following prenatal tobacco/nicotine exposure, there is also an associated increased susceptibility to respiratory infections [41, 94]. As childhood pneumonia has been independently associated with decreased lung function in adulthood, it further heightens the risk of CLD later in life [95]. Although the exact mechanism is not yet determined, based upon a number of animal models and human studies, the increased risk of respiratory infections likely stems from nicotine's effects on the fetus' innate and adaptive immune responses [96, 97]. The normal development of a fetus' immune system is essential for protection against infections not only postnatally but also prenatally during the period of exposure to maternal alloantigens. Prenatal nicotine exposure can affect the early differentiation of white blood cells (WBCs), with a predominance of lymphocytes in circulation along with a decrease in neutrophils [98, 99]. B6C3F1 mice exposed to cigarette smoke prenatally were found to have increased WBC and lymphocytes in circulation at 2-1/2 months of age, although no difference was found in any subsets of lymphoid origin [100]. Prenatal cigarette exposure also resulted in a decrease in T-cell proliferation as well as suppression in innate immune cell-mediated inflammation in offspring. Maternal mononuclear cells from cord blood in mothers who smoked produced higher levels of IL13 after antigen exposure [101, 102]. Additionally, suppressed toll-like receptor (TLR) immune response in these offspring was also noted [101, 102].

Normally, upon delivery, the newborn's immune system shifts T-helper (Th) cell production into predominant Th1. Animal models have demonstrated, however, that after prenatal and postnatal tobacco smoke exposure, an increase in Th2 cells occurs, resulting in an increased risk of subsequent respiratory infections in the offspring [103]. A decrease in the normal increase in Th1 cells results in a subsequent decrease in interferon-γ levels after prenatal smoke exposure, which persists through age 11 if postnatal exposure persists [97, 104]. This decrease contributes to increased infection risk, allergies (also evidenced by elevated IgE and IgD levels postexposure) [105], and asthma. Mice models of prenatal nicotine exposure showed increased M2 phenotype in macrophages in alveoli, which is consistent with the predominance of the Th2 pathway following exposure to nicotine [62]. Although there are only limited human data, primate models have corroborated that prenatal and postnatal smoke exposure results in a decreased production of Th1 and a decreased expression of interferon-γ genes [106].

3.6 Genes and Signaling Pathways Involved in Early-Life Tobacco Smoke/Nicotine-Induced Lung Phenotype

Nicotinic acetylcholine receptors (nAChRs) are extensively expressed in the developing lung [94]. Fetal nicotine exposure causes α7 nAChR upregulation, leading to an increase in collagen and a decrease in elastin [52, 107]. Also, the effect of nicotine on the developing lung is lost in α7 nAChR knockout mice [63]. Lung hypoplasia and higher α7 nAChR immunostaining in the lungs were noted in a study of lung tissues from fetal and infant sudden death cases [108]. Mediated via nicotine's effects on nAChRs, perinatal smoke/nicotine exposure upregulates Wnt signaling and downregulates airway and alveolar PPARγ signaling [54, 109, 110].

Evidence showed that oxidative stress was caused by smoke/nicotine exposure both in vitro and in vivo [111–113]. Nicotine and smoking have been shown to stimulate the hypothalamic pituitary adrenal (HPA) axis, leading to the release of adrenocorticotropic hormone (ACTH) from the anterior pituitary. Increased ACTH results in increased circulating cortisol levels [114–116], which increases blood glucose levels. Glucose, an essential energy source for the lungs [117], is important for its development [118–120].

Several recent studies have focused on epigenetic programming and perinatal smoke/nicotine exposure. For example, DNA methylation changes have been found in the placenta, fetus, and cord blood after prenatal smoke exposure [121–124]. Alterations on specific loci persist even up to adolescence [125–127]. Some of these changes at specific loci can result in tissue-specific morbidities, such as an increased risk of asthma [128, 129]. Specific genes in cord blood studies that may play a role in childhood respiratory morbidities include *AHRR, GF1, FOXP3, CYP1A1, and RUNX* [122, 128–133]. Interestingly, RUNX transcription factors play a critical role in lung development [131, 133]. Airway hyper-responsiveness and asthma have been directly linked to *RUNX1* polymorphisms. Following in utero nicotine exposure, its expression increases in the human embryonic lung [128]. Hypermethylation in RUNX1 and RUNX3 was noted in the placenta and cord samples of tobacco-exposed pregnant mothers [122, 132]. Hypomethylation in AHRR loci has been observed in the cord blood of human neonates, correlating with maternal levels of cotinine, and these changes persisted up to 18 months of age [126, 134, 135]. Lastly, increased risk of asthma and sensitivity of the fetus to maternal smoking have been demonstrated to involve structural polymorphisms or deletions in CYP1A1 and GSTT1 enzymes, which are involved in detoxification and metabolism processes of the toxic metabolites of tobacco products [125, 136].

4 Early-Life Tobacco Smoke/Nicotine Exposure and Offspring Weight

One of the most prevalent consequences of prenatal smoke exposure is a reduction in fetal growth and LBW (2–3 times increased risk for LBW, 200–400 g decrease in birth weight) [7, 137, 138]. LBW likely results from poor fetal growth, prematurity, or a combination of both, possibly resulting from decreased uterine blood flow, nicotine-induced placental vasoconstriction, higher levels of fetal carboxyhemoglobin and the resultant fetal hypoxia, adverse maternal nutrient intake, and elevated fetal stress hormones. While CYP1A1 and GSTs polymorphisms have been previously suggested to be key determinants of maternal smoke exposure-associated LBW, recent work suggests CYP1A1 and GSTs gene polymorphisms to be merely modifiers, while prenatal smoke exposure being the prime determinant [2]. Therefore, it is not surprising that if a woman stops smoking by the end of the first trimester, she is no more likely to have an LBW infant than a woman who never smoked. Smoking cessation even during the third trimester can improve fetal growth. It is important to note that in contrast to the reduction in birth weight, increased risk of overweight/obesity has been observed later in life in prenatally smoke-exposed offspring [139, 140]. Experimentally, rats prenatally exposed to nicotine have been found to gain more weight postnatally compared to controls that persist into adulthood [141]. This is likely mediated by the effect of nicotine on endocrine system's control of body weight through the hypothalamus (center for appetite regulation) [142, 143], which is known to have nAChRs [144]. Supporting this, macaques prenatally exposed to nicotine had altered expression of two hypothalamic peptides that help to regulate satiety and appetite, proopiomelanocortin (POMC) mRNA, and neuropeptide Y [145]. Rat models with similar exposure had increased levels of POMC mRNA, an effect, blocked by dihydro-β-erythroidine (a nAChR antagonist) [146].

5 Early-Life Tobacco Smoke/Nicotine Exposure and Offspring Neurobehavior

Prenatal smoke exposure is linked to offspring disruptive behavior, attention deficits, decreased ability to self-regulate, and altered motor activity [147–149]. Although the mechanism underlying these effects remains unclear, a rigorous meta-analysis revealed the substantial and unique impact of prenatal tobacco smoke exposure on the placental methylome with more than 1200 CpGs being affected, of which more than 25% have been linked to infant outcomes [150].

6 Early-Life Tobacco Smoke/Nicotine Exposure and Offspring Diabetes

In addition to its effects on obesity, evidence shows that prenatal smoke exposure can independently lead to increased risk for type 2 diabetes mellitus (DM) [151–153]. For middle-aged women, prenatal maternal smoking had a stronger association with DM risk than prenatal paternal smoking, and this association persisted even after adjusting for parental race, employment, and diabetes. Furthermore, the effect of parental smoking remained unchanged under adjustment for daughters' birth weight or current body mass index [153]. The risk of type II DM seems to result from a decrease in the pancreas' ability to produce insulin and maintain glucose homeostasis as well as an increased resistance to insulin itself [154]. In particular, decreased insulin production due to a decrease in beta cell numbers, beta cells that secrete insulin abnormally and a reduction in insulin receptor in peripheral tissues have been demonstrated following prenatal and neonatal nicotine exposure to the developing pancreas [155]. Nicotine's interactions with nAChRs expressed on beta cells resulted in increased reactive oxygen species (ROS) production as well as oxidative damage to the mitochondrial proteins in the pancreas of the nicotine-exposed neonates [113]. Interestingly, it may be worth noting that children with maternal smoking during pregnancy tend to undergo a lower risk of type 1 diabetes [156].

7 Early-Life Tobacco Smoke/Nicotine Exposure and Offspring Fertility

Decreased fertility is well known in both men and women who smoke [157, 158]. However, the effects of prenatal cigarette smoke exposure on offspring fertility are inconsistent. For example, some epidemiological studies reported a decrease in the fecundability of women exposed to cigarette smoke in utero [159–162], whereas others reported no association [163, 164]. Animal models have also suggested a potential decreased fertility in offspring prenatally exposed to nicotine due to altered follicle function and impaired regulation of ovarian steroidogenesis [165]. In addition, after progression into adulthood, changes such as increased ovarian cell apoptosis, reduced granulosa cell production, and decreased ovarian angiogenesis have been noted [166]. In contrast, male offspring fertility issues appear to be less significant than those seen in female counterparts, but the effects are considered to be yet unclear.

8 Early-Life Tobacco Smoke/Nicotine Exposure and the Developing Heart

In a rat model of perinatal nicotine exposure, increased susceptibility to cardiac ischemia/reperfusion injury, i.e., an increase in left ventricular infarct size and attenuation of postischemic recovery, has been reported [167]. In addition to the altered cardiac injury repair, in a number of animal [168, 169] and human studies [170–172], perinatal smoke/nicotine exposure has been associated with systemic hypertension with genetic background, sex, and the timing/dose of nicotine exposure being important determinants [173–175]. The exact mechanism, however, is not understood, although endothelial cell dysfunction [176], changes in renal function [177], and alterations in perivascular adipose tissue along with an impairment in its ability to attenuate contraction in blood vessels [141, 174] have been implicated. Furthermore, following prenatal nicotine exposure, intolerance to hypoxia, i.e., bradycardia instead of the usual tachycardia response, has been reported in a neonatal rat model [178]. Lastly, in an embryonic zebrafish model, exposure to nicotine-containing vapors has been recently shown to impact the heart development negatively, with cigarette smoke having a great impact vs e-cig vapors [179].

9 Effects of Prenatal Tobacco Smoke/Nicotine Exposure on Craniofacial Development

Using both self-reports of smoke exposure and serum cotinine levels during pregnancy, evidence has accumulated that there is association between smoking during pregnancy and increased risk of oral clefts [180, 181]. Additionally, it has been recently reported that direct exposure of *Xenopus laevis* embryos to flavored vapors, with and without nicotine, caused significant defects in craniofacial development, demonstrating potentially negative implications for embryonic development due to vapor exposure, even in the absence of nicotine [182]; however, the developmental defects were more significant in those vapors that contained nicotine, indicating that nicotine may be interacting with other components of the vapor to produce effects on craniofacial development.

10 Effects of E-cig Flavorings on Developing Organs

The addition of flavorings to e-cigs is ubiquitous [183] and the concentrations in e-liquids range from 1% to 4% (10–40 mg/mL) [184]. The generally higher likelihood of toxicity to developing systems, lower fetal plasma binding protein concentration, decreased biliary and renal excretion, and greater in utero accumulation of water-soluble compounds in the amniotic fluid predispose to the likely cellular toxicity of e-cig flavorings to the developing fetus [185]. Although e-cig manufacturers argue that e-cig flavorings are "food grade" and are "generally recognized as safe" (GRAS), it is important to realize that the GRAS certification pertains only to ingestion and not inhalation. Moreover, GRAS classification does not consider the heat-induced changes in flavorings' compositions during vaping [49, 186]. A number of cultured systems including endothelial cells, cardiomyocytes, and lung epithelial cells and fibroblasts exposed to commonly used e-cig flavorings show evidence of toxicity and altered gene expression of several key functionally relevant genes [187–189]. Studies focusing on the specific flavoring components of e-liquids indicate the potential for specific negative health effects associated with specific flavoring constituents in e-vapors. For example, some vaping liquids are flavored with diacetyl (artificial butter flavor) which has been implicated in the development of bronchiolitis obliterans, also known as "popcorn lung" [190]. Another common flavoring chemical, cinnamaldehyde (cinnamon flavor), is both genotoxic and cytotoxic to human respiratory cells [191], and 2,5-dimethylpyrazine (chocolate flavor) has cytotoxic effects on both human and mouse respiratory epithelial cells in vitro [192]. Results of these studies indicate that the flavoring components themselves may contribute to the potential health effects caused by vaping.

11 Early-Life Tobacco Smoke/Nicotine Exposure and the Risk of Sudden Infant Death Syndrome (SIDS)

The risk of SIDS is well established in the offspring of parents who smoke during pregnancy and the risk is greater when the mother smokes versus when the father smokes [193]. The predominant effect from maternal smoking comes from the in utero exposure of the fetus to tobacco smoke. Altered central autonomic nervous system development and peripheral physiological responses have been documented in in utero smoke-exposed infants to explain the association with SIDS. For example, experimentally, alterations in the lung [194] and cardiovascular [195] responses and a decreased release of catecholamines during hypoxic periods [196] in in utero nicotine-exposed animal models have been demonstrated. In fact, decreased levels of catecholamines were also found in the cord blood of smokers compared to nonsmokers [197].

12 Early-Life Tobacco Smoke/Nicotine Exposure and Later Risk of Malignancies

Prenatal nicotine exposure has been linked to upward risk of carcinomas such as leukemias, lymphomas, and brain tumors [198]. Nicotine and its metabolites have been known to initiate and stimulate tumor growth [199]. Nicotine can be metabolized to a carcinogenic component, tobacco-specific nitrosamine (TSNA) 4-(methylnitrosamino)-1-(3-pyridyl)-1- butanone (NNK) (also see section on THS). NNK has been found in the urine of neonates exposed prenatally to nicotine [200]. In a hamster model, offspring prenatally exposed to NNK developed tumors in various locations, such as the liver, adrenal glands, lungs, and pancreas [201, 202].

13 Perinatal Tobacco Smoke/Nicotine Exposure and Transgenerational Effect

13.1 Tobacco Smoke/Nicotine Exposure and the Transgenerational Transmission Phenomenon

Numerous studies have shown that not only are first-generation offspring at risk following maternal exposure to smoke/nicotine during pregnancy, but a transgenerational transmission occurs of the pulmonary phenotype to the subsequent-generation offspring as well. For example, in a telephonic survey in Southern California, it was determined that tobacco smoke consumption during pregnancy has potential effects on the lung development of the grandchild, regardless of the mother's smoking status during pregnancy [203]. Similar association was seen in grandchildren developing asthma, who had grandmothers that smoked during their pregnancies [204]. Experimentally, in a rat model, it was convinced that methacholine-induced airway contractility proteins and airway constriction were increased not only in the exposed first-generation offspring but also in subsequent second- and third-generation offspring, without any subsequent exposure to nicotine beyond the F0 generation [31, 32].

13.2 Mechanism Underlying Smoke/Nicotine-Induced Transgenerational Transmission of Pulmonary Phenotype

While the exact mechanism(s) underlying this phenomenon are still unclear, it is relevant to note, that nicotine-induced transgenerational inheritance of other phenotypic and molecular traits has been described in other models [205, 206]. Although the general consensus is that most epigenetic changes induced by environmental exposures are purged at every generation, organisms can demonstrate varying degrees of germline reprogramming [207, 208]. Examples of environmentally induced epigenetic markers across generations being retained have been documented [209–213]. It is safe to say that for transgenerational inheritance of nicotine-induced pulmonary phenotype to occur, the exposure has to occur early in embryonic development, although this remains to be proven [31, 32, 214]. However, other studies have questioned the occurrence of transgenerational asthma following prenatal smoke exposure. For example, no conclusive evidence was found to correlate prenatal smoking of grandmothers with any effect on subsequent offspring in the Avon Longitudinal Study of Parents and Children (ALSPAC) [93].

14 Early-Life Secondhand Smoke/Nicotine Exposure and Respiratory Outcome

14.1 Secondhand Smoke Exposure Sources, Epidemiology, and Health Risks

There is convincing evidence of children's exposure to SHS and its potential harms [215]. SHS is derived from not only exhaled smoke from a smoker but also the sidestream smoke from burning tobacco products, such as cigarettes, pipes, and cigars [135–138]. It is well established that there is no risk-free SHS exposure [215]. Any level or duration of exposure may be harmful. The most common source of SHS exposure to children is the home, but other sources include schools, childcare, transportation, and other public places [216]. SHS exposure results in increased respiratory and ear infections, allergy and asthma, and SIDS in children [137]. One study even reported a 20% increase in the incidence of asthma with SHS exposure [217]. Although there was a brisk drop in the prevalence of SHS exposure to nonsmokers in the US from 1988 to 2014 from 87.5% to 25.2%, there were still 58 million people exposed to SHS from 2013 to 2014. Of these 58 million people, 14 million were children [218]. This tremendous decrease is suspected to be secondary to increased awareness and marketing on its dangers, the initiation of smoke-free laws prohibiting smoking in workplaces and in many public places, the increasing number of voluntary smoke-free homes, and decreased cigarette smoking [219]. Despite this improvement in prevalence, SHS is still thought to be the cause of about 603,000 deaths each year of both children and adults as well as 1% of mortality worldwide [220].

14.2 Mechanism Underlying Respiratory Morbidity Following SHS Exposure

The mechanisms underlying increased risk of allergies including asthma following SHS exposure are likely to be the same as those following direct prenatal exposure, i.e., a shift toward the Th2 phenotype, which results in worsening inflammation and sensitization [221]. SHS also promotes the release of interleukin (IL)-17A, a known proinflammatory cytokine linked to asthma [222], and an increase in IgE levels [223]. Numerous studies, investigating SHS effects on the development of allergic rhinitis, have found increased eotaxin-1 immunoreactive cells, eosinophils, as well as an increase in the production of ROS, lipopolysaccharide, and TLR4 [224, 225]. SHS exposure can also result in a cascade of elastic fiber and collagen degeneration, ultimately resulting in atopic dermatitis [226, 227]. In addition to childhood respiratory diseases, SHS has been linked to the development of CLD in adulthood from the chronic damage incurred from childhood [228]; in fact, SHS exposure in childhood has been found to increase CLD risk by double in adulthood [229].

15 Early-Life Thirdhand Smoke Exposure and Long-Term Outcome

Thirdhand smoke exposure presents a hidden but widespread risk [15, 230]. THS becomes more toxic during its aging process [231], reflecting a dynamic change in its composition. It is recognized that children are the frailest populations to THS exposure, but the adverse effects on their health remain largely unclear. Recent studies using mouse models convinced that exposure to THS during early life can cause changes to many organs, affect behavior and immunity [232, 233], and increase risk for lung cancer later in life [234].

15.1 Sources of THS

THS evolves from SHS and many of the toxic components in SHS are gradually being discovered in THS pollution [15]. One of the main advantages in THS study is the discovery of toxic TSNAs and oxidation products generated de novo from the reaction of surface-bound nicotine, the main constituent in THS, with indoor pollutants [235, 236]. This sheds light on why THS becomes progressively more toxic with time. These TSNAs include NNK, 4-(methylnitrosamino)-4-(3-pyridyl)butanal (NNA) and *N′*-nitrosonornicotine (NNN). NNK and NNN are carcinogens, while NNA is specific to THS as it is not commonly found in fresh smoke [15]. It should be noted that children are often exposed to mixtures of THS and SHS in the real world, which makes analyzing both the THS exposure and its unique health impact difficult.

15.2 Children's Early-Life Exposure

As a distinct entity, the concept of THS which poses health risks for small children has developed only in recent years. In 2004, Matt et al. reported elevated levels of nicotine on household surfaces, in dust, on the smoking mothers' hands, and in homes of the smoking mothers of infants with and without indoor smoking bans [237]. Additionally, compared to infants in homes without smoking allowed, urine cotinine levels of infants whose parents smoked indoors were much higher [237]. It was also reported that nicotine on the hands of children increases with indoor smoking [238]. The 4-(methylnitrosamino)-1-(3-pyridyl)-1-butanol (NNAL)/cotinine ratio represents the biomarker for exposure to NNK and nicotine [15]. The urinary NNAL/cotinine ratio of children was higher than that of adult nonsmokers exposed to SHS [239–241], indicating that THS is another important source of environmental tobacco smoke exposure. Even in places where smoking bans are strictly enforced, such as neonatal intensive care units in hospitals, THS can be found by measuring urinary cotinine and NNAL in infants [242].

15.3 Animal Studies on THS Effects

There are several confounders in humans, such as SHS, which make it difficult for us to reach definitive conclusions on the health impact of THS. On the contrary, animal models offer advantages for assessing such effects as they allow control of the environmental components of the risk, such as exposure to THS only [243].

Various rodent models have been developed and utilized under conditions that mimic exposure of humans. In one of the earliest studies to determine the effect of THS on the developing lung, we exposed fetal rat lung explants to NNA and NNK, the two main TSNA constituents of THS, and determined that this resulted in the breakdown of the alveolar epithelial-mesenchymal cross-talk similar to that caused by nicotine. Later, in a mouse model, Martins-Green et al. found that exposure to THS from 3 weeks to 6 months of age led to pathological alterations in multiple organ systems, including hepatic steatosis, lipid abnormalities, insulin resistance diabetes, lung fibrosis and metabolic syndrome, delayed wound healing, and behavior hyperactivity [233, 244]. Furthermore, we found that early-life exposure to THS could result in developmental changes and persistent impaired immunity in C57BL/6 mice [232]. We also reported that short-term early-life THS exposure using the A/J mouse model led to a significant increase in lung cancer incidence [234]. In these experiments [232, 234], the concentrations of constituents in the THS material were measured and estimated to be comparable to the ingestion exposure of a toddler.

To explore the toxicological effects of THS exposure, many studies using in vitro (cell lines) or ex vivo systems were carried out in various laboratories in the past years. Our own studies first demonstrated evidence for the genotoxicity of THS including the formation of DNA strand breaks, oxidative DNA damage, and NNA-DNA adducts in vitro [234, 245, 246]. In addition, numerous changes have been observed at molecular, cellular, and tissue levels, including inhibited cell proliferation, metabolomic alteration of pathways, fragmentation of cells, and damaged mitochondria [15, 230].

15.4 Human Risks of THS Exposure

So far, little is known about the THS health impact in humans, especially the magnitude of its health risk during early-life exposure. As discussed above, many of the THS components could result in adverse health effects potentially; a critical question is whether their quantities in environments are sufficient to do so. Ramirez et al. found that the calculated cancer risk from THS exposure increases in children from 1 to 6 years old via analyzing nicotine and nitrosamines/TSNAs in house samples [247]. Mahabee-Gittens et al. reported that there may be an association between high hand nicotine and complaints of cough/congestion in children [12].

THS pollution is a new concept and worldwide issue, with infants and young children being the most vulnerable. However, its effects on children health remain unclear. Recent progress on the health effects of early-life exposure to THS in animal models suggests that THS is indeed a potential threat to young children. Attempts should be made on improving awareness by families and the general public [248, 249].

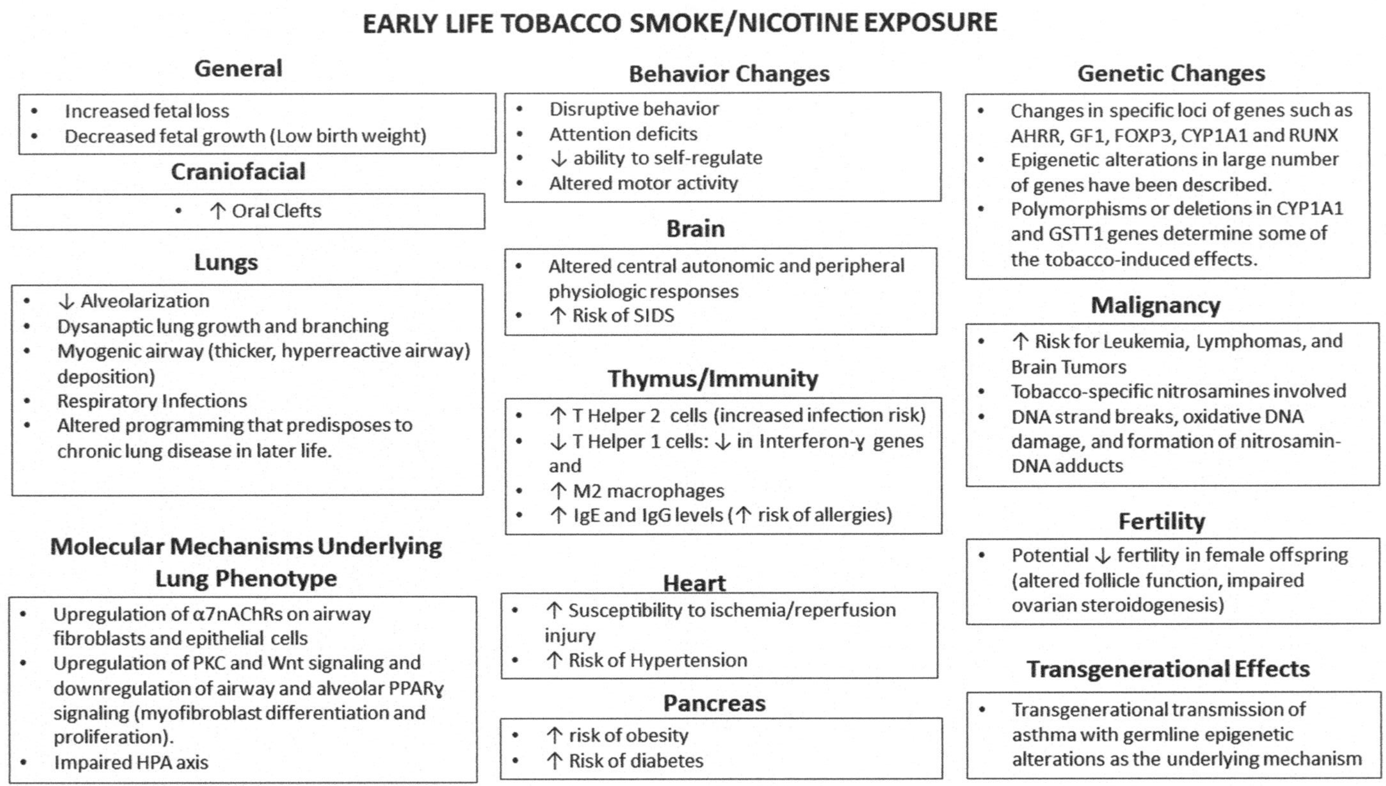

Fig. 1 Effects of tobacco smoke exposure on various organ systems. This figure depicts the numerous effects of early-life tobacco smoke/nicotine exposure from in utero to childhood and adulthood, and even transgenerationally

16 Conclusions

Tobacco smoke/nicotine exposure remains a serious global health concern regardless of over five decades of campaigning on its dangers. Prenatal smoke/nicotine exposure in various forms leads to pulmonary molecular, structural, and functional changes, consistent with asthma in the exposed offspring, as well as its risks for respiratory infections and CLD. In addition to the effects on the lungs, prenatal exposure to smoke/nicotine can also affect the developing heart, brain, and immune systems, oxygen sensing ability, metabolic milieu, fertility, and cancer risk. SHS and THS exposure to the developing lung and other organs is also of concern, as that could be as or even more hazardous than firsthand smoke/nicotine exposure. There is also evidence that some of these effects may not be confined to the exposed offspring but are also transmitted transgenerationally. Novel disease preventive strategies supported by data from the on-going experimental and epidemiological studies are necessary to educate health practitioners, families, and the public regarding the potential risks of early-life environmental tobacco smoke/nicotine exposure; it should be useful for developing strategies for remediation and further preventing children's exposure (Fig. 1).

Acknowledgments This work was supported by grants from the NIH HL127137 and HD071731 (VKR) and the TRDRP 23RT-0018 and 27IP-0050 (VKR) and 24RT-0038 and 28PT-0076 (BH).

References

1. https://www.who.int/news-room/facts-in-pictures/detail/children's-environmental-health
2. Alberg AJ, Shopland DR, Cummings KM (2014 Feb 15) The 2014 Surgeon General's report: commemorating the 50th anniversary of the 1964 report of the Advisory Committee to the US Surgeon General and updating the evidence on the health consequences of cigarette smoking. Am J Epidemiol 179(4):403–412
3. http://www.who.int/tobacco/publications/surveillance/rep_mortality_attributable/en/
4. Jamal A, King BA, Neff LJ et al (2016 Nov 11) Current cigarette smoking among adults – United States, 2005–2015. MMWR Morb Mortal Wkly Rep 65(44):1205–1211
5. Scherman A, Tolosa JE, McEvoy C (2018 Aug) Smoking cessation in pregnancy: a continuing challenge in the United States. Ther Adv Drug Saf 9(8):457–474
6. Shipton D, Tappin DM, Vadiveloo T et al (2009 Oct 29) Reliability of self reported smoking status by pregnant women for estimating smoking prevalence: a retrospective, cross sectional study. BMJ 339:b4347
7. Dietz PM, England LJ, Shapiro-Mendoza CK et al (2010 July) Infant morbidity and mortality attributable to prenatal smoking in the U.S. Am J Prev Med 39(1):45–52
8. Salihu HM, Aliyu MH, Pierre-Louis BJ et al (2003 Dec) Levels of excess infant deaths attributable to maternal smoking during pregnancy in the United States. Matern Child Health J 7(4):219–227
9. Aguirre CG, Bello MS, Andrabi N et al (2016 Jan) Gender, ethnicity, and their intersectionality in the prediction of smoking outcome expectancies in regular cigarette smokers. Behav Modif 40(1–2):281–302

10. Rahmanian SD, Diaz PT, Wewers ME (2011 Mar) Tobacco use and cessation among women: research and treatment-related issues. J Women's Health (Larchmt) 20(3):349–357
11. Stoddard JJ, Gray B (1997 Feb) Maternal smoking and medical expenditures for childhood respiratory illness. Am J Public Health 87(2):205–209
12. Mahabee-Gittens EM, Matt GE, Hoh E et al (2019 May 2) Contribution of thirdhand smoke to overall tobacco smoke exposure in pediatric patients: study protocol. BMC Public Health 19 (1):491
13. Rehan VK, Sakurai R, Torday JS (2011 July) Thirdhand smoke: a new dimension to the effects of cigarette smoke on the developing lung. Am J Phys Lung Cell Mol Phys 301(1):L1–L8
14. Tong VT, Dietz PM, Morrow B et al (2013 Nov 8) Trends in smoking before, during, and after pregnancy – pregnancy risk assessment monitoring system, United States, 40 sites, 2000–2010. MMWR Surveill Summ 62(6):1–19
15. Jacob P 3rd, Benowitz NL, Destaillats H et al (2017 Jan 17) Thirdhand smoke: new evidence, challenges, and future directions. Chem Res Toxicol 30(1):270–294
16. Stepanov I, Jensen J, Hatsukami D et al (2008 Dec) New and traditional smokeless tobacco: comparison of toxicant and carcinogen levels. Nicotine Tob Res 10(12):1773–1782
17. McMillen R, Maduka J, Winickoff J (2012) Use of emerging tobacco products in the United States. J Environ Public Health 2012:989474
18. Mangan D (2013) E-cigarette sales are smoking hot, set to hit $1.7 billion. CNBC Healthcare (2013 August 28)
19. Baeza-Loya S, Viswanath H, Carter A et al (2014 Summer) Perceptions about e-cigarette safety may lead to e-smoking during pregnancy. Bull Menn Clin 78(3):243–252
20. Kahr MK, Padgett S, Shope CD et al (2015 Dec 21) A qualitative assessment of the perceived risks of electronic cigarette and hookah use in pregnancy. BMC Public Health 15:1273
21. Li G, Saad S, Oliver BG et al (2018 Aug) Heat or burn? Impacts of intrauterine tobacco smoke and E-cigarette vapor exposure on the offspring's health outcome. Toxics 1:6(3)
22. Nguyen KH, Tong VT, Marynak KL et al (2016 Dec 22) US Adults' perceptions of the harmful effects during pregnancy of using electronic vapor products versus smoking cigarettes, styles survey, 2015. Prev Chronic Dis 13:E175
23. Oncken C, Ricci KA, Kuo CL et al (2017 May 1) Correlates of electronic cigarettes use before and during pregnancy. Nicotine Tob Res 19(5):585–590
24. Wapner RJ, Sorokin Y, Mele L et al (2007 Sept 20) Long-term outcomes after repeat doses of antenatal corticosteroids. N Engl J Med 357(12):1190–1198
25. Redner R (ed) (2018) Tobacco and nicotine delivery product use in a US national sample of women of reproductive age. Society for Research on Nicotine and Tobacco, Baltimore
26. Farsalinos KE, Spyrou A, Stefopoulos C et al (2015 June 17) Nicotine absorption from electronic cigarette use: comparison between experienced consumers (vapers) and naive users (smokers). Sci Rep 5:11269
27. Marsot A, Simon N (2016 Mar–Apr) Nicotine and cotinine levels with electronic cigarette: a review. Int J Toxicol 35(2):179–185
28. Maritz GS, Harding R (2011 Mar) Life-long programming implications of exposure to tobacco smoking and nicotine before and soon after birth: evidence for altered lung development. Int J Environ Res Public Health 8(3):875–898
29. Tager IB, Segal MR, Speizer FE et al (1988 Oct) The natural history of forced expiratory volumes. Effect of cigarette smoking and respiratory symptoms. Am Rev Respir Dis 138 (4):837–849
30. Upton MN, Smith GD, McConnachie A et al (2004 Feb 15) Maternal and personal cigarette smoking synergize to increase airflow limitation in adults. Am J Respir Crit Care Med 169 (4):479–487
31. Rehan VK, Liu J, Naeem E et al (2012 Oct 30) Perinatal nicotine exposure induces asthma in second generation offspring. BMC Med 10:129
32. Rehan VK, Liu J, Sakurai R et al (2013 Oct 1) Perinatal nicotine-induced transgenerational asthma. Am J Phys Lung Cell Mol Phys 305(7):L501–L507

33. Gilliland FD, Berhane K, Li YF et al (2003 Mar 15) Effects of early onset asthma and in utero exposure to maternal smoking on childhood lung function. Am J Respir Crit Care Med 167 (6):917–924
34. Guerra S, Stern DA, Zhou M et al (2013 Nov) Combined effects of parental and active smoking on early lung function deficits: a prospective study from birth to age 26 years. Thorax 68(11):1021–1028
35. Hanrahan JP, Tager IB, Segal MR et al (1992 May) The effect of maternal smoking during pregnancy on early infant lung function. Am Rev Respir Dis 145(5):1129–1135
36. Tager IB, Ngo L, Hanrahan JP (1995 Sept) Maternal smoking during pregnancy. Effects on lung function during the first 18 months of life. Am J Respir Crit Care Med 152(3):977–983
37. Tanaka K, Miyake Y (2011 June) Association between prenatal and postnatal tobacco smoke exposure and allergies in young children. J Asthma 48(5):458–463
38. Cunningham J, Dockery DW, Speizer FE (1994 June 15) Maternal smoking during pregnancy as a predictor of lung function in children. Am J Epidemiol 139(12):1139–1152
39. Lodrup Carlsen KC, Jaakkola JJ, Nafstad P et al (1997 Aug) In utero exposure to cigarette smoking influences lung function at birth. Eur Respir J 10(8):1774–1779
40. Tager IB, Hanrahan JP, Tosteson TD et al (1993 Apr) Lung function, pre- and post-natal smoke exposure, and wheezing in the first year of life. Am Rev Respir Dis 147(4):811–817
41. McEvoy CT, Spindel ER (2017 Jan) Pulmonary effects of maternal smoking on the Fetus and child: effects on lung development, respiratory morbidities, and life long lung health. Paediatr Respir Rev 21:27–33
42. Sheikh S, Goldsmith LJ, Howell L et al (1999 July) Comparison of lung function in infants exposed to maternal smoking and in infants with a family history of asthma. Chest 116 (1):52–58
43. Jensen RP, Luo W, Pankow JF et al (2015 Jan 22) Hidden formaldehyde in e-cigarette aerosols. N Engl J Med 372(4):392–394
44. Laino T, Tuma C, Curioni A et al (2011 Apr 21) A revisited picture of the mechanism of glycerol dehydration. J Phys Chem A 115(15):3592–3595
45. Laino T, Tuma C, Moor P et al (2012 May 10) Mechanisms of propylene glycol and triacetin pyrolysis. J Phys Chem A 116(18):4602–4609
46. Dinakar C, O'Connor GT (2016 Oct 6) The health effects of electronic cigarettes. N Engl J Med 375(14):1372–1381
47. Hess CA, Olmedo P, Navas-Acien A et al (2017 Jan) E-cigarettes as a source of toxic and potentially carcinogenic metals. Environ Res 152:221–225
48. cco-containing cigarettes: comparison of emission rates and secondhand exposure (2014) Environ Sci Process Impacts 16(10):2259–2267
49. Cheng T (2014) Chemical evaluation of electronic cigarettes. Tob Control 23(Suppl 2):ii11–ii17
50. Dempsey DA, Benowitz NL (2001) Risks and benefits of nicotine to aid smoking cessation in pregnancy. Drug Saf 24(4):277–322
51. Eriksen M, Mackay J, Ross H. The tobacco atlas: World Lung Foundation. Available from: http://www.tobaccoatlas.org
52. Spindel ER, McEvoy CT (2016 Mar 1) The role of nicotine in the effects of maternal smoking during pregnancy on lung development and childhood respiratory disease. Implications for dangers of E-cigarettes. Am J Respir Crit Care Med 193(5):486–494
53. Pierce RA, Nguyen NM (2002 Jan) Prenatal nicotine exposure and abnormal lung function. Am J Respir Cell Mol Biol 26(1):10–13
54. Rehan VK, Asotra K, Torday JS (2009 Sept-Oct) The effects of smoking on the developing lung: insights from a biologic model for lung development, homeostasis, and repair. Lung 187 (5):281–289
55. Sekhon HS, Jia Y, Raab R et al (1999 Mar) Prenatal nicotine increases pulmonary alpha7 nicotinic receptor expression and alters fetal lung development in monkeys. J Clin Invest 103 (5):637–647

56. Sekhon HS, Keller JA, Benowitz NL et al (2001 Sept 15) Prenatal nicotine exposure alters pulmonary function in newborn rhesus monkeys. Am J Respir Crit Care Med 164(6):989–994
57. Maritz GS, Thomas RA (1995 Apr) Maternal nicotine exposure: response of type II pneumocytes of neonatal rat pups. Cell Biol Int 19(4):323–331
58. Roman J, Ritzenthaler JD, Gil-Acosta A et al (2004 Sept) Nicotine and fibronectin expression in lung fibroblasts: implications for tobacco-related lung tissue remodeling. FASEB J 18 (12):1436–1438
59. Wuenschell CW, Zhao J, Tefft JD et al (1998 Jan) Nicotine stimulates branching and expression of SP-A and SP-C mRNAs in embryonic mouse lung culture. Am J Phys 274(1): L165–L170
60. Sandberg KL, Pinkerton KE, Poole SD et al (2011 Apr 30) Fetal nicotine exposure increases airway responsiveness and alters airway wall composition in young lambs. Respir Physiol Neurobiol 176(1–2):57–67
61. Sekhon HS, Proskocil BJ, Clark JA et al (2004 June) Prenatal nicotine exposure increases connective tissue expression in foetal monkey pulmonary vessels. Eur Respir J 23(6):906–915
62. Wongtrakool C, Wang N, Hyde DM et al (2012 May) Prenatal nicotine exposure alters lung function and airway geometry through alpha7 nicotinic receptors. Am J Respir Cell Mol Biol 46(5):695–702
63. Wongtrakool C, Roser-Page S, Rivera HN et al (2007 Sept) Nicotine alters lung branching morphogenesis through the alpha7 nicotinic acetylcholine receptor. Am J Phys Lung Cell Mol Phys 293(3):L611–L618
64. Burri PH (1984) Fetal and postnatal development of the lung. Annu Rev Physiol 46:617–628
65. Herring MJ, Putney LF, Wyatt G et al (2014 Aug 15) Growth of alveoli during postnatal development in humans based on stereological estimation. Am J Phys Lung Cell Mol Phys 307 (4):L338–L344
66. Smith LJ, McKay KO, van Asperen PP et al (2010 Sept) Normal development of the lung and premature birth. Paediatr Respir Rev 11(3):135–142
67. World Health Organization ICD-10 (1992) International statistical classification of diseases and health related problems. WHO, Geneva
68. Schittny J, Burri P (2003) Morphogenesis of the mammalian lung, aspects of structure and extracellular matrix components. In: Massaro D, Massaro G, Chambon P (eds) Lung development and regeneration. Dekker, New York, pp 275–317
69. Carlsten C, Dimich-Ward H, DyBuncio A et al (2012 Dec 5) Cotinine versus questionnaire: early-life environmental tobacco smoke exposure and incident asthma. BMC Pediatr 12:187
70. Neuman A, Hohmann C, Orsini N et al (2012 Nov 15) Maternal smoking in pregnancy and asthma in preschool children: a pooled analysis of eight birth cohorts. Am J Respir Crit Care Med 186(10):1037–1043
71. Brewer BG, Roberts AM, Rowell PP (2004 Aug 16) Short-term distribution of nicotine in the rat lung. Drug Alcohol Depend 75(2):193–198
72. Suzuki K, Horiguchi T, Comas-Urrutia AC et al (1974 May 15) Placental transfer and distribution of nicotine in the pregnant rhesus monkey. Am J Obstet Gynecol 119(2):253–262
73. Luck W, Nau H (1984 July) Nicotine and cotinine concentrations in serum and milk of nursing smokers. Br J Clin Pharmacol 18(1):9–15
74. Matta SG, Balfour DJ, Benowitz NL et al (2007 Feb) Guidelines on nicotine dose selection for in vivo research. Psychopharmacology 190(3):269–319
75. Onuki M, Yokoyama K, Kimura K et al (2003 May) Assessment of urinary cotinine as a marker of nicotine absorption from tobacco leaves: a study on tobacco farmers in Malaysia. J Occup Health 45(3):140–145
76. Andres RL, Day MC (2000 Aug) Perinatal complications associated with maternal tobacco use. Semin Neonatol 5(3):231–241
77. Benowitz N (1998) Nicotine safety and toxicity. Oxford University Press, New York. (Tobacco SfRoNa, editor.)

78. Lambers DS, Clark KE (1996 Apr) The maternal and fetal physiologic effects of nicotine. Semin Perinatol 20(2):115–126
79. Szuts T, Olsson S, Lindquist NG et al (1978 July) Long-term fate of [14C]nicotine in the mouse: retention in the bronchi, melanin-containing tissues and urinary bladder wall. Toxicology 10(3):207–220
80. Sastry BV, Chance MB, Hemontolor ME et al (1998 Aug) Formation and retention of cotinine during placental transfer of nicotine in human placental cotyledon. Pharmacology 57 (2):104–116
81. Luck W, Nau H, Hansen R et al (1985) Extent of nicotine and cotinine transfer to the human fetus, placenta and amniotic fluid of smoking mothers. Dev Pharmacol Ther 8(6):384–395
82. Maritz GS, Windvogel S (2003 June) Is maternal copper supplementation during alveolarization protecting the developing rat lung against the adverse effects of maternal nicotine exposure? A morphometric study. Exp Lung Res 29(4):243–260
83. Maritz GS (2013 Mar) Perinatal exposure to nicotine and implications for subsequent obstructive lung disease. Paediatr Respir Rev 14(1):3–8
84. Martinez FD (2016 Sept 1) Early-life origins of chronic obstructive pulmonary disease. N Engl J Med 375(9):871–878
85. Goksor E, Amark M, Alm B et al (2007 July) The impact of pre- and post-natal smoke exposure on future asthma and bronchial hyper-responsiveness. Acta Paediatr 96 (7):1030–1035
86. Blacquière MJ, Timens W, Melgert BN et al (2009) Maternal smoking during pregnancy induces airway remodelling in mice offspring. Eur Respir J 33(5):1133
87. Collins MH, Moessinger AC, Kleinerman J et al (1985 Apr) Fetal lung hypoplasia associated with maternal smoking: a morphometric analysis. Pediatr Res 19(4):408–412
88. Maritz GS, Dennis H (1998) Maternal nicotine exposure during gestation and lactation interferes with alveolar development in the neonatal lung. Reprod Fertil Dev 10(3):255–261
89. Maritz GS, Matthews HL, Aalbers J (2000) Maternal copper supplementation protects the neonatal rat lung against the adverse effects of maternal nicotine exposure. Reprod Fertil Dev 12(1–2):97–103
90. Sandberg K, Poole SD, Hamdan A et al (2004 Sept) Altered lung development after prenatal nicotine exposure in young lambs. Pediatr Res 56(3):432–439
91. Li YF, Langholz B, Salam MT et al (2005 Apr) Maternal and grandmaternal smoking patterns are associated with early childhood asthma. Chest 127(4):1232–1241
92. Maritz GS, Mutemwa M (2014 Jan) The effect of grand maternal nicotine exposure during gestation and lactation on lung integrity of the F2 generation. Pediatr Pulmonol 49(1):67–75
93. Miller LL, Henderson J, Northstone K et al (2014 June) Do grandmaternal smoking patterns influence the etiology of childhood asthma? Chest 145(6):1213–1218
94. Gibbs K, Collaco JM, McGrath-Morrow SA (2016 Feb) Impact of tobacco smoke and nicotine exposure on lung development. Chest 149(2):552–561
95. Chan JY, Stern DA, Guerra S et al (2015 Apr) Pneumonia in childhood and impaired lung function in adults: a longitudinal study. Pediatrics 135(4):607–616
96. Haberg SE, Stigum H, Nystad W et al (2007 Sept 15) Effects of pre- and postnatal exposure to parental smoking on early childhood respiratory health. Am J Epidemiol 166(6):679–686
97. Macaubas C, de Klerk NH, Holt BJ et al (2003 Oct 11) Association between antenatal cytokine production and the development of atopy and asthma at age 6 years. Lancet 362 (9391):1192–1197
98. Almanzar G, Eberle G, Lassacher A et al (2013 Apr 18) Maternal cigarette smoking and its effect on neonatal lymphocyte subpopulations and replication. BMC Pediatr 13:57
99. Paganelli R, Ramadas D, Layward L et al (1979 May) Maternal smoking and cord blood immunity function. Clin Exp Immunol 36(2):256–259
100. Harrison KL (1979 Aug) The effect of maternal smoking on neonatal leucocytes. Aust N Z J Obstet Gynaecol 19(3):166–168

101. Noakes PS, Hale J, Thomas R et al (2006 Oct) Maternal smoking is associated with impaired neonatal toll-like-receptor-mediated immune responses. Eur Respir J 28(4):721–729
102. Noakes PS, Holt PG, Prescott SL (2003 Oct) Maternal smoking in pregnancy alters neonatal cytokine responses. Allergy 58(10):1053–1058
103. Singh SP, Gundavarapu S, Pena-Philippides JC et al (2011 Nov 1) Prenatal secondhand cigarette smoke promotes Th2 polarization and impairs goblet cell differentiation and airway mucus formation. J Immunol 187(9):4542–4552
104. Tebow G, Sherrill DL, Lohman IC et al (2008 June) Effects of parental smoking on interferon gamma production in children. Pediatrics 121(6):e1563–e1569
105. Magnusson CG (1986 Nov) Maternal smoking influences cord serum IgE and IgD levels and increases the risk for subsequent infant allergy. J Allergy Clin Immunol 78(5 Pt 1):898–904
106. Wang L, Joad JP, Zhong C et al (2008) Effects of environmental tobacco smoke exposure on pulmonary immune response in infant monkeys. J Allergy Clin Immunol 122(2):400–406. 406 e1–5
107. Sekhon HS, Keller JA, Proskocil BJ et al (2002 Jan) Maternal nicotine exposure upregulates collagen gene expression in fetal monkey lung. Association with alpha7 nicotinic acetylcholine receptors. Am J Respir Cell Mol Biol 26(1):31–41
108. Lavezzi AM, Corna MF, Alfonsi G et al (2014 Feb 1) Possible role of the alpha7 nicotinic receptors in mediating nicotine's effect on developing lung – implications in unexplained human perinatal death. BMC Pulm Med 14:11
109. Liu J, Naeem E, Tian J et al (2013 Jan) Sex-specific perinatal nicotine-induced asthma in rat offspring. Am J Respir Cell Mol Biol 48(1):53–62
110. Torday JS, Rehan VK (2006 Oct) Up-regulation of fetal rat lung parathyroid hormone-related protein gene regulatory network down-regulates the Sonic Hedgehog/Wnt/betacatenin gene regulatory network. Pediatr Res 60(4):382–388
111. Noakes PS, Thomas R, Lane C et al (2007 Aug) Association of maternal smoking with increased infant oxidative stress at 3 months of age. Thorax 62(8):714–717
112. Orhon FS, Ulukol B, Kahya D et al (2009 Aug) The influence of maternal smoking on maternal and newborn oxidant and antioxidant status. Eur J Pediatr 168(8):975–981
113. Bruin JE, Petre MA, Lehman MA et al (2008 June 1) Maternal nicotine exposure increases oxidative stress in the offspring. Free Radic Biol Med 44(11):1919–1925
114. Ji B, Zhao GZ, Sakurai R et al (2016 Aug) Effect of maternal electroacupuncture on perinatal nicotine exposure-induced lung phenotype in offspring. Lung 194(4):535–546
115. Matta SG, Beyer HS, McAllen KM et al (1987 Oct) Nicotine elevates rat plasma ACTH by a central mechanism. J Pharmacol Exp Ther 243(1):217–226
116. Xue Y, Morris M, Ni L et al (2010 Apr) Venous plasma nicotine correlates of hormonal effects of tobacco smoking. Pharmacol Biochem Behav 95(2):209–215
117. O'Neil JJ, Tierney DF (1974 Apr) Rat lung metabolism: glucose utilization by isolated perfused lungs and tissue slices. Am J Phys 226(4):867–873
118. Bourbon J, Jost A (1982 Jan) Control of glycogen metabolism in the developing fetal lung. Pediatr Res 16(1):50–56
119. Post M, Copeland L (2002) Overview of lung development. Acta Pharmacol Sin 23:S4–S7
120. Maritz G (1986 July) Pre- and postnatal carbohydrate metabolism of rat lung tissue. The effect of maternal nicotine exposure. Arch Toxicol 59(2):89–93
121. Chhabra D, Sharma S, Kho AT et al (2014 Nov) Fetal lung and placental methylation is associated with in utero nicotine exposure. Epigenetics 9(11):1473–1484
122. Joubert BR, Haberg SE, Nilsen RM et al (2012 Oct) 450K epigenome-wide scan identifies differential DNA methylation in newborns related to maternal smoking during pregnancy. Environ Health Perspect 120(10):1425–1431
123. Lehmann M, Baarsma HA, Konigshoff M (2016 Dec) WNT signaling in lung aging and disease. Ann Am Thorac Soc 13(Suppl 5):S411–S416

124. Nielsen CH, Larsen A, Nielsen AL (2016 Feb) DNA methylation alterations in response to prenatal exposure of maternal cigarette smoking: a persistent epigenetic impact on health from maternal lifestyle? Arch Toxicol 90(2):231–245
125. Breton CV, Byun HM, Wang X et al (2011 July 15) DNA methylation in the arginase-nitric oxide synthase pathway is associated with exhaled nitric oxide in children with asthma. Am J Respir Crit Care Med 184(2):191–197
126. Novakovic B, Ryan J, Pereira N et al (2014 Mar) Postnatal stability, tissue, and time specific effects of AHRR methylation change in response to maternal smoking in pregnancy. Epigenetics 9(3):377–386
127. Richmond RC, Simpkin AJ, Woodward G et al (2015 Apr 15) Prenatal exposure to maternal smoking and offspring DNA methylation across the lifecourse: findings from the Avon Longitudinal Study of Parents and Children (ALSPAC). Hum Mol Genet 24(8):2201–2217
128. Haley KJ, Lasky-Su J, Manoli SE et al (2011 Nov) RUNX transcription factors: association with pediatric asthma and modulated by maternal smoking. Am J Phys Lung Cell Mol Phys 301(5):L693–L701
129. Morales E, Bustamante M, Vilahur N et al (2012 May 1) DNA hypomethylation at ALOX12 is associated with persistent wheezing in childhood. Am J Respir Crit Care Med 185(9):937–943
130. Hinz D, Bauer M, Roder S et al (2012 Mar) Cord blood Tregs with stable FOXP3 expression are influenced by prenatal environment and associated with atopic dermatitis at the age of one year. Allergy 67(3):380–389
131. Lee JM, Kwon HJ, Lai WF et al (2014 May) Requirement of Runx3 in pulmonary vasculogenesis. Cell Tissue Res 356(2):445–449
132. Suter M, Abramovici A, Showalter L et al (2010 Oct) In utero tobacco exposure epigenetically modifies placental CYP1A1 expression. Metabolism 59(10):1481–1490
133. Voon DC, Hor YT, Ito Y (2015 Dec) The RUNX complex: reaching beyond haematopoiesis into immunity. Immunology 146(4):523–536
134. Joubert BR, Haberg SE, Bell DA et al (2014 June) Maternal smoking and DNA methylation in newborns: in utero effect or epigenetic inheritance? Cancer Epidemiol Biomark Prev 23 (6):1007–1017
135. Monick MM, Beach SR, Plume J et al (2012 Mar) Coordinated changes in AHRR methylation in lymphoblasts and pulmonary macrophages from smokers. Am J Med Genet B Neuropsychiatr Genet 159B(2):141–151
136. Wenten M, Li YF, Lin PC et al (2009 May) In utero smoke exposure, glutathione S-transferase P1 haplotypes, and respiratory illness-related absence among schoolchildren. Pediatrics 123 (5):1344–1351
137. U.S. Department of Health and Human Services (2014) The health consequences of Smoking—50 years of progress: a report of the surgeon general Atlanta: U.S. Department of Health and Human Services, Centers for Disease Control and Prevention, National Center for Chronic Disease Prevention and Health Promotion, Office on Smoking and Health
138. Hammoud AO, Bujold E, Sorokin Y et al (2005) Smoking in pregnancy revisited: findings from a large population-based study. Am J Obstet Gynecol 192(6):1856–1862. discussion 1862-3
139. da Silva Magalhaes EI, Peixoto Lima N, Baptista Menezes AM et al (2019 June 12) Maternal smoking during pregnancy and offspring body composition in adulthood: results from two birth cohort studies. BMJ Open 9(6):e023852
140. Harris HR, Willett WC, Michels KB (2013 Oct) Parental smoking during pregnancy and risk of overweight and obesity in the daughter. Int J Obes 37(10):1356–1363
141. Gao YJ, Holloway AC, Zeng ZH et al (2005 Apr) Prenatal exposure to nicotine causes postnatal obesity and altered perivascular adipose tissue function. Obes Res 13(4):687–692
142. Hillebrand JJ, de Wied D, Adan RA (2002 Dec) Neuropeptides, food intake and body weight regulation: a hypothalamic focus. Peptides 23(12):2283–2306
143. Wilding JP (2002 Aug) Neuropeptides and appetite control. Diabet Med 19(8):619–627

144. Li MD, Kane JK, Konu O (2003) Nicotine, body weight and potential implications in the treatment of obesity. Curr Top Med Chem 3(8):899–919
145. Grove KL, Sekhon HS, Brogan RS et al (2001 Nov) Chronic maternal nicotine exposure alters neuronal systems in the arcuate nucleus that regulate feeding behavior in the newborn rhesus macaque. J Clin Endocrinol Metab 86(11):5420–5426
146. Huang LZ, Winzer-Serhan UH (2007 Feb 15) Nicotine regulates mRNA expression of feeding peptides in the arcuate nucleus in neonatal rat pups. Dev Neurobiol 67(3):363–377
147. Cornelius MD, Day NL (2009 Apr) Developmental consequences of prenatal tobacco exposure. Curr Opin Neurol 22(2):121–125
148. Stroud LR, Papandonatos GD, Rodriguez D et al (2014 Oct) Maternal smoking during pregnancy and infant stress response: test of a prenatal programming hypothesis. Psychoneuroendocrinology 48:29–40
149. Wakschlag LS, Keenan K (2001 June) Clinical significance and correlates of disruptive behavior in environmentally at-risk preschoolers. J Clin Child Psychol 30(2):262–275
150. Everson T, Vives-Usano M, Sevve E (2019) Placental DNA methylation signatures of maternal smoking during pregnancy and potential impacts on fetal growth. bioRxiv
151. Bao W, Michels KB, Tobias DK et al (2016 Feb) Parental smoking during pregnancy and the risk of gestational diabetes in the daughter. Int J Epidemiol 45(1):160–169
152. Chang CH, Chuang LM (2016 July) Fetal exposure to parental smoking and the risk of type 2 diabetes: are lifestyle-related factors more important? J Diabetes Investig 7(4):472–475
153. La Merrill MA, Cirillo PM, Krigbaum NY et al (2015 June) The impact of prenatal parental tobacco smoking on risk of diabetes mellitus in middle-aged women. J Dev Orig Health Dis 6 (3):242–249
154. Butler AE, Janson J, Bonner-Weir S et al (2003 Jan) Beta-cell deficit and increased beta-cell apoptosis in humans with type 2 diabetes. Diabetes 52(1):102–110
155. Bruin JE, Kellenberger LD, Gerstein HC et al (2007 July) Fetal and neonatal nicotine exposure and postnatal glucose homeostasis: identifying critical windows of exposure. J Endocrinol 194 (1):171–178
156. Magnus MC, Tapia G, Olsen SF et al (2018 Nov) Parental smoking and risk of childhood-onset type 1 diabetes. Epidemiology 29(6):848–856
157. Augood C, Duckitt K, Templeton AA (1998 June) Smoking and female infertility: a systematic review and meta-analysis. Hum Reprod 13(6):1532–1539
158. Kunzle R, Mueller MD, Hanggi W et al (2003 Feb) Semen quality of male smokers and nonsmokers in infertile couples. Fertil Steril 79(2):287–291
159. Jensen TK, Henriksen TB, Hjollund NH et al (1998 Nov 15) Adult and prenatal exposures to tobacco smoke as risk indicators of fertility among 430 Danish couples. Am J Epidemiol 148 (10):992–997
160. Jensen TK, Joffe M, Scheike T et al (2006 Dec) Early exposure to smoking and future fecundity among Danish twins. Int J Androl 29(6):603–613
161. Weinberg CR, Wilcox AJ, Baird DD (1989 May) Reduced fecundability in women with prenatal exposure to cigarette smoking. Am J Epidemiol 129(5):1072–1078
162. Ye X, Skjaerven R, Basso O et al (2010 Nov) In utero exposure to tobacco smoke and subsequent reduced fertility in females. Hum Reprod 25(11):2901–2906
163. Baird DD, Wilcox AJ (1986 Sept) Future fertility after prenatal exposure to cigarette smoke. Fertil Steril 46(3):368–372
164. Joffe M, Barnes I (2000 Nov) Do parental factors affect male and female fertility? Epidemiology 11(6):700–705
165. Holloway AC, Kellenberger LD, Petrik JJ (2006 Oct) Fetal and neonatal exposure to nicotine disrupts ovarian function and fertility in adult female rats. Endocrine 30(2):213–216
166. Petrik JJ, Gerstein HC, Cesta CE et al (2009 Oct) Effects of rosiglitazone on ovarian function and fertility in animals with reduced fertility following fetal and neonatal exposure to nicotine. Endocrine 36(2):281–290

167. Spreafico G, Sartori F, Roviaro GC et al (1975 Jan-Feb) Bronchiolo-alveolar carcinoma. Arch Chir Torac Cardiovasc 32(1–2):107–140
168. Pausova Z, Paus T, Sedova L et al (2003 Sept) Prenatal exposure to nicotine modifies kidney weight and blood pressure in genetically susceptible rats: a case of gene-environment interaction. Kidney Int 64(3):829–835
169. Tao H, Rui C, Zheng J et al (2013 June) Angiotensin II-mediated vascular changes in aged offspring rats exposed to perinatal nicotine. Peptides 44:111–119
170. Beratis NG, Panagoulias D, Varvarigou A (1996 June) Increased blood pressure in neonates and infants whose mothers smoked during pregnancy. J Pediatr 128(6):806–812
171. Geerts CC, Grobbee DE, van der Ent CK et al (2007) Tobacco smoke exposure of pregnant mothers and blood pressure in their newborns: results from the wheezing illnesses study Leidsche Rijn birth cohort. Hypertension (Dallas, Tex: 1979) 50(3):572–578
172. Morley R, Leeson Payne C, Lister G et al (1995 Feb) Maternal smoking and blood pressure in 7.5 to 8 year old offspring. Arch Dis Child 72(2):120–124
173. Brion MJ, Leary SD, Smith GD et al (2007) Similar associations of parental prenatal smoking suggest child blood pressure is not influenced by intrauterine effects. Hypertension (Dallas, Tex: 1979) 49(6):1422–1428
174. Gao YJ, Holloway AC, Su LY et al (2008 Aug 20) Effects of fetal and neonatal exposure to nicotine on blood pressure and perivascular adipose tissue function in adult life. Eur J Pharmacol 590(1–3):264–268
175. Law CM, Barker DJ, Bull AR et al (1991 Nov) Maternal and fetal influences on blood pressure. Arch Dis Child 66(11):1291–1295
176. Xiao D, Huang X, Lawrence J et al (2007 Feb) Fetal and neonatal nicotine exposure differentially regulates vascular contractility in adult male and female offspring. J Pharmacol Exp Ther 320(2):654–661
177. Mao C, Wu J, Xiao D et al (2009 Apr) The effect of fetal and neonatal nicotine exposure on renal development of AT(1) and AT(2) receptors. Reprod Toxicol 27(2):149–154
178. Slotkin TA, Saleh JL, McCook EC et al (1997 Mar) Impaired cardiac function during postnatal hypoxia in rats exposed to nicotine prenatally: implications for perinatal morbidity and mortality, and for sudden infant death syndrome. Teratology 55(3):177–184
179. Palpant NJ, Hofsteen P, Pabon L et al (2015) Cardiac development in zebrafish and human embryonic stem cells is inhibited by exposure to tobacco cigarettes and e-cigarettes. PLoS One 10(5):e0126259
180. Little J, Cardy A, Munger RG (2004 Mar) Tobacco smoking and oral clefts: a meta-analysis. Bull World Health Organ 82(3):213–218
181. Shaw GM, Carmichael SL, Vollset SE et al (2009 Jan) Mid-pregnancy cotinine and risks of orofacial clefts and neural tube defects. J Pediatr 154(1):17–19
182. Kennedy AE, Kandalam S, Olivares-Navarrete R et al (2017) E-cigarette aerosol exposure can cause craniofacial defects in Xenopus laevis embryos and mammalian neural crest cells. PLoS One 12(9):e0185729
183. Morean ME, Butler ER, Bold KW et al (2018) Preferring more e-cigarette flavors is associated with e-cigarette use frequency among adolescents but not adults. PLoS One 13(1):e0189015
184. Tierney PA, Karpinski CD, Brown JE et al (2016 Apr) Flavour chemicals in electronic cigarette fluids. Tob Control 25(e1):e10–e15
185. Makri A, Goveia M, Balbus J et al (2004 Nov-Dec) Children's susceptibility to chemicals: a review by developmental stage. J Toxicol Environ Health B Crit Rev 7(6):417–435
186. Grana R, Benowitz N, Glantz SA (2014 May 13) E-cigarettes: a scientific review. Circulation 129(19):1972–1986
187. Fetterman JL, Weisbrod RM, Feng B et al (2018 July) Flavorings in tobacco products induce endothelial cell dysfunction. Arterioscler Thromb Vasc Biol 38(7):1607–1615
188. Gerloff J, Sundar IK, Freter R et al (2017 Mar 1) Inflammatory response and barrier dysfunction by different e-cigarette flavoring chemicals identified by gas chromatography-mass

spectrometry in e-liquids and e-Vapors on human lung epithelial cells and fibroblasts. Appl In Vitro Toxicol 3(1):28–40
189. Keith RJ, Fetterman JL, Riggs DW et al (2018 Mar 30) Protocol to assess the impact of tobacco-induced volatile organic compounds on cardiovascular risk in a cross- sectional cohort: cardiovascular injury due to tobacco use study. BMJ Open 8(3):e019850
190. Allen JG, Flanigan SS, LeBlanc M et al (2016 June) Flavoring chemicals in E-cigarettes: diacetyl, 2,3-pentanedione, and acetoin in a sample of 51 products, including fruit-, candy-, and cocktail-Flavored E-cigarettes. Environ Health Perspect 124(6):733–739
191. Behar RZ, Luo W, Lin SC et al (2016) Distribution, quantification and toxicity of cinnamaldehyde in electronic cigarette refill fluids and aerosols. Tob Control 25(Suppl 2): ii94–ii102
192. Sherwood CL, Boitano S (2016 May 17) Airway epithelial cell exposure to distinct e-cigarette liquid flavorings reveals toxicity thresholds and activation of CFTR by the chocolate flavoring 2,5-dimethypyrazine. Respir Res 17(1):57
193. Mitchell EA, Milerad J (2006 Apr-June) Smoking and the sudden infant death syndrome. Rev Environ Health 21(2):81–103
194. Sandberg KL, Poole SD, Hamdan A et al (2007 June 15) Prenatal nicotine exposure transiently alters the lung mechanical response to hypoxia in young lambs. Respir Physiol Neurobiol 156 (3):283–292
195. Hafstrom O, Milerad J, Sundell HW (2002 Dec 15) Prenatal nicotine exposure blunts the cardiorespiratory response to hypoxia in lambs. Am J Respir Crit Care Med 166(12 Pt 1):1544–1549
196. Slotkin TA, Lappi SE, McCook EC et al (1995) Loss of neonatal hypoxia tolerance after prenatal nicotine exposure: implications for sudden infant death syndrome. Brain Res Bull 38 (1):69–75
197. Oncken CA, Kranzler HR (2003 June) Pharmacotherapies to enhance smoking cessation during pregnancy. Drug Alcohol Rev 22(2):191–202
198. Sasco AJ, Vainio H (1999 Apr) From in utero and childhood exposure to parental smoking to childhood cancer: a possible link and the need for action. Hum Exp Toxicol 18(4):192–201
199. Martin JW, Mousa SS, Shaker O et al (2009 June) The multiple faces of nicotine and its implications in tissue and wound repair. Exp Dermatol 18(6):497–505
200. Lackmann GM, Salzberger U, Tollner U et al (1999 Mar 3) Metabolites of a tobacco-specific carcinogen in urine from newborns. J Natl Cancer Inst 91(5):459–465
201. Schuller HM, Jorquera R, Lu X et al (1994) Transplacental carcinogenicity of low doses of 4-(methylnitrosamino)-1-(3-pyridyl)-1-butanone administered subcutaneously or intratracheally to hamsters. J Cancer Res Clin Oncol 120(4):200–203
202. Schuller HM, Jorquera R, Reichert A et al (1993 June 1) Transplacental induction of pancreas tumors in hamsters by ethanol and the tobacco-specific nitrosamine 4-(methylnitrosamino)-1-(3-pyridyl)-1-butanone. Cancer Res 53(11):2498–2501
203. Li YF, Gilliland FD, Berhane K et al (2000 Dec) Effects of in utero and environmental tobacco smoke exposure on lung function in boys and girls with and without asthma. Am J Respir Crit Care Med 162(6):2097–2104
204. Magnus MC, Haberg SE, Karlstad O et al (2015 Mar) Grandmother's smoking when pregnant with the mother and asthma in the grandchild: the Norwegian mother and child cohort study. Thorax 70(3):237–243
205. McCarthy DM, Morgan TJ Jr, Lowe SE et al (2018 Oct) Nicotine exposure of male mice produces behavioral impairment in multiple generations of descendants. PLoS Biol 16(10): e2006497
206. Taki FA, Pan X, Lee MH et al (2014 Dec 17) Nicotine exposure and transgenerational impact: a prospective study on small regulatory microRNAs. Sci Rep 4:7513
207. Daxinger L, Whitelaw E (2012 Jan 31) Understanding transgenerational epigenetic inheritance via the gametes in mammals. Nat Rev Genet 13(3):153–162

208. Monk M, Boubelik M, Lehnert S (1987 Mar) Temporal and regional changes in DNA methylation in the embryonic, extraembryonic and germ cell lineages during mouse embryo development. Development 99(3):371–382
209. Dias BG, Ressler KJ (2014 Jan) Parental olfactory experience influences behavior and neural structure in subsequent generations. Nat Neurosci 17(1):89–96
210. Heard E, Martienssen RA (2014 Mar 27) Transgenerational epigenetic inheritance: myths and mechanisms. Cell 157(1):95–109
211. Iqbal K, Tran DA, Li AX et al (2015 Mar 27) Deleterious effects of endocrine disruptors are corrected in the mammalian germline by epigenome reprogramming. Genome Biol 16:59
212. Morgan HD, Sutherland HG, Martin DI et al (1999 Nov) Epigenetic inheritance at the agouti locus in the mouse. Nat Genet 23(3):314–318
213. Seong KH, Li D, Shimizu H et al (2011 June 24) Inheritance of stress-induced, ATF-2-dependent epigenetic change. Cell 145(7):1049–1061
214. Skinner MK (2015 Apr 26) Environmental epigenetics and a unified theory of the molecular aspects of evolution: a neo-Lamarckian concept that facilitates neo-Darwinian evolution. Genome Biol Evol 7(5):1296–1302
215. US Department of Health and Human Services (2006) The health consequences of involuntary exposure to tobacco smoke: a report of the Surgeon General Washington, DC: US Department of Health and Human Services. Available from: https://www.surgeongeneral.gov/library/reports/secondhandsmoke/fullreport.pdf
216. Hwang SH, Hwang JH, Moon JS et al (2012 Feb) Environmental tobacco smoke and children's health. Korean J Pediatr 55(2):35–41
217. Burke H, Leonardi-Bee J, Hashim A et al (2012 Apr) Prenatal and passive smoke exposure and incidence of asthma and wheeze: systematic review and meta-analysis. Pediatrics 129 (4):735–744
218. Tsai J, Homa DM, Gentzke AS et al (2018 Dec 7) Exposure to secondhand smoke among nonsmokers – United States, 1988–2014. MMWR Morb Mortal Wkly Rep 67(48):1342–1346
219. American Nonsmokers' Rights Foundation (2018) Summary of 100% smokefree state laws and population protected by 100% U.S. smokefree laws Berkeley, CA: American Nonsmokers' Rights Foundation. Available from: http://no-smoke.org/wp-content/uploads/pdf/SummaryUSPopList.pdf
220. Oberg M, Jaakkola MS, Woodward A et al (2011 Jan) Worldwide burden of disease from exposure to second-hand smoke: a retrospective analysis of data from 192 countries. Lancet 377(9760):139–146
221. Strzelak A, Ratajczak A, Adamiec A et al (2018 May) Tobacco smoke induces and alters immune responses in the lung triggering inflammation, allergy, Asthma and Other Lung Diseases: a mechanistic review. Int J Environ Res Public Health 21:15(5)
222. Bozinovski S, Seow HJ, Chan SP et al (2015 Nov) Innate cellular sources of interleukin-17A regulate macrophage accumulation in cigarette- smoke-induced lung inflammation in mice. Clin Sci (Lond) 129(9):785–796
223. Baena-Cagnani CE, Gomez RM, Baena-Cagnani R et al (2009 Apr) Impact of environmental tobacco smoke and active tobacco smoking on the development and outcomes of asthma and rhinitis. Curr Opin Allergy Clin Immunol 9(2):136–140
224. Huang CC, Wang CH, Fu CH et al (2016 Nov) Association between cigarette smoking and interleukin-17A expression in nasal tissues of patients with chronic rhinosinusitis and asthma. Medicine (Baltimore) 95(47):e5432
225. Pace E, Ferraro M, Di Vincenzo S et al (2014 Mar) Oxidative stress and innate immunity responses in cigarette smoke stimulated nasal epithelial cells. Toxicol in Vitro 28(2):292–299
226. Kantor R, Kim A, Thyssen JP et al (2016 Dec) Association of atopic dermatitis with smoking: a systematic review and meta-analysis. J Am Acad Dermatol 75(6):1119–1125 e1
227. Puri P, Nandar SK, Kathuria S et al (2017 July–Aug) Effects of air pollution on the skin: a review. Indian J Dermatol Venereol Leprol 83(4):415–423

228. Vanker A, Gie RP, Zar HJ (2017 Aug) The association between environmental tobacco smoke exposure and childhood respiratory disease: a review. Expert Rev Respir Med 11(8):661–673
229. Johannessen A, Bakke PS, Hardie JA et al (2012 Apr) Association of exposure to environmental tobacco smoke in childhood with chronic obstructive pulmonary disease and respiratory symptoms in adults. Respirology 17(3):499–505
230. Matt GE, Quintana PJ, Destaillats H et al (2011 Sept) Thirdhand tobacco smoke: emerging evidence and arguments for a multidisciplinary research agenda. Environ Health Perspect 119 (9):1218–1226
231. Schick SF, Glantz SA (2006 Dec) Sidestream cigarette smoke toxicity increases with aging and exposure duration. Tob Control 15(6):424–429
232. Hang B, Snijders AM, Huang Y et al (2017 Feb) Early exposure to thirdhand cigarette smoke affects body mass and the development of immunity in mice. Sci Rep 7:41915
233. Martins-Green M, Adhami N, Frankos M et al (2014) Cigarette smoke toxins deposited on surfaces: implications for human health. PLoS One 9(1):e86391
234. Hang B, Wang Y, Huang Y et al (2018 Feb) Short-term early exposure to thirdhand cigarette smoke increases lung cancer incidence in mice. Clin Sci (Lond) 132(4):475–488
235. Destaillats H, Singer BC, Lee SK et al (2006 Mar) Effect of ozone on nicotine desorption from model surfaces: evidence for heterogeneous chemistry. Environ Sci Technol 40(6):1799–1805
236. Sleiman M, Gundel LA, Pankow JF et al (2010 Apr) Formation of carcinogens indoors by surface-mediated reactions of nicotine with nitrous acid, leading to potential thirdhand smoke hazards. Proc Natl Acad Sci U S A 107(15):6576–6581
237. Matt GE, Quintana PJ, Hovell MF et al (2004 Mar) Households contaminated by environmental tobacco smoke: sources of infant exposures. Tob Control 13(1):29–37
238. Mahabee-Gittens EM, Merianos AL, Hoh E et al (2019) Nicotine on children's hands: limited protection of smoking bans and initial clinical findings. Tob Use Insights 12:1179173X18823493
239. Chao MR, Cooke MS, Kuo CY et al (2018 Nov) Children are particularly vulnerable to environmental tobacco smoke exposure: evidence from biomarkers of tobacco-specific nitrosamines, and oxidative stress. Environ Int 120:238–245
240. Hovell MF, Zakarian JM, Matt GE et al (2009 Dec) Counseling to reduce children's secondhand smoke exposure and help parents quit smoking: a controlled trial. Nicotine Tob Res 11 (12):1383–1394
241. Jacob P, Havel C, Yu L et al (eds) (2015) Assessing exposure to Thirdhand Smoke (THS) in humans: the need for a comprehensive approach. Tobacco control, Research and education: joining forces to address new challenges, 2015 October 27–29. Sacramento CA, USA
242. Northrup TF, Khan AM, Jacob P 3rd, et al (2016) Thirdhand smoke contamination in hospital settings: assessing exposure risk for vulnerable pediatric patients. Tob Control 25(6):619–623
243. Hang B, Wang P, Zhao Y et al (2017 Apr) Adverse health effects of Thirdhand smoke: from cell to animal models. Int J Mol Sci 28:18(5)
244. Dhall S, Alamat R, Castro A et al (2016 July) Tobacco toxins deposited on surfaces (third hand smoke) impair wound healing. Clin Sci (Lond) 130(14):1269–1284
245. Hang B, Lavarone A, Havel C, et al (eds) (2014) NNA, a Thirdhand smoke constituent, induces DNA damage in vitro and in human cells. 247th national meeting of the American Chemical Society (ACS) with press release. Dallas, TX USA
246. Hang B, Sarker AH, Havel C et al (2013 July) Thirdhand smoke causes DNA damage in human cells. Mutagenesis 28(4):381–391
247. Ramirez N, Ozel MZ, Lewis AC et al (2014 Oct) Exposure to nitrosamines in thirdhand tobacco smoke increases cancer risk in non-smokers. Environ Int 71:139–147
248. Drehmer JE, Walters BH, Nabi-Burza E et al (2017 Dec) Guidance for the clinical management of thirdhand smoke exposure in the child health care setting. J Clin Outcomes Manag 24 (12):551–559
249. Samet JM, Chanson D, Wipfli H (2015 Sept) The challenges of limiting exposure to THS in vulnerable populations. Curr Environ Health Rep 2(3):215–225

Prenatal Pesticide Exposure and Child Health

Monica K. Silver and John D. Meeker

1 Introduction

Fetuses are rapidly developing, making them highly vulnerable to the long-lasting effects of pesticide exposure. Important windows of susceptibility occur in utero and exposure during these highly vulnerable periods, even to low levels that might not affect adults, may have the potential to lead to long-term health effects [1–3]. Fetal susceptibility to pesticides is further augmented by the fact that many pesticides can cross the placenta [4]. Fetuses also have lower levels of detoxifying enzymes to metabolize pesticides [5] and immature metabolic pathways, which results in slow excretion [6].

This chapter provides an overview of the human evidence for associations between prenatal exposure to some common pesticides and adverse impacts on child health and development, focusing specifically on neurodevelopment, obesity, preterm birth (PTB)/fetal growth, congenital abnormalities (CAs), and childhood cancers as the health end points of interest. This chapter is not meant to be an exhaustive review of all health effects that have been associated with early life pesticide exposure, but rather a compilation of some of the most notable findings for common childhood morbidities. Contemporary review and primary research articles are referenced here, and readers are directed toward those for additional details. For further information regarding specific biological mechanisms of prenatal pesticide exposure and child health outcomes, interested readers are encouraged to explore the related toxicology literature.

M. K. Silver · J. D. Meeker (✉)
Department of Environmental Health Sciences, University of Michigan School of Public Health, Ann Arbor, MI, USA
e-mail: meekerj@umich.edu

Y. Xia (ed.), *Early-life Environmental Exposure and Disease*,
https://doi.org/10.1007/978-981-15-3797-4_3

2 Assessment of Prenatal Pesticide Exposure

Assessment of prenatal pesticide exposure typically falls into one of two categories, biomarker or ecological/environmental assessment (Fig. 1). Exposure assessment using biomarkers is preferred as it can provide a more precise measurement of exposure, as well as capture all routes of exposure. Two examples of biomarkers sometimes used to determine prenatal pesticide exposures are maternal blood during pregnancy and umbilical cord blood. These can provide direct evidence of prenatal exposure during pregnancy, though pesticide levels in blood tend to be low, particularly for the contemporary pesticides with short half-lives, which can make detection difficult [7]. Collection of maternal blood during pregnancy is also invasive and therefore not always the best choice. One of the most common biomarkers for assessing prenatal exposure is the measurement of pesticide metabolites in maternal urine samples taken during pregnancy. Urine collection is simple and noninvasive, making collection at multiple time points more feasible. A disadvantage of using urinary metabolites is that they are often class specific, but not necessarily pesticide specific. For example, the majority of organophosphate pesticides (OPs) are excreted in urine as dialkylphosphate (DAP) metabolites. While DAPs do reflect exposure to OPs, they are not specific to any single pesticide and may also represent exposure to the DAPs themselves, which are nontoxic, as OPs degrade into DAPs naturally in the environment [8]. Other less commonly seen biomarkers include amniotic fluid collection during pregnancy or placental tissue extraction at birth. Meconium, the infant's first stool, can also provide a measurement of prenatal pesticide exposure. It contains materials ingested by the fetus in the last half of gestation and can provide information about fetal exposure for up to 20 weeks. The alternative way of assessing exposure is known as ecological exposure assessment. It tends to be less

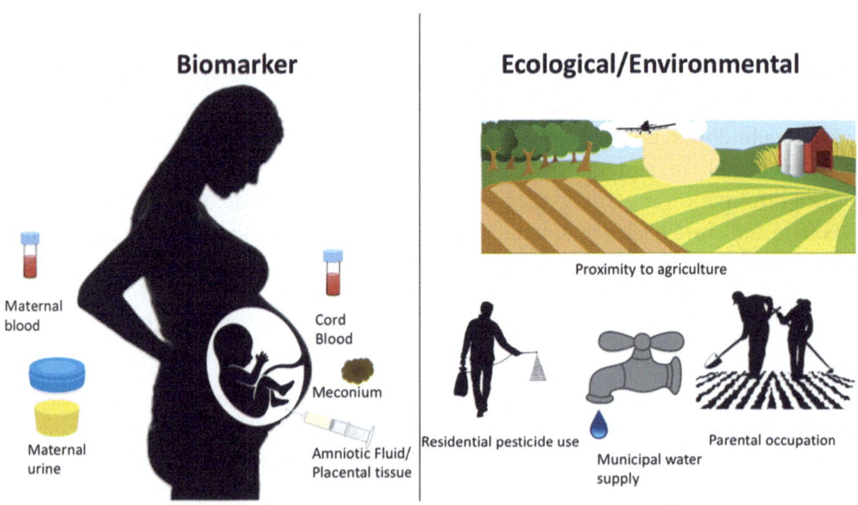

Fig. 1 Most common methods of determining prenatal exposure to pesticides

precise, in general, but is common in studies where biomarkers of exposure are not used.

Common types of ecological/environmental prenatal exposure assessment include residential proximity to agriculture or pesticide use sites during gestation. While pesticide application records may be accurate, it is difficult to determine the level of individual exposure. Living near an agricultural site does not necessarily result in consistent exposure to pesticide spray drift. Parental occupation during pregnancy or around conception is also often used to estimate exposure to certain pesticides, as are residential use surveys. Residential use surveys seek to determine what types of pesticides may have been used in or around the home during pregnancy. While these less precise methods of exposure assessment tend to be much less expensive than a biomarker study because there are no laboratory expenses for analysis or storage, they tend to rely on recall, which can be problematic. Recall bias may occur when parents whose children have a health problem may be more likely to or incorrectly recall using pesticides during their pregnancy than parents of healthy children, thereby potentially biasing study results.

3 Persistent Versus Nonpersistent Pesticides

The vast majority of pesticides in use today are classified as "nonpersistent," meaning that they generally have relatively short half-lives (hours to days) in the environment and the human body. These chemicals are largely believed to be "safer" than their more persistent counterparts, which tend to have much longer half-lives (months to years). Persistent pesticides, such as the organochlorines (OCs) dichlorodiphenyltrichloroethane (DDT), aldrin, dieldrin, and endrin, favored for their broad-spectrum activity and low cost, were heavily used in the 1940s for controlling a wide variety of pests affecting agriculture and human health [9]. Overuse of these pesticides was common and resulted in harmful effects on nontarget species and the development of genetic resistance to pesticides in some target species. Concerns of widespread health effects led many countries to shift to more nonpersistent pesticides in the 1970s. In addition to faster breakdown times, the nonpersistent pesticides also tend to be more "pest specific" and therefore believed to be safer for nontarget species. In 2001, the Stockholm Convention went so far as to mandate a global ban on nine persistent pesticides: aldrin, chlordane, DDT, dieldrin, endrin, heptachlor, hexachlorobenzene (HCB), mirex, and toxaphene [10]. Endosulfan, chlordecone, and lindane have since been added to the banned list as well. Despite the phasing out of these persistent pesticides, exposure remains a public health problem because of their persistence in the environment and continued exempted uses in some countries. For example, while banned for agricultural use, DDT is still used as an effective way to control mosquitos in countries with high malaria prevalence.

Most pesticides in use today are nonpersistent and designed to break down quickly. However, it has been shown that even nonpersistent pesticides can remain for years after application in homes and other indoor environments where they are protected from moisture, sunlight, and other degradation mechanisms. Common classes of nonpersistent pesticides include OPs, carbamates, and pyrethroids. These pesticides were all considered "safe" when introduced into the market; however, similarities between insect and human nervous systems can lead to shared toxicity [9]. This book chapter largely focuses on the most common nonpersistent pesticides in use today and also touches on the persistent pesticides of the past.

4 Health Outcomes

4.1 Neurodevelopment

Neurobehavioral disorders, such as autism spectrum disorder (ASD) and/or attention-deficit/hyperactivity disorder (ADHD), appear to be on the rise globally [11]. Nearly ubiquitous exposure to pesticides in the environment may play a role in the global uptick of these disorders [11]. Pesticides are neurotoxic by design and rapidly developing fetal brains may be an unintended target. Comprehensive reviews and numerous epidemiologic studies across countries, populations, and settings have reported significant associations between prenatal OP exposures and deficits in cognitive, behavioral, and social development in childhood [12–14]. Affected outcomes include deficits in memory, processing speed, verbal comprehension, perceptual reasoning, and IQ, as well as mental and motor delays, abnormal reflexes, and increased risk of developing ASD and/or ADHD [15]. Recent studies continue to support the notion that early life exposure to OPs is detrimental to the developing brain. Children born to residences in proximity to agricultural fields where OPs are applied have a higher likelihood of ASD diagnosis [16] and a reduction in IQ [17]. Impaired neurodevelopment was greater among children of farmworkers [18]. OP metabolite concentrations in maternal urine during pregnancy were also associated with ASD traits in adolescence [19], while cord blood concentrations were associated with arm tremors in children [20]. While recent studies also report no association between agricultural OPs and developmental delay [16] or maternal OP metabolites with intelligence test scores in urban settings [21, 22], the overall body of evidence that prenatal OP exposure can adversely affect neurodevelopment in children is convincing.

The effects of prenatal exposure to other nonpersistent pesticides, such as pyrethroids, on child neurodevelopment are less well studied. Recent studies have reported that pyrethroid metabolites in maternal urine during pregnancy were associated with ADHD symptoms [23], internalizing difficulties [24], and a variety of behavioral problems and poorer executive functioning deficits [25] in children and mental functioning in infants [26] and poorer social-emotional [27], language [27], and mental development [28] in toddlers. However, other studies have reported no significant associations between prenatal pyrethroid metabolites and motor functioning in infants [26] or cognitive scores in children [29].

Studies of persistent pesticides, such as the OC DDT, are also limited and have mixed results. Cord blood levels of DDT have been associated with deficits in cognitive skills in preschoolers (verbal and memory tests) [30]. DDT and/or its metabolite, dichlorodiphenyldichloroethylene (DDE), measured in maternal serum during pregnancy were also associated with a significant reduction in psychomotor development in infants in one study [31], but not neurodevelopmental deficits in infants [32] or toddlers [27, 33] in three others.

4.2 Obesity

The rapidly increasing prevalence of overweight and obesity worldwide may result from environmental chemical obesogens [34, 35], altering lipid homeostasis to accelerate lipid accumulation and adipogenesis. There have been studies investigating the possible role of prenatal pesticides as environmental obesogens with outcomes in childhood such as obesity and BMI. Unfortunately, there is a dearth of epidemiological research concerning prenatal nonpersistent pesticide exposure and childhood obesity. One study examined the effects of prenatal dialkylphosphate (DAP) metabolites measured in maternal urine during pregnancy on markers of glucose metabolism, adiponectin, and insulin, in umbilical cord blood serum. Insulin levels were associated with higher urinary DAPs, but adiponectin levels were not [36]. A research assessed prenatal nonpersistent pesticide exposure by employment of pregnant women in a greenhouse and found that pregnant women who were the most highly exposed to pesticides may lead to increased skinfold thickness, BMI, and percentage of body fat in children [37].

Most contemporary research about persistent pesticide exposure during pregnancy and childhood obesity and other health outcomes have focused on DDT and/or DDE and few other OCs and have yielded mixed results. Studies have found that DDT and DDE in either maternal serum or cord blood are positively associated with waist circumference, BMI, and risk of obesity (for DDT and DDE) significantly [38] and risk of overweight (for DDT) [39]. Multiple studies have reported that prenatal DDE was associated with overweight [39], increased waist circumference [40], and BMI [40, 41] in girls, while another study reported a decrease in insulin and adiponectin levels in umbilical cord blood with increased levels of DDE, only in girls [36]. One additional study found that prenatal DDT and DDE were associated with adiposity measures and BMI in boys, but not girls [42]. Other studies have reported no associations between prenatal DDT/DDE [43, 44] and other organochlorine pesticides [43] and increased risk of obesity, overweight, or increased BMI in children.

4.3 Preterm Birth/Fetal Growth

Preterm birth (PTB), defined as delivery prior to 37 weeks of gestation, occurs in approximately 10% of pregnancies and is one of the strongest predictors of neonatal mortality and morbidity worldwide [45]. Likewise, extremely low or high birth weight is also a well-known risk factor for neonatal mortality and morbidities in infancy and childhood [46]. Investigations of nonpersistent pesticides and preterm birth (PTB) are limited. Until recently, they have mainly focused on OPs and the herbicide atrazine [47]. No associations were reported between maternal exposure to OPs and PTB [48, 49] and studies of atrazine, measured in drinking water, are similarly inconclusive [50–53]. One additional study similarly found no associations between individual or total urinary pyrethroid levels and length of gestation [54]. A more recent study examined prenatal exposure to 17 agricultural pesticides and three nonpersistent pesticide classes (OPs, pyrethroids, and carbamates) and their associations with PTB. Pesticide exposure that occurred in the first or second trimester of pregnancy and exposure to multiple pesticides (two or more) were associated with an increased risk for PTB; results were strongest for girls [55].

Contemporary review studies examining the strength of evidence for associations between prenatal exposure to nonpersistent pesticides and measures of fetal growth have reported mixed results [46]. The bulk of epidemiological research has been focused on OPs, with exposures typically measured using maternal urinary metabolites during pregnancy [46]. Overall, results were largely null, though a few studies yielded significant findings, particularly in some subpopulations of interest. Maternal urinary DAPs were associated with lower birth weight [56, 57], smaller head circumference [58, 59], and birth length (non-Hispanic black women only) [60], while a metabolite specific to parathion and methyl parathion was also associated with birth length [48]. In addition to OPs, a few studies have also examined maternal urinary metabolites of other nonpersistent pesticides with mixed results [54, 61–63]. 3-Phenoxybenzoic acid (3-PBA), a commonly studied pyrethroid metabolite, has been associated with smaller birth size [61], while total pyrethroid metabolites were associated with birth weight, but not birth length [54]. The herbicide atrazine was similarly associated with decreased birth weight and head circumference, while metolachlor levels were inversely associated with head circumference [52]. An additional study measured nonpersistent pesticides in the umbilical cord and found reduced birth weight in newborns with higher total number of pesticides detected [64]. Several others used less precise methods of assessing exposure, such as maternal occupation during pregnancy [37] and residential proximity to agricultural pesticides during pregnancy [55]. Newborns whose mothers had high occupational exposure during pregnancy had lower birth weights [37], yet residential exposure to agricultural pesticides was not associated with low birth weight for all but one (myclobutanil, a fungicide) of 17 pesticides studied [55].

Current studies of prenatal exposure to persistent OCs and PTB reveal a possible association. Umbilical cord serum levels of hexachlorocyclohexanes (HCHs) [65] and HCB [66], and maternal serum levels of chlordecone [67], were associated with shortened gestational age. Women who delivered preterm had significantly higher placental levels of HCHs, DDE, and DDT compared to those with term deliveries [68], and total placental OCs were significantly associated with increased risk of PTB [69]. In contrast, another study found no association between a number of OCs in maternal serum and preterm birth [70].

For persistent pesticides, total OCs detected in placental tissues were significantly associated with increased risk of low birth weight [69], while hexachlorobenzene (HCB) measured in maternal serum was inversely associated with indices of fetal growth and higher odds of being small for gestational age [71]. HCB in umbilical cord serum was also associated with reduced abdominal circumference growth in early pregnancy (as a measure of fetal growth), as estimated by ultrasound, though no associations were observed for DDE with any of the longitudinal fetal growth curves [72].

4.4 Congenital Abnormalities

According to the World Health Organization, congenital abnormalities (CAs), sometimes referred to as birth defects, resulted in the death of over 2.5 million infants within their first month of life between the years 2000 and 2015 [73]. Here we discuss the evidence concerning the associations between prenatal exposure to pesticides and CAs of the urogenital, musculoskeletal, and cardiovascular systems, as well as neural tube defects (NTDs).

Cryptorchidism, when one or both testes are undescended, and hypospadias, when the opening of the urethra is on the bottom of the penis instead of the tip, are the most common urogenital CAs. Review studies of the associations between nonpersistent pesticides, measured directly using biomarkers, and urogenital CAs were inconclusive [74]. However, positive associations were observed for persistent OCs measured in breast milk [75] and placental tissue [76] in relation to cryptorchidism [75, 76] and hypospadias [76]. Several studies linked hypospadias and/or cryptorchidism with specific pesticides including mirex and lindane in the placenta [76], hexachlorobenzene [77], and DDT and metabolites [78] in maternal serum, and trans-chlordane in breast milk [75]. When ecological measures of overall pesticide exposure were used to define prenatal exposure, associations with hypospadias and cryptorchidism were largely positive [74]. Studies revealed that county-level estimates of atrazine exposure during pregnancy were associated with the risk of hypospadias and cryptorchidism [79], as well as an increased risk of hypospadias [80, 81] and cryptorchidism [80] in boys whose parents self-reported occupational exposure to pesticides during the pregnancy.

The most common musculoskeletal abnormalities (MSAs), or CAs of the skeletal and muscular system, are gastroschisis and reduction defects of the upper limbs. Studies of associations between these MSAs and prenatal exposure to pesticides appear to be limited to a few studies with only ecological assessments of exposure. Review studies indicate an overall positive association between occupational/

environmental prenatal pesticide exposure and MSAs [74]. Women who worked in the agriculture industry [82], as well as those with self-reported occupational exposure to insecticides, herbicides, and fungicides [83], during pregnancy had an elevated risk of having offspring with limb defects. Environmental atrazine exposure (residential proximity) was also associated with increased risk of gastroschisis [84, 85].

Cardiovascular abnormalities (CVAs) are the leading CA-related cause of death in newborns [86]. Though only a handful of studies have assessed prenatal pesticide exposure and CVAs, a general positive association is observed overall [74]; however, results should be interpreted with caution given the sole use of ecological exposure assessments. Residential proximity to the agricultural application of a variety of pesticides was found to be associated with a number of CVAs [87]. For example, increased odds of pulmonary valve stenosis and ventricular septal defects were observed with exposure to OPs and pyrethroids, respectively [87]. Maternal residential use of herbicides and rodenticides during pregnancy was associated with an increased risk of transposition of the great arteries in their newborns [88], while maternal occupational exposure to insecticides, herbicides, and fungicides was associated with an increased risk for other CVAs, such as tetralogy of Fallot [89].

Neural tube defects (NTDs), CAs of the brain, spine, or spinal cord, occur during the first month of pregnancy. The few available studies are suggestive of a positive association between prenatal pesticide exposure and NTDs, though exposure was assessed indirectly for most of the studies, so results should be interpreted with caution. Maternal exposure to persistent OCs, measured in serum, was associated with an increased risk of NTD occurrence in offspring [90]. Several other studies showed positive associations between parental occupational exposure during pregnancy to unspecified pesticides and anencephaly and spina bifida, the two most common NTDs, as well as others [91–93].

4.5 Childhood Cancers

The overall body of research suggests that prenatal pesticide exposure may be associated to the development of leukemia and brain tumors in childhood, though, in general, these studies tend to be limited by their assessment of prenatal exposure, making it hard to draw definitive conclusions. Review articles [94] and meta-analyses reveal associations between prenatal pesticide exposure and childhood leukemia. For example, several meta-analyses have reported that residential pesticide exposure in the few months before conception [95] and during pregnancy [95–97] was associated with an increased risk of childhood leukemias. Another large meta-analysis found a significantly increased risk of lymphoma and leukemia in children whose mothers were exposed to personal household use or professionally applied pesticides during the prenatal period [98]. Maternal prenatal exposure was also associated with a significantly increased risk of childhood brain tumors (CBTs) among offspring, for both agricultural [99] and residential pesticide exposures

[99, 100]. Interestingly, two meta-analyses have also revealed increased risks of childhood brain tumors (CBT) [99] or brain cancer [98] with paternal prenatal or preconception pesticide exposure.

5 Conclusions

Here we have summarized some epidemiological evidence that prenatal exposure to contemporary-use pesticides may be associated with alterations in infant and child health and development, specifically neurodevelopment, obesity, pre-term birth/fetal growth, congenital abnormalities, and childhood cancers (Table 1). Perhaps the strongest evidence is for the effects of early life exposure to pesticides on neurodevelopment. Pesticides are neurotoxic by design, each with a prescribed mechanism of toxicity and target organism(s). While the effects of high exposures in humans often mirror those seen for target organisms, low-dose effects in humans seem to disrupt alternative pathways, such as through endocrine or thyroid disruption, oxidative stress, interference with signaling pathways, or epigenetic changes.

Table 1 Summary of the health effects in children related to prenatal pesticide exposure and research needs

Health outcome	Summary of findings	Research needs
Neurodevelopment	Nonpersistent OPs adversely impact neurodevelopment; persistent OCs may be associated with neurodevelopment	Additional studies of other common nonpersistent pesticides; additional longitudinal studies and mixture analyses
Obesity	Few studies of nonpersistent pesticides; persistent OCs may be associated with obesity-related health outcomes	Studies of nonpersistent pesticides; longitudinal studies and mixture analyses
Pre-term Birth/fetal growth	Nonpersistent pesticides do not appear to be associated with PTB but may be with reduced fetal growth; persistent pesticides may be associated with PTB/fetal growth	Additional studies of nonpersistent pesticides; longitudinal studies and mixture analyses; measurements of fetal growth using ultrasound
Congenital abnormalities	Persistent pesticides may be associated with urogenital CAs; pesticides may be associated with MSAs, CVAs, and NTDs	Studies of nonpersistent pesticides and urogenital CAs; biomarker studies of specific persistent and nonpersistent pesticides and MSAs, CVAs, and NTDs; longitudinal studies and mixture analyses
Childhood cancer	Pesticides may be associated with childhood leukemia and brain tumors	Biomarker studies of specific persistent and nonpersistent pesticides and leukemia and brain tumors; longitudinal studies and mixture analyses

Perturbation of these pathways at critical times of growth could potentially lead to downstream health effects.

While much of the literature reviewed in this chapter supports a growing body of evidence that pesticides may adversely affect child health and development, more work needs to be carried out before any conclusions regarding causation can be drawn with certainty. The strongest evidence presented here comes from studies where biomarkers of exposure were measured, such as maternal urine or blood or umbilical cord blood, especially those that assessed exposure at multiple time points. Exposure biomarkers, as opposed to more ecological measures of exposure, such as proximity to agriculture, or self-reported residential/occupational exposures, which may be subject to recall bias, provide direct evidence of exposure from any source. Studies that collected exposure biomarkers at multiple time points throughout pregnancy are also preferred over those that collected only measurement. Using only one time point to estimate prenatal exposure may be problematic, especially for nonpersistent pesticides. Exposure at one point in time may not necessarily be representative of exposure over the course of the pregnancy. It cannot capture temporal or intraindividual variability in exposure or allow for identification of the sensitive windows of susceptibility during gestation. Further, epidemiological studies should be used in conjunction with toxicology/animal studies to help establish the causality and elucidate specific biological mechanisms, individual susceptibility factors, and sensitive windows of exposure. Additionally, research exploring the health effects following exposure to multiple pesticides simultaneously is also needed. More studies are beginning to account for multiple exposures to real-life mixtures, though these can make interpretation (e.g., risk assessment, risk management, and regulation) challenging.

Given all these factors and the large variability across epidemiological studies, it is problematic to determine whether there are "safe" levels of gestational exposure to pesticides. Although many of the risk estimates reported in the literature seem small on an individual level, even a seemingly small shift in the population distribution could be important in a public health perspective. Given the nearly ubiquitous exposure to pesticides among the general population, the vulnerability of fetuses, and the potential for long-term effects on health and development, efforts to reduce pesticide exposure as a precaution among pregnant women are warranted.

In conclusion, this chapter presents studies that indicate that prenatal pesticide exposure may adversely affect child health and development. Many of the current studies are limited by nonspecific exposure assessments and cross-sectional study designs that do not account for temporal variability in pesticide exposure, especially for nonpersistent pesticides, or identify sensitive windows of susceptibility during gestation. Additional well-designed longitudinal studies that measure exposure at multiple potentially sensitive time points and exposure to multiple pesticides simultaneously are needed, as well as the development of novel, noninvasive biomarkers for measuring these exposures. Still, given the range of potentially serious developmental effects and widespread exposure in the population, efforts to reduce pesticide exposure as a precaution among pregnant women are likely prudent.

References

1. Landrigan PJ, Miodovnik A (2011) Children's health and the environment: an overview. Mt Sinai J Med 78(1):1–10
2. Garcia SJ, Seidler FJ, Slotkin TA (2005) Developmental neurotoxicity of chlorpyrifos: targeting glial cells. Environ Toxicol Pharmacol 19(3):455–461. S1382-6689(04)00268-6 [pii]
3. Grandjean P, Landrigan PJ (2014) HHS public access neurobehavioural effects of developmental toxicity. Lancet 13(3):330–338
4. Bradman A, Barr DB, Claus Henn BG, Drumheller T, Curry C, Eskenazi B (2003) Measurement of pesticides and other toxicants in amniotic fluid as a potential biomarker of prenatal exposure: a validation study. Environ Health Perspect 111(14):1779–1782
5. Eskenazi B, Rosas LG, Marks AR et al (2008) Pesticide toxicity and the developing brain. Basic Clin Pharmacol Toxicol 102(2):228–236. PTO171 [pii]
6. Rauh VA, Margolis AE (2016) Research review: environmental exposures, neurodevelopment, and child mental health – new paradigms for the study of brain and behavioral effects. J Child Psychol Psychiatry 57(7):775–793
7. Barr DB, Barr JR, Driskell WJ et al (1999) Strategies for biological monitoring of exposure for contemporary-use pesticides. Toxicol Ind Health 15(1-2):168–179
8. Sudakin DL, Stone DL (2011) Dialkyl phosphates as biomarkers of organophosphates: the current divide between epidemiology and clinical toxicology. Clin Toxicol (Phila) 49 (9):771–781
9. Abreu-Villaça Y, Levin ED (2017) Developmental neurotoxicity of succeeding generations of insecticides. Environ Int 99:55–77
10. Secretariat of the Stockholm Convention (2001) Paper presented at Stockholm convention on persistent organic pollutants. Geneva, Switzerland
11. Grandjean P, Landrigan PJ (2014) Neurobehavioural effects of developmental toxicity. Lancet Neurol 13(3):330–338. S1474-4422(13)70278-3 [pii]
12. Gonzalez-Alzaga B, Lacasana M, Aguilar-Garduno C et al (2014) A systematic review of neurodevelopmental effects of prenatal and postnatal organophosphate pesticide exposure. Toxicol Lett 230(2):104–121. S0378-4274(13)01425-2 [pii]
13. Koureas M, Tsakalof A, Tsatsakis A, Hadjichristodoulou C (2012) Systematic review of biomonitoring studies to determine the association between exposure to organophosphorus and pyrethroid insecticides and human health outcomes. Toxicol Lett 210(2):155–168
14. Munoz-Quezada MT, Lucero BA, Barr DB et al (2013) Neurodevelopmental effects in children associated with exposure to organophosphate pesticides: a systematic review. Neurotoxicology 39:158–168
15. Hertz-Picciotto I, Sass JB, Engel S et al (2018) Organophosphate exposures during pregnancy and child neurodevelopment: recommendations for essential policy reforms. PLoS Med 15 (10):e1002671
16. Shelton JF, Geraghty EM, Tancredi DJ et al (2014) Neurodevelopmental disorders and prenatal residential proximity to agricultural pesticides: the CHARGE study. Environ Health Perspect 122(10):1103–1109
17. Gunier RB, Bradman A, Harley KG, Kogut K, Eskenazi B (2017) Prenatal residential proximity to agricultural pesticide use and IQ in 7-year-old children. Environ Health Perspect 125(5):57002
18. Engel SM, Bradman A, Wolff MS et al (2016) Prenatal Organophosphorus pesticide exposure and child neurodevelopment at 24 months: an analysis of four birth cohorts. Environ Health Perspect 124(6):822–830
19. Sagiv SK, Harris MH, Gunier RB et al (2018) Prenatal organophosphate pesticide exposure and traits related to autism spectrum disorders in a population living in proximity to agriculture. Environ Health Perspect 126(4):047012
20. Rauh VA, Garcia WE, Whyatt RM, Horton MK, Barr DB, Louis ED (2015) Prenatal exposure to the organophosphate pesticide chlorpyrifos and childhood tremor. Neurotoxicology 51:80

21. Donauer S, Altaye M, Xu Y et al (2016) An observational study to evaluate associations between low-level gestational exposure to organophosphate pesticides and cognition during early childhood. Am J Epidemiol 184(5):410
22. Cartier C, Warembourg C, Le Maner-Idrissi G et al (2016) Organophosphate insecticide metabolites in prenatal and childhood urine samples and intelligence scores at 6 years of age: results from the mother-child PELAGIE cohort (France). Environ Health Perspect 124(5)
23. Dalsager L, Fage-Larsen B, Bilenberg N et al (2019) Maternal urinary concentrations of pyrethroid and chlorpyrifos metabolites and attention deficit hyperactivity disorder (ADHD) symptoms in 2-4-year-old children from the Odense Child Cohort. Environ Res 176:108533
24. Viel J-F, Rouget F, Warembourg C et al (2017) Behavioural disorders in 6-year-old children and pyrethroid insecticide exposure: the PELAGIE mother–child cohort. Occup Environ Med 74(4):275–281
25. Furlong MA, Barr DB, Wolff MS, Engel SM (2017) Prenatal exposure to pyrethroid pesticides and childhood behavior and executive functioning. Neurotoxicology 62:231–238
26. Fluegge KR, Nishioka M, Wilkins JR, Wilkins JR 3rd (2016) Effects of simultaneous prenatal exposures to organophosphate and synthetic pyrethroid insecticides on infant neurodevelopment at three months of age. J Environ Toxicol Public Health 1:60–73
27. Eskenazi B, An S, Rauch SA et al (2018) Prenatal exposure to DDT and pyrethroids for malaria control and child neurodevelopment: the VHEMBE cohort, South Africa. Environ Health Perspect 126(4):047004
28. Watkins DJ, Fortenberry GZ, Sanchez BN et al (2016) Urinary 3-phenoxybenzoic acid (3-PBA) levels among pregnant women in Mexico City: distribution and relationships with child neurodevelopment. Environ Res 147:307–313. S0013-9351(16)30069-X [pii]
29. Viel J-F, Warembourg C, Le Maner-Idrissi G et al (2015) Pyrethroid insecticide exposure and cognitive developmental disabilities in children: the PELAGIE mother–child cohort. Environ Int 82:69–75
30. Ribas-Fitó N, Torrent M, Carrizo D et al (2006) In utero exposure to background concentrations of DDT and cognitive functioning among Preschoolers. Am J Epidemiol 164 (10):955–962
31. Torres-Sánchez L, Rothenberg SJ, Schnaas L et al (2007) In utero p, p′-DDE exposure and infant neurodevelopment: a perinatal cohort in Mexico. Environ Health Perspect 115 (3):435–439
32. Bahena-Medina LA, Torres-Sánchez L, Schnaas L et al (2011) Neonatal neurodevelopment and prenatal exposure to dichlorodiphenyldichloroethylene (DDE): a cohort study in Mexico. J Expo Sci Environ Epidemiol 21(6):609–614
33. Torres-Sánchez L, Schnaas L, Cebrián ME et al (2009) Prenatal dichlorodiphenyldichloroethylene (DDE) exposure and neurodevelopment: a follow-up from 12 to 30 months of age. Neurotoxicology 30(6):1162–1165
34. La Merrill M, Birnbaum LS (2011) Childhood obesity and environmental chemicals. Mt Sinai J Med 78(1):22–48
35. Wang Y, Lobstein T (2006) Worldwide trends in childhood overweight and obesity. Int J Pediatr Obes 1(1):11–25
36. Debost-Legrand A, Warembourg C, Massart C et al (2016) Prenatal exposure to persistent organic pollutants and organophosphate pesticides, and markers of glucose metabolism at birth. Environ Res 146:207–217
37. Wohlfahrt-Veje C, Main KM, Schmidt IM et al (2011) Lower birth weight and increased body fat at school age in children prenatally exposed to modern pesticides: a prospective study. Environ Health 10(1):79
38. Warner M, Wesselink A, Harley KG, Bradman A, Kogut K, Eskenazi B (2014) Prenatal exposure to dichlorodiphenyltrichloroethane and obesity at 9 years of age in the CHAMACOS study cohort. Am J Epidemiol 179(11):1312–1322. kwu046 [pii]

39. Valvi D, Mendez MA, Martinez D et al (2012) Prenatal concentrations of polychlorinated biphenyls, DDE, and DDT and overweight in children: a prospective birth cohort study. Environ Health Perspect 120(3):451–457
40. Tang-Peronard JL, Heitmann BL, Andersen HR et al (2014) Association between prenatal polychlorinated biphenyl exposure and obesity development at ages 5 and 7 y: a prospective cohort study of 656 children from the Faroe Islands. Am J Clin Nutr 99(1):5–13. ajcn.113.066720 [pii]
41. Verhulst SL, Nelen V, Hond ED et al (2009) Intrauterine exposure to environmental pollutants and body mass index during the first 3 years of life. Environ Health Perspect 117(1):122–126
42. Warner M, Ye M, Harley K, Kogut K, Bradman A, Eskenazi B (2017) Prenatal DDT exposure and child adiposity at age 12: the CHAMACOS study. Environ Res 159:606–612
43. Cupul-Uicab LA, Klebanoff MA, Brock JW, Longnecker MP (2013) Prenatal exposure to persistent Organochlorines and childhood obesity in the U.S. collaborative perinatal project. Environ Health Perspect 121(9):1103–1109
44. Warner M, Aguilar Schall R, Harley KG, Bradman A, Barr D, Eskenazi B (2013) In utero DDT and DDE exposure and obesity status of 7-year-old Mexican-American children in the CHAMACOS cohort. Environ Health Perspect 121(5):631–636
45. Behrman R, Butler A (2007) Preterm birth: causes, consequences, and prevention. National Academies Press, Washington, DC
46. Kamai EM, McElrath TF, Ferguson KK (2019) Fetal growth in environmental epidemiology: mechanisms, limitations, and a review of associations with biomarkers of non-persistent chemical exposures during pregnancy. Environ Health 18(1):43
47. Ferguson KK, Chin HB (2017) Environmental chemicals and preterm birth: biological mechanisms and the state of the science. Curr Epidemiol Report 4(1):56–71
48. Eskenazi B, Harley K, Bradman A et al (2004) Association of in utero organophosphate pesticide exposure and fetal growth and length of gestation in an agricultural population. Environ Health Perspect 112(10):1116–1124
49. Sathyanarayana S, Basso O, Karr CJ et al (2010) Maternal pesticide use and birth weight in the agricultural health study. J Agromedicine 15(2):127–136
50. Ochoa-Acuña H, Frankenberger J, Hahn L, Carbajo C (2009) Drinking-water herbicide exposure in Indiana and prevalence of small-for-gestational-age and preterm delivery. Environ Health Perspect 117(10):1619–1624
51. Villanueva CM, Durand G, Coutte MB, Chevrier C, Cordier S (2005) Atrazine in municipal drinking water and risk of low birth weight, preterm delivery, and small-for-gestational-age status. Occup Environ Med 62(6):400–405. 62/6/400 [pii]
52. Chevrier C, Limon G, Monfort C et al (2011) Urinary biomarkers of prenatal atrazine exposure and adverse birth outcomes in the PELAGIE birth cohort. Environ Health Perspect 119 (7):1034–1041
53. Rinsky JL, Hopenhayn C, Golla V, Browning S, Bush HM (2012) Atrazine exposure in public drinking water and preterm birth. Public Health Rep 127(1):72–80
54. Ding G, Cui C, Chen L et al (2015) Prenatal exposure to pyrethroid insecticides and birth outcomes in rural Northern China. J Expo Sci Environ Epidemiol 25(3):264–270
55. Ling C, Liew Z, von Ehrenstein OS et al (2018) Prenatal exposure to ambient pesticides and preterm birth and term low birthweight in agricultural regions of California. Toxics 6(3). https://doi.org/10.3390/toxics6030041
56. Huang YF, Pan WC, Tsai YA et al (2017) Concurrent exposures to nonylphenol, bisphenol A, phthalates, and organophosphate pesticides on birth outcomes: a cohort study in Taipei, Taiwan. Sci Total Environ 607-608:1126–1135. S0048-9697(17)31796-5 [pii]
57. Rauch SA, Braun JM, Barr DB et al (2012) Associations of prenatal exposure to organophosphate pesticide metabolites with gestational age and birth weight. Environ Health Perspect 120 (7):1055–1060
58. Wolff MS, Engel S, Berkowitz G et al (2007) Prenatal pesticide and PCB exposures and birth outcomes. Pediatr Res 61(2):243–250

59. Liu P, Wu C, Chang X, Qi X, Zheng M, Zhou Z (2016) Adverse associations of both prenatal and postnatal exposure to organophosphorous pesticides with infant neurodevelopment in an agricultural area of Jiangsu Province, China. Environ Health Perspect 124(10):1637–1643
60. Harley KG, Engel SM, Vedar MG et al (2016) Prenatal exposure to organophosphorous pesticides and fetal growth: pooled results from four longitudinal birth cohort studies. Environ Health Perspect 124(7):1084–1092
61. Zhang J, Yoshinaga J, Hisada A et al (2014) Prenatal pyrethroid insecticide exposure and thyroid hormone levels and birth sizes of neonates. Sci Total Environ (488–489):275–279
62. Dalsager L, Christensen LE, Kongsholm MG et al (2018) Associations of maternal exposure to organophosphate and pyrethroid insecticides and the herbicide 2,4-D with birth outcomes and anogenital distance at 3 months in the Odense Child Cohort. Reprod Toxicol 76:53–62. S0890-6238(17)30339-8 [pii]
63. Berkowitz GS, Wetmur JG, Birman-Deych E et al (2004) In utero pesticide exposure, maternal paraoxonase activity, and head circumference. Environ Health Perspect 112(3):388–391
64. Wickerham EL, Lozoff B, Shao J, Kaciroti N, Xia Y, Meeker JD (2012) Reduced birth weight in relation to pesticide mixtures detected in cord blood of full-term infants. Environ Int 47:80–85. S0160-4120(12)00134-1 [pii]
65. Fang J, Liu H, Zhao H, Zhou Y, Xu S, Cai Z (2019) Association of in utero hexachlorocyclohexane exposure with gestational age. Ecotoxicol Environ Saf 174:263–269
66. Dallaire R, Dewailly É, Ayotte P et al (2013) Exposure to organochlorines and mercury through fish and marine mammal consumption: associations with growth and duration of gestation among Inuit newborns. Environ Int 54:85–91
67. Kadhel P, Monfort C, Costet N et al (2014) Chlordecone exposure, length of gestation, and risk of preterm birth. Am J Epidemiol 179(5):536–544. kwt313 [pii]
68. Anand M, Singh L, Agarwal P, Saroj R, Taneja A (2019) Pesticides exposure through environment and risk of pre-term birth: a study from Agra city. Drug Chem Toxicol 42 (5):471–477
69. Toichuev RM, Zhilova LV, Paizildaev TR et al (2018) Organochlorine pesticides in placenta in Kyrgyzstan and the effect on pregnancy, childbirth, and newborn health. Environ Sci Pollut Res 25(32):31885–31894
70. Basterrechea M, Lertxundi A, Iniguez C et al (2014) Prenatal exposure to hexachlorobenzene (HCB) and reproductive effects in a multicentre birth cohort in Spain. Sci Total Env 466–467:770–776. S0048-9697(13)00821-8 [pii]
71. Lauritzen HB, Larose TL, Øien T et al (2017) Maternal serum levels of perfluoroalkyl substances and organochlorines and indices of fetal growth: a Scandinavian case–cohort study. Pediatr Res 81(1):33–42
72. Lopez-Espinosa M-J, Murcia M, Iñiguez C et al (2016) Organochlorine compounds and ultrasound measurements of fetal growth in the INMA cohort (Spain). Environ Health Perspect 124(1):157–163
73. World Health Organization (2016) Congenital Anomalies Fact Sheet. Geneva, Switzerland. https://www.who.int/en/news-room/fact-sheets/detail/congenital-anomalies. Accessed 24 Oct 2019
74. Kalliora C, Mamoulakis C, Vasilopoulos E et al (2018) Association of pesticide exposure with human congenital abnormalities. Toxicol Appl Pharmacol 346:58–75
75. Damgaard IN, Skakkebaek NE, Toppari J et al (2006) Persistent pesticides in human breast milk and cryptorchidism. Environ Health Perspect 114(7):1133–1138
76. Fernandez MF, Olmos B, Granada A et al (2007) Human exposure to endocrine-disrupting chemicals and prenatal risk factors for cryptorchidism and hypospadias: a nested case–control study. Environ Health Perspect 115(Suppl 1):8–14
77. Giordano F, Abballe A, De Felip E et al (2010) Maternal exposures to endocrine disrupting chemicals and hypospadias in offspring. Birth Defects Res Part A Clin Mol Teratol 88(4):241–250

78. Longnecker MP, Gladen BC, Cupul-Uicab LA et al (2007) In utero exposure to the antiandrogen 1,1-dichloro-2,2-bis(p-chlorophenyl)ethylene (DDE) in relation to anogenital distance in male newborns from Chiapas, Mexico. Am J Epidemiol 165(9):1015–1022. kwk109 [pii]
79. Agopian AJ, Lupo PJ, Canfield MA, Langlois PH (2013) Case-control study of maternal residential atrazine exposure and male genital malformations. Am J Med Genet A 161A (5):977–982
80. Gaspari L, Paris F, Jandel C et al (2011) Prenatal environmental risk factors for genital malformations in a population of 1442 French male newborns: a nested case-control study. Hum Reprod 26(11):3155–3162. der283 [pii]
81. Rocheleau CM, Romitti PA, Dennis LK (2009) Pesticides and hypospadias: a meta-analysis. J Pediatr Urol 5(1):17–24. S1477-5131(08)00378-1 [pii]
82. Engel LS, O'Meara ES, Schwartz SM (2000) Maternal occupation in agriculture and risk of limb defects in Washington state, 1980–1993. Scand J Work Environ Health 26(3):193–198
83. Kielb C, Lin S, Herdt-Losavio M et al (2014) Maternal periconceptional occupational exposure to pesticides and selected musculoskeletal birth defects. Int J Hyg Environ Health 217 (2–3):248–254
84. Agopian AJ, Langlois PH, Cai Y, Canfield MA, Lupo PJ (2013) Maternal residential atrazine exposure and gastroschisis by maternal age. Matern Child Health J 17(10):1768–1775
85. Waller SA, Paul K, Peterson SE, Hitti JE (2010) Agricultural-related chemical exposures, season of conception, and risk of gastroschisis in Washington State. Am J Obstet Gynecol 202 (3):241.e1-6
86. Yang Q, Chen H, Correa A, Devine O, Mathews TJ, Honein MA (2006) Racial differences in infant mortality attributable to birth defects in the United States, 1989-2002. Birth Defects Res A Clin Mol Teratol 76(10):706–713
87. Carmichael SL, Yang W, Roberts E et al (2014) Residential agricultural pesticide exposures and risk of selected congenital heart defects among offspring in the San Joaquin Valley of California. Environ Res 135:133–138
88. Loffredo CA, Silbergeld EK, Ferencz C, Zhang J (2001) Association of transposition of the great arteries in infants with maternal exposures to herbicides and rodenticides. Am J Epidemiol 153(6):529–536
89. Rocheleau CM, Bertke SJ, Lawson CC et al (2015) Maternal occupational pesticide exposure and risk of congenital heart defects in the National Birth Defects Prevention Study. Birth Defects Res A Clin Mol Teratol 103(10):823–833
90. Kalra S, Dewan P, Batra P, Sharma T, Tyagi V, Banerjee BD (2016) Organochlorine pesticide exposure in mothers and neural tube defects in offsprings. Reprod Toxicol 66:56–60
91. Brender JD, Felkner M, Suarez L, Canfield MA, Henry JP (2010) Maternal pesticide exposure and neural tube defects in Mexican Americans. Ann Epidemiol 20(1):16–22
92. Fear NT, Hey K, Vincent T, Murphy M (2007) Paternal occupation and neural tube defects: a case-control study based on the Oxford record linkage study register. Paediatr Perinat Epidemiol 21(2):163–168
93. Lacasaña M, Vázquez-Grameix H, Borja-Aburto VH et al (2006) Maternal and paternal occupational exposure to agricultural work and the risk of anencephaly. Occup Environ Med 63(10):649–656
94. Kim KH, Kabir E, Jahan SA (2017) Exposure to pesticides and the associated human health effects. Sci Total Environ 575. https://doi.org/10.1016/j.scitotenv.2016.09.009
95. Bailey HD, Infante-Rivard C, Metayer C et al (2015) Home pesticide exposures and risk of childhood leukemia: findings from the childhood leukemia international consortium. Int J Cancer 137(11):2644–2663
96. Van Maele-Fabry G, Gamet-Payrastre L, Lison D (2019) Household exposure to pesticides and risk of leukemia in children and adolescents: updated systematic review and meta-analysis. Int J Hyg Environ Health 222(1):49–67

97. Turner MC, Wigle DT, Krewski D (2011) Residential pesticides and childhood leukemia: a systematic review and meta-analysis. Cien Saude Colet 16(3):1915–1931
98. Vinson F, Merhi M, Baldi I, Raynal H, Gamet-Payrastre L (2011) Exposure to pesticides and risk of childhood cancer: a meta-analysis of recent epidemiological studies. Occup Environ Med 68(9):694–702
99. Kunkle B, Bae S, Singh KP, Roy D (2014) Increased risk of childhood brain tumors among children whose parents had farm-related pesticide exposures during pregnancy. JP J Biostat 11 (2):89–101
100. Vidart d'Egurbide Bagazgoïtia N, Bailey HD, Orsi L et al (2018) Maternal residential pesticide use during pregnancy and risk of malignant childhood brain tumors: a pooled analysis of the ESCALE and ESTELLE studies (SFCE). Int J Cancer 142(3):489–497

Prenatal Metal Exposure and Child Health

Binafsha Manzoor Syed

1 Introduction

Metals are fundamental elements of the Earth's crust; thus, human interaction with metals is a natural phenomenon. Some of these elements are essential for normal human development and body functions such as sodium, potassium, calcium, magnesium, and zinc, while others are not required and do not come in contact that often. Although another group of metals are not required by the human body, when exposed, they cause detrimental effects on the development and produce both short-term and long-term effects after birth. The effects of exposure and its detrimental effects are influenced by the trimester (i.e., the first trimester having organogenesis being highly vulnerable) and dose and duration of the metal exposure (i.e., high-dose acute exposure and low-dose chronic exposure both produce poor effects).

As metals are components of the Earth's crust, they are widely expressed in nature though some have rare interaction with human subjects, while others interact quite frequently. Essential metals are required to be part of daily diet (Fig. 1). Nonessential or toxic metals interact with human subjects by ingestions (i.e., eating vegetables, meat, fish, and lentils having high concentration of the toxic metals), drinking (water contamination), inhalation (air pollutant metals), and topical exposure (absorption through skin). A number of metals and metalloids including lead, cadmium, mercury, and arsenic have been labeled as carcinogenic even at low dose. Ten chemicals, which include arsenic, cadmium, lead, and mercury, have been labeled as a major public health concern by the World Health Organization (WHO) due to their detrimental effects on child health [1]. The first 1000 days of

B. M. Syed (✉)
Medical Research Centre, Liaquat University of Medical & Health Sciences, Jamshoro, Pakistan

Pakistan Health Research Council, LUMHS Centre, Liaquat University of Medical & Health Sciences, Jamshoro, Pakistan
e-mail: binafsha.syed@lumhs.edu.pk

Y. Xia (ed.), *Early-life Environmental Exposure and Disease*,
https://doi.org/10.1007/978-981-15-3797-4_4

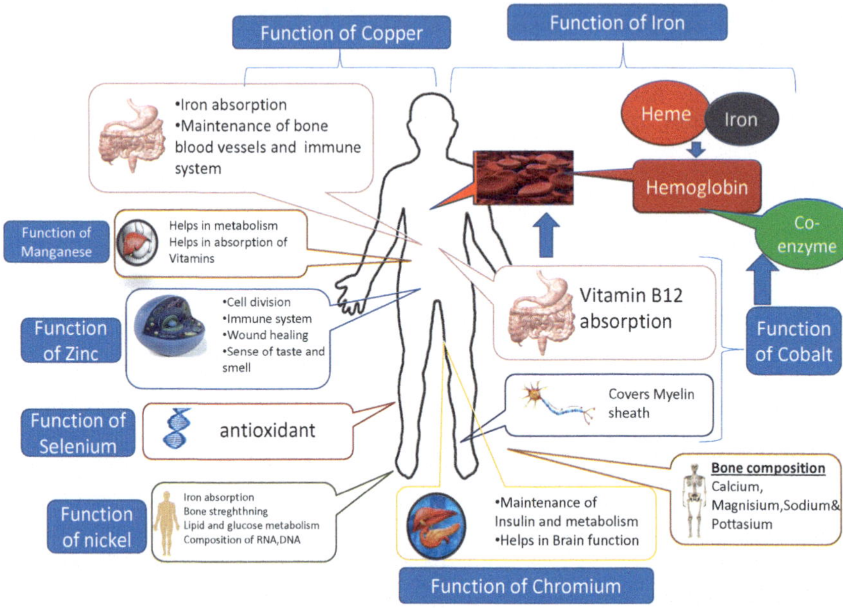

Fig. 1 Schematic diagram of the physiological functions of metals on the human body

a human's life starting from the day of conception till the second birthday are the most critical period as all the development and differentiation occur during this time [2]. The first trimester remains highly vulnerable due to organogenesis; thus, exposure during the first trimester results in most teratological effects and afterward functional disorders and deformities.

Epigenetic mechanisms are particularly involved in normal development and thus get affected in response to toxic metals [3]. The effects start as early as conception and continue throughout the prenatal period and can also occur at the postnatal period. After birth the most vulnerable system is reported to be the immune system as it continues to grow [3]. It is also an interesting finding that the direct effects on the growing fetus are obvious, but the epigenetic changes that occur in parents can be transferred to the offspring and produce transgenerational effects. These results involve environmental toxin exposure. The other most vulnerable system that remains at high risk during the developmental phase is the nervous system. However, the brain of the growing fetus has a double protection including the placental barrier from the mother, which prevents the entry of environmental toxins into the fetal environment and the blood brain barrier of the fetus, which then protects the growing brain from toxins that cross the placenta, but there still remain a number of factors that cross these barriers and produce their effects which might remain there before it becomes apparent years later [3].

In many regions of the world, exposure to toxic metals such as lead, mercury, cadmium, chromium, and arsenic has raised public health concern not only during pregnancy but also afterward with increased burden of morbidity and mortality due to functional and morphological defects. A hospital-based case control study from Pearl River Delta was conducted to evaluate the effects of metals. Lead, chromium, cadmium, copper, mercury, and selenium were measured from maternal blood and correlated with congenital heart defects. The results suggested that the cases had a significantly higher concentration of lead and cadmium but a significantly lower concentration of copper, mercury, and selenium. However it is difficult to assess if copper, mercury, and selenium deficiency is involved in the development of congenital heart defects or they provide antagonistic effects on the toxicity of lead and cadmium [4]. Another population-based study from Sweden linked high concentration of aluminum, cadmium, lithium, lead, and mercury with autoimmune juvenile arthritis in early life [5]. Thus, metal exposure in the prenatal period appears to be significant for child health. This chapter discusses evidence on the exposure to metals and their effects on early life (i.e., the first 1000 days).

2 Metals Crossing the Placenta

The placenta is a natural shield to protect the developing human embryo from toxic elements, e.g., drugs and metals, and allows essential nutrients to reach the fetal environment. However, the placental barrier has limitation to allow some toxic compounds, including heavy metals and metalloids such as mercury, lead, and arsenic, which not only produce toxic effects during prenatal life but also have shown long-term effects after birth. The toxic substances get entry into maternal circulation by inhalation or ingestion (i.e., food and drinking water) or by absorption from skin exposure. The essential metals including iron, copper, zinc, selenium, sodium, potassium, calcium, magnesium, cobalt, and chromium needed for normal development in trace amount are collectively called as trace elements.

There are a number of studies on animals and human subjects that attempted to explore the transport of metals from maternal blood to the fetuses. These studies analyzed maternal blood for concentration and compared it with cord blood. The placental barrier allows these metals through active transport, facilitated transport, and passive diffusion. In order to understand the mechanism of transport of metals from the mother to the fetus, a study was conducted, where trace metals were measured in maternal serum, umbilical cord serum, and colostrums. The results were suggestive of active transport mechanism for manganese, calcium, rubidium, and zinc. The study showed that cesium, lithium and strontium get transported by concentration gradient, while arsenic and copper use blocking action [6].

3 Essential Metals Required for Normal Development

Metals including iron, zinc, and copper are required for normal human development and a small quantity is essential as part of dietary requirement for the maintenance of normal physiological functions (Fig. 1). There was a study on the concentration of metals including aluminum, arsenic, calcium, chromium, copper, iron, lead, magnesium, nickel, potassium, rubidium, selenium, silver strontium, and zinc from the amniotic fluid, which compared it with the fetal growth seen on the fifth and ninth month ultrasounds. The results of the study suggested that calcium has a positive association with biparietal diameter. Head circumference showed a positive association with nickel and copper, while femur length showed a positive association with selenium. Arsenic is shown to have a negative impact on fetal weight [7].

4 Teratogenic Effects of Toxic Metals

4.1 Lithium (Li)

Lithium is a soft silvery alkali metal, widely used in the industry in manufacturing batteries, heat-resistant glass, ceramic, and lithium-grease lubricants. It is utilized by the human body in trace amount. It is found in vegetables, grains, and drinking water where humans can be exposed. In addition, it is used in medication as a mood stabilizer and in bipolar disorders. Lithium crosses the placental barrier radially and the concentration fluctuates during pregnancy, where it decreases during the first trimester, starts to increase in the second trimester, and considerably increases during the third trimester [8]. It also shows a slight increase in the postpartum period. The literature suggests a significant difference in cardiovascular anomalies and abortions in the lithium-exposed group during pregnancy; however, there was a nonsignificant pattern of other genetic and cytogenetic anomalies in the offspring [9]. A systematic review was conducted including 72 studies on lithium and antipsychotic exposure during gestational period [10]. Out of them, seven preclinical studies and three clinical studies looked at the effects of lithium. The preclinical studies were conducted on rats, mice, and zebrafish. The studies showed slow brain responses in preclinical experiments; however, there was limited research on human subjects, which did not show any significant effects. Nevertheless, based on limited data, dose adjustment on lithium is recommended for women if they conceive. Another detailed review was conducted exclusively on lithium, and the cardiovascular anomalies were reported to be associated with lithium exposure; the Ebstein anomaly (tricuspid valve defect) has been reported by a number of studies, while some studies negated the association [9, 11, 12].There is literature showing a low 1-min APGAR score, high rate of jaundice, and longer hospital stay during the neonatal period [13]. Small case reports have also shown evidence of slow brain responses like hypotonia, lethargy, etc., though there is inadequate robust data confirming this finding.

Given the association of lithium exposure with slow brain development in animal models had not addressed the genetic predisposition to neurodevelopmental growth, the mother having bipolar disorder or depression and the child having slow mental growth and reflexes could be a genetic link rather than an influence of lithium. Table 1 summarizes the recent studies on lithium exposure and its effects on human development and early life. Nonetheless it has been advised to have a careful fetal monitoring during pregnancy when there is lithium exposure (Fig. 2).

4.2 Aluminum (Al)

It is one of the most commonly occurring metals in the Earth's crust and human beings get exposed to the metal quite often. It is widely used in the transportation industry, aerospace technology, and the construction industry. It has been reported to be noncarcinogenic and less likely to be accumulated in the body in normal physiological mechanisms for its excretion in urine and feces. Aluminum toxicity commonly occurs due to high intake in the form of medication (i.e., patients on parenteral nutrition) or decreased excretion (as it is excreted by kidneys, i.e., patients with compromised renal function) [14]. Premature neonates are also among the high-risk population. Aluminum used to be considered a nontoxic inert element until recently when animal data showed its toxic effects on genetic make-up and metabolic bone disease due to the inhibition of bone mineralization, by competing with calcium [14]. It is also reported to compete with Vitamin D. A detailed review on effects of aluminum in animals including mice and rats showed that prenatal exposure causes low but considerable effect on growth and is associated with delayed bone ossification and even malformations [15]. A recent study on humans was conducted to assess mitochondrial DNA copy number (mtDNAcn) in fetus in association with maternal urinary aluminum. A summary of the studies is given in Table 1. There is literature suggesting the neurotoxicity of aluminum in rats and mice. However oral aluminum intake has not been linked with any detrimental effects.

4.3 Technetium (Tc)

Technetium is a silvery grey transition metal, most commonly occurring as technetium 99 (99Tc). It is widely used in nuclear imaging as a radioactive tracer due to its penetration to many organs and clear metabolism. It is also used in the industry but human exposure mainly occurs while imaging. The study was conducted to assess the safe dose for workers in the radiology department dealing with CT using 99Tc [16]. The study suggested to limit the radiation exposure to 1.3 mSv corresponding to six adult studies on 99Tc CT scans. In a study on intrauterine death of the fetus, Tc99 was evaluated to be deposited in the brain, liver, and kidneys [17]. Older studies have also suggested the excretion of Tc99 in milk [18]. The technetium binds

Table 1 Summary of the studies on the prenatal exposure of toxic metals

S No	Author	Study type	Exposure type	Key findings		
Lithium						
01	Kindgren E et al. (2019) [5]	Registry-based prospective cohort study	Lithium was assessed in cord blood and correlated with juvenile idiopathic arthritis	High lithium concentration was significantly associated with development of autoimmune juvenile idiopathic arthritis		
02	Fosberg L et al. (2018) [47]	Retrospective cohort	1. Maternal mood disorder only	No significant association was found between lithium and children's intelligent quotient		
			2. Lithium exposure			
			3. No MMD no lithium			
03	Diav-Citrin O et al. (2014) [9]	Prospective comparative study	1. Lithium exposure group	Outcome measure	Exposed	Nonexposed
			2. Nonexposed	Miscarriages	9.3%	2.0%
				Cardiovascular anomalies	4.1%	0.6%
				Non-cardiovascular anomalies	13.7%	6.0%
04	Harari F et al. (2012) [48]	Prospective population-based cohort study	Blood and urine concentration of lithium was measured and compared with fetal size on ultrasound during the 2nd and 3rd trimesters	Increased serum lithium concentration was associated with shorter size of the fetus		
Aluminum						
01	Kindgren E et al. (2019) [5]	Registry-based prospective cohort study	Aluminum was assessed in cord blood and correlated with juvenile idiopathic arthritis	High aluminum concentration was significantly associated with development of autoimmune juvenile idiopathic arthritis		
02	Bingqing Liu et al. (2019) [49]	Prospective cohort study	Urinary aluminum was measured in all three trimesters and fetal cord blood was assessed for mtDNAcn	Rise in urinary aluminum in the second and third trimesters was associated with increased mtDNAcn		
03	Liu Z et al. (2018) [50]	Multicenter hospital-based case control study	Aluminum was measured in umbilical cord serum	High aluminum level was associated with cardiac anomalies		
Technetium						

01	Schaefer C et al. (2009) [20]	Prospective cohort study	Fetal outcome of the pregnant women had 99Tc scans with those who were not exposed	There was no significant pattern of birth defects or additional abnormality was found in the exposed group
Cadmium				
01	Kindgren E et al. (2019) [5]	Registry-based prospective cohort study	Cadmium was assessed in cord blood and correlated with juvenile idiopathic arthritis	High cadmium concentration was significantly associated with development of autoimmune juvenile idiopathic arthritis
02	Wang Y et al. (2015) [51]	Prospective cohort study	Maternal blood was collected at the time of delivery and cord blood was collected for assessment of brain-derived neurotrophic factor (BDNF) and Gesell Developmental Schedules (GDS)	Maternal blood cadmium level showed negative association with fetal GDS scores and BDNF
03	Xu X et al. (2015) [52]	Prospective cohort study	KISS1 gene was analyzed in the cord blood	Low birth weight was associated with cadmium exposure and overexpressed KISS 1 gene
04	Yanqiu Ou et al. (2017) [4]	Hospital-based case control study	Cadmium level was measured in maternal blood and correlated with congenital heart defects	Significantly higher level of cadmium was found in cases as compared to controls
Vanadium				
01	Jie Hu et al. (2018) [53]	Prospective cohort study	Urine samples for vanadium concentration and fetal ultrasound at 16, 24 and 31 weeks	High concentration of vanadium during the first trimester, early second trimester, and late third trimester was associated with restricted fetal growth
02	Jie Hu et al. (2017) [54]	Population-based cohort study (healthy baby cohort)	Urinary vanadium and creatinine levels were measured	High risk of preterm and early term delivery, low birth weight, and smaller babies for gestational age were associated with vanadium exposure
03	Minmin Jiang et al. (2016) [55]	Nested case-control study	Urinary vanadium measured at delivery (i.e., 39 weeks)	A pattern was observed with high maternal urinary vanadium concentration with low birth weight

(continued)

Table 1 (continued)

S No	Author	Study type	Exposure type	Key findings
Lead				
01	Pi X et al. (2018) [56]	Case control study	Concentration of lead in placental tissue was measured and correlated with orofacial clefts	High concentration was associated with high risk of orofacial cleft
02	Yanqiu Ou et al. (2017) [4]	Hospital-based case control study	Lead level was measured in maternal blood and correlated with congenital heart defects	Significantly higher level of lead was found in cases as compared to controls
03	Silver MK et al. (2016) [57]	Prospective cohort study	Prenatal maternal blood lead during pregnancy and from cord blood were correlated with visual and auditory maturation	Exposure to lead during late pregnancy appears to be associated with delayed visual and auditory maturation
04	Shah-Kulkarni S et al. (2016) [58]	Prospective cohort study	Prenatal maternal blood lead level was measured and children's neurodevelopment was assessed at 6, 12, 24, and 36 months	Lead exposure in particular at late pregnancy produce detrimental effects on cognitive function
05	Liu Z et al. (2015) [50]	Case control study	Maternal hair lead measurement in cases and controls was compared with congenital heart defects	The high level of maternal lead was associated with subtypes of congenital heart defects
06	Hong YC et al. (2014) [59]	Prospective cohort study	Maternal blood levels were measured and correlated with child growth at 6, 12, and 24 months	Lead exposure in late pregnancy was associated with reduced infantile growth at 2 years
07	Mohsin Vigeh et al. (2014) [60]	Prospective cohort study	Blood lead level measured during pregnancy (each trimester), cord blood and early childhood development in pre-school children	Maternal lead level in the first trimester was inversely proportional to developmental scores
Thorium				
01	Wei Y (2019) [61]	Case control study	Scalp hair concentration at periconceptional (3 months before to 3 months after pregnancy) period	High thorium concentration showed strong association with high risk of orofacial clefts
Molybdenum				
01	Vazquez-Salas RA et al. (2014) [62]	Prospective cohort study	Apparently healthy women with normal pregnancy were chosen. Urinary molybdenum was assessed during pregnancy and correlated with neurodevelopmental and mental development indices up to 30 months of age	High urinary molybdenum was significantly negatively associated with infant neurodevelopment

Cesium				
01	Callan AC et al. (2016) [63]	Cross-sectional study	Maternal urinary samples were collected 2 weeks before delivery and fetal outcome details were recorded from medical record of the time of birth (i.e., Baby book)	Cesium was associated with low birth weight in female fetuses
Barium				
01	Pi X et al. (2019) [64]	Case control study	Barium concentration was measured from placental tissue and correlated with the orofacial cleft	There was significant association of barium concentration and orofacial clefts
02	Zhang N et al. (2018) [65]	Case control study	Barium concentration was measured from the mother's hair and fetal placenta and correlated with congenital heart defects	There was significant difference in the presence of septal defects, conotruncal defects, right and left ventricular outflow track obstruction, and abnormal pulmonary venous system
03	Callan AC et al. (2016) [63]	Cross-sectional study	Maternal urinary samples were collected 2 weeks before delivery and fetal outcome details were recorded from medical record of the time of birth (i.e., Baby book)	Barium was associated with increased birth length and proportional of optimal birth weight and reduction ponderal index in male fetuses
04		In vitro study	Colostrum phagocytes were evaluated for the effects of barium contamination	Increased apoptosis and superoxide release and decreased viability
05	Han BH (2011) [66]	Prospective cohort study	Fetal outcome was correlated with the inadvertent use of barium and ionizing radiation during pregnancy and controls were not exposed	No significant difference in the fetal outcome of cases and controls
06	Han BH et al. (2010) [67]	Prospective cohort study	Women exposed to barium and ionizing radiation	There was no significant teratogenic effect of barium
Mercury				
01	Kindgren E et al. (2019) [5]	Registry-based prospective cohort study	Mercury was assessed in cord blood and correlated with juvenile idiopathic arthritis	High mercury concentration was significantly associated with development of autoimmune juvenile idiopathic arthritis
02	Yanqiu Ou et al. (2017) [4]	Hospital-based case control study	Mercury level was measured in maternal blood and correlated with congenital heart defects	Significantly lower level of mercury was found in cases as compared to controls
03	Pi X et al. (2019) [64]	Case control study	Mercury concentration was measured from placental tissue and correlated with the orofacial cleft	There was borderline significant association of mercury concentration and orofacial clefts

(continued)

Table 1 (continued)

S No	Author	Study type	Exposure type	Key findings
04	Barbone F et al. (2019) [68]	Cohort study	Total mercury level was measured as sum of the hair, maternal blood, cord blood, and milk and correlated with neurodevelopment	The higher total mercury concentration was associated with lower neuronal development of the child at 18 months age
05	Kim Y et al. (2018) [69]	Cohort study	Mercury concentration in maternal and cord blood was measured and correlated with neurocognitive development of child	Mercury concentration was associated with neurocognitive development of child
Thallium				
01	Qi J et al. (2019) [70]	Prospective cohort study	Maternal blood samples were collected at the first and second trimesters and cord blood sample was collected at birth	Umbilical cord concentration of thallium was negatively association with weight of the fetus according to age
Arsenic				
01	Mullin AM et al. (2019) [71]	Prospective cohort study	Maternal arsenic level was measured in the second and third trimesters, at delivery, and from cord blood and correlated with fetal weight	High arsenic concentration at the third trimester was associated with low birth weight
02	Suhl J et al. (2018) [72]	Case control study	Interview-based information collected for arsenic exposure and correlated with orofacial clefts	Significant association was found between arsenic exposure and cleft palate in infants
03	Wang B et al. (2018) [73]	Cross-sectional study	Arsenic was measured from umbilical cord blood and correlated with neurodevelopment at the 3rd day of life	There was inverse relationship of arsenic concentration with neurodevelopment of newborn
04	Liao KW et al. (2018) [74]	Cohort study	Arsenic concentration was measured in maternal urine and correlated with fetal growth features	High arsenic concentration was associated with low birth weight and head and chest circumference
05	Huyck KL et al. (2007) [75]	Cohort study	Arsenic concentration was measured in maternal hair, toenail, and drinking water samples and correlated with birth weight	High arsenic concentration was associated with low birth weight

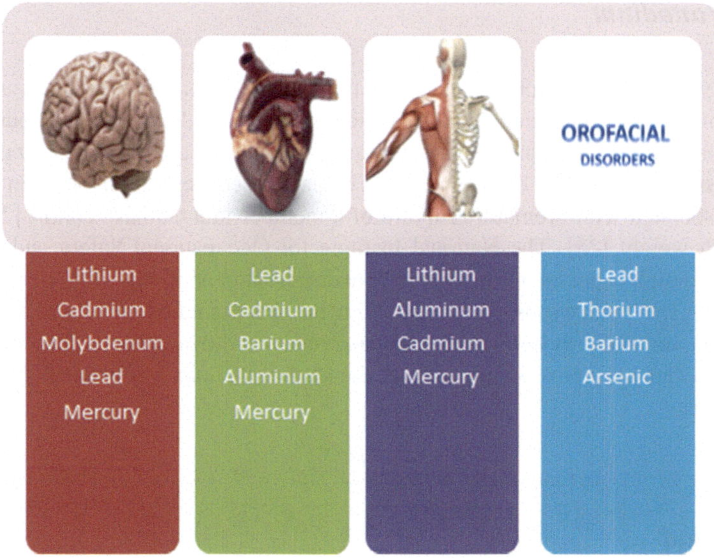

Fig. 2 Summary of the systemic toxic effects of prenatal metal exposures

to the placenta and a small amount crosses to reach the growing fetus, where it is suggested to be deposited mainly in the liver and to some extent in the brain tissue and kidneys [19]. Nonetheless it is reported to be safe [20] (Table 1).

4.4 Cadmium (Cd)

Cadmium is a silvery white metal, commonly used for manufacturing batteries, pigments, coating, and electroplating. It is also used in laboratories with helium to produce blue ultraviolet laser light. The common exposure to human occurs by inhalation. There is limited literature available that suggests its carcinogenic effects, as well as cardiotoxic (i.e., congenital heart defects) and bone effects (juvenile idiopathic arthritis). In younger children cadmium was associated with adiposity in girls [21]. Rat models have shown increased breast buds and enhanced mammary gland development as a result of cadmium exposure [22]. Preschool children have shown negative association with the mother's urinary cadmium concentration during pregnancy [23]. A summary of the studies is given in Table 1.

4.5 Vanadium

It is a silvery grey transition metal, used in the industry in making steel alloy and stab zig titanium and combining lithium, which are then used for different purposes. Vanadium is an essential trace element required in a small quantity (i.e., 10 μg/day) and consumed from olive oil, peanuts, etc. Vanadium concentration has been shown to be associated with premature rupture of a member in a Chinese cohort [24] and low birth weight [25]. The National Institute for Occupational Safety and Health considered high exposure to be toxic and made a limit over 35 mg/m^3 to be injurious to health. The fetal exposure of vanadium has been studied in rats showing its effects on the body systems, including nervous, cardiovascular, respiratory, and musculoskeletal systems. A summary of the studies on human subjects is presented in Table 1.

4.6 Lead

It is a silvery grey post-transition metal. Lead is an essential trace element. Adults can only accumulate 1% of lead which then mainly gets stored in bones, while in children half of the lead is stored. However, when the developing fetus is exposed to a higher concentration (i.e., ≥5.0 μg/dl of maternal blood), it poses risk of mental and behavioral abnormalities. It readily crosses the placenta and gets accumulated in the developing fetus, given that the developing fetus has a less developed system for excretion. Studies have also shown the association of lead exposure with low birth weight and preterm labor [26, 27]; however, confounding factors were not appropriately addressed. Lead exposure is also linked with difficult temperament in toddlers (i.e., 24 months) [28]. Cognitive impairment and high blood pressure have been reported in exposed children [29, 30]. A summary of the studies is presented in Table 1.

4.7 Thorium

It is a silvery and tarnish black actinide metal found in large quantities in the Earth's crust. It is highly radioactive. The most common source of exposure is ingestion and the skeleton is the likely site for deposition. There is limited literature available studying the effects of thorium on human subjects. A small case control study linked high thorium concentration with orofacial cleft; however, further substantial evidence is still awaited (Table 1).

4.8 Molybdenum

It is a silvery transition metal considered to be an essential trace element in the human body. However limited literature is available to associate its high prenatal exposure with development issues in the nervous system. A summary is given in Table 1.

4.9 Cesium (Cs)

It is a silvery golden alkali metal, nearly liquid at room temperature. Cesium is most widely used in drilling of earth. The radioactive form cesium^{137} has uses in the industry including medical applications in radiotherapy for the treatment of cancer. The research activities conducted after the Chernobyl accident in April 1986, where there was a huge release of radioactive substances in the environment, including cesium^{137} showed that immediately after the accident, the contamination was high but with passage of time, it was reduced to a low dose. The women were exposed to cesium by eating vegetables and fruits and drinking contaminated water [31]. However the data from registries for the entry of the congenital defects and developmental anomalies did not appear to show any rise attributable to the accident [32]. The animal studies on rats showed that fetal and after birth continuous exposure to cesium disturbs cholesterol metabolism at the genetic level [33]. Fort M et al. studied the concentration level of a number of alkali metals and showed that cesium concentration was high in the first trimester as compared to the third trimester [34]. A small cross-sectional showed association of cesium exposure with low birth weight (Table 1).

4.10 Barium (Ba)

It is a silvery white alkaline earth metal. Barium sulfate in insoluble form is used as a contrast medium for imaging of the gastrointestinal tract. Barium in insoluble form does not cause any harmful effects but in soluble form at low dose acts as a muscle stimulant while at high concentration is neurotoxic. However, there is data available suggesting barium as a safe contrast medium during pregnancy though low-dose chronic barium exposure causes toxic effects. Table 1 summarizes the studies exploring the exposure of barium during pregnancy. Some studies have shown its exposure in pregnancy to be linked with orofacial defects and congenital cardiac anomalies.

4.11 *Mercury (Hg)*

It is silvery grey in color and the only liquid metal. It comes in contact in two forms: inorganic and organic. Inorganic mercury interacts via dental amalgam which is used for dental fillings while organic forms including methyl and ethyl forms interact via sea food and medical preparations, respectively. The toxicity from mercury occurs by inhalation and ingestion in any form. A summary of the recent studies is presented in Table 1 suggesting its association with cognitive and neurodevelopment. It has been linked with genetic methylation resulting in cognitive effects. Mercury exposure has been reported to be linked with low birth weight and growth restrictions. However, the evidence is not that strong but it is recommended that pregnant women should avoid mercury exposure.

4.12 *Thallium (Tl)*

It is a grey post-transition metal. Its isoform thalium^{201} is used for cardiography to evaluate the risk of coronary artery disease. It is labeled as an extremely toxic element and has been linked with carcinogenesis. There is evidence available suggesting low birth weight when exposed during pregnancy (Table 1). In animal models there is suggestion of achondroplasia but there is a lack of substantial evidence in human subjects.

4.13 *Titanium*

It is a silver transition metal, which is used with other metals, including iron, which is then used in aerospace technology. It is also used in making medical implants (orthopedic and dental) and sports stuff and the mobile industry. It is also used in making paints, papers, toothpastes, and plastics. Given its noncorrosive property, it is used to store nuclear material for a long time. Titanium oxide nanoparticles were evaluated for toxicity in human fetal lung fibroblasts and showed its toxic effects causing mitochondrial dysfunction, morphological changes, and eventual apoptosis [35]. Most of the studies were conducted on mice, rats, and zebrafish showing its association with genetic expression alterations and phototoxicity [36, 37]. Mouse model studies have also shown its influence on inhibiting central nervous system development by using nanoparticles by altering gene expression [38].

4.14 *Boron (B)*

It is a black-brown metalloid, rarely occurring element in the Earth's crust. The highest quantity of boron is found in Turkey. It is used in fiberglass, polymer, and the ceramic industry. It has insecticidal and mild antimicrobial properties. Given its plant cell strengthening properties, it is used in small amount as fertilizer but there is a lack of substantial evidence to suggest its essential role in the human body. It is suggested to be required for bones in wound healing. It has been reported to have antioxidant property as well. Its higher maternal serum concentration has been observed to be associated with smaller and low-birth-weight babies [39]. The main source of boron exposure is drinking water. Small boronated particles are widely used in the industry, agriculture, and even cosmetics. There is no evidence to suggest its mutagenic effects but there is some evidence suggesting its association with developmental defects such as testicular toxicity [40].

4.15 *Arsenic (As)*

It is a metalloid, grey-colored chemical commonly used in the industry. It is also found in yellow and black colors. It is used in car batteries and ammunition with lead. Arsenic contamination is a major health issue in many countries such as Pakistan, China, and Bangladesh. It is toxic to many bacteria, viruses, and fungi and thus has become famous for wood preservation. Arsenic is a trace element required for some functions in the human body; however, its higher exposure in particular food and drinks results in many harmful effects on the body. It has been labeled as carcinogenic. An interesting study was reported from Chile where there was a particular pattern of bladder cancer. Eventually it was found that the patients were exposed in arsenic in utero. Arsenic has been reported to be associated with DNA damage in a cohort study [41]. There has been a strong association of arsenic exposure in prenatal life and development of cancer and diabetes later in life [42, 43]. A summary of the studies on arsenic is presented in Table 1. There has been association with still birth and high mortality. Due to the low birth weight, small size, and less developed immunity of babies, they are at higher risk of infections resulting in high mortality and morbidity among infants.

4.16 *Indium (In)*

It is a silvery white post-transition metal used in the industry. It gets entry into the human body by injection, ingestion, and inhalation. There is no known physiological role of indium but it is used as indium 111 in radiotracer for the movement of labeled proteins in white blood cells. Mostly the exposure is occupational; as a result of its potential toxic effects, the per day work limit is restricted to 8 hours. There is limited data available on human subjects but studies on rats showed inhibitory effects of indium on chondrogenic ossification of the bones. In addition a study also suggested that the concentration of indium in the fetus was half of the mother's due to the placental barrier [44].

5 Metals with Limited Evidence of Effects on Human Intrauterine Development and Body Functions

There are some rarely occurring metals which do not come in contact with human beings and even rarer when it comes to pregnant women. These metals are listed in Table 2. The available literature on these metals is mainly derived from animal studies including mice, rats, and zebrafish. Some studies also used goats, frogs, and shrimps as well. The evidence of their effects on growing humans is rare. Moscovium is a synthetic short-lived element produced in the laboratory. It is a manmade element without much of known uses. Livermorium (Lv) is a highly radioactive synthetic element made from shower curium on calcium. It is very short lived (61 ms) and is produced in the laboratory; thus, there is a thin chance of exposure in prenatal life. Polonium is measured in the placenta (i.e., 27.8 pg/100 gm), 80 times higher than the recommended concentration when diet taken is high in polonium. The main source of polonium is animal meat. Antimony has shown an inverse relationship between umbilical cord blood level and birth weight. Gold was studied on mice and rats which have shown toxicity of gold on reproductive organs (i.e., ovary and uterus) [45]. Gold nanoparticle exposure at early pregnancy was associated with abortions in mice [46]. Germanium is a grayish white metalloid commonly used as transistor in making electronic items. It is not considered to be used in human body systems and it is reported to be toxic to the kidneys when orally ingested in soluble form. In Japan it is used in making polyethylene terephthalate (PET) bottles. As naturally occurring germanium is found in small quantity, less likely exposure at mass is expected. However, its synthetic compounds such as germanium chloride irritate the eyes and skin on exposure, and when inhaled, it causes irritation of the throat and lungs.

Silicon is the most commonly occurring metalloid in the Earth's crust, with a blue-grey crystal solid texture. It is used in the construction industry and making of electronic devices. It is considered as an essential trace element in the human body because of its use in bone strengthening and the formation of elastin and cartilage which is a key component of major vessels (i.e., aorta). This is the most widely occurring element and exposure is very common. Inhaled silicon causes lung irritation resulting in silicosis, an occupational disease. However, exposure in utero is less well studied. Cerium is a soft silvery white, rare-earth metal. Cerium oxide is widely distributed in nature and humans get easily exposed. A number of studies have been conducted to explore the effects of growing fetuses. However, the studies used animals including mice to study contact. There are studies suggesting

Table 2 Summary of metals with limited evidence on human subjects

(a) Metals with toxicity evidence from animal and in vitro studies			
S#	Name of metal	Tissues studied	Target organ/system
01	Beryllium	Chicken, human lung cell lines	Inhibits fibroblast in lung tissue
			Affects in vitro phalangeal growth of chicken
02	Californium	Mouse, rats	Carcinogenesis
03	Antimony	Fetal urine concentration	High fetal urine concentration was seen in pre-mature infants
04	Scandium	Nothing	
05	Titanium	Mouse, zebrafish	Increased risk of phototoxicity, genotoxicity, brain developmental anomalies
06	Gallium	Mouse, zebrafish, pulmonary cell lines	Limited evidence on zebrafish embryo toxicity
07	Polonium	Guinea pig, goat, rat, mice	Polonium crosses the placenta
08	Ruthenium (Ru)	Limited information	Used in diagnostic and treatment process but no studies on its effects on developing human
09	Palladium (Pd)	Cell lines, zebrafish	1. Anti-angiogenic activity
			2. Zebrafish embryo showed expression of metal-induced genes and antioxidant enzyme downregulation
(b) Metals with no evidence of toxicity on humans			
01	Rubidium		
02	Strontium		
03	Rhodium		
04	Praseodymium		
05	Neodymium		
06	Holmium		
07	Erbium		
08	Lutetium		
09	Hafnium		
10	Rhenium		
11	Iridium		
12	Platinum		
13	Francium		
14	Radium		
15	Actinium		
16	Protactinium		
17	Uranium		
18	Plutonium		

toxic effects on testicular development and impairment of lung development. However, its rare occurrence indicates less exposure to human beings; therefore, it is less likely to cause toxic effects in masses. Gadolinium is a silvery white earth metal used as a contrast medium for MRI. The pure form is highly toxic but the toxicity of the chelated form is negligible. Although there is limited data available suggesting the toxicity of gadolinium in developing human beings or pregnant women, the FDA recommends its use with caution due to the risk of gadolinium deposition disease.

6 Conclusion

Metals have various effects on the human body ranging from normal physiological effects to detrimental effects on body systems. Lead, aluminum, mercury, lithium, arsenic, cadmium, and vanadium are reported to be toxic when a fetus is exposed. They not only have effects on the fetus by reducing birth weight but also produce long-term effects. The nervous system appears to be the most affected system in utero followed by the cardiovascular system. Other systems such as gastrointestinal, biliary, genitourinary, endocrine, and immune are not well studied.

The expanding exposure of metals during prenatal period and the working environment making pregnant women exposed to rarer metals warrant further research not only on frequently occurring metals but also on rarer elements to predict their detrimental effects and make strategies for prevention.

References

1. World Health Organisation (2010) Ten chemicals of major public health concern, P.H.a. Environment, Editor. WHO, Geneva
2. Schwarzenberg SJ, Georgieff MK (2018) Advocacy for improving nutrition in the first 1000 days to support childhood development and adult health. Pediatrics 141(2):e20173716
3. Moore T et al (2017) Getting it right in the first 1000 Days Initiative, C.f.C.C. Health, Editor. Murdoch Children's Research Institute, Parkville
4. Ou Y et al (2017) Associations between toxic and essential trace elements in maternal blood and fetal congenital heart defects. Environ Int 106:127–134
5. Kindgren E, Guerrero-Bosagna C, Ludvigsson J (2019) Heavy metals in fish and its association with autoimmunity in the development of juvenile idiopathic arthritis: a prospective birth cohort study. Pediatr Rheumatol Online J 17(1):33
6. Krachler M, Rossipal E, Micetic-Turk D (1999) Trace element transfer from the mother to the newborn – investigations on triplets of colostrum, maternal and umbilical cord sera. Eur J Clin Nutr 53(6):486–494
7. Jalali LM, Koski KG (2018) Amniotic fluid minerals, trace elements, and prenatal supplement use in humans emerge as determinants of fetal growth. J Trace Elem Med Biol 50:139–145
8. Wesseloo R et al (2017) Lithium dosing strategies during pregnancy and the postpartum period. Br J Psychiatry 211(1):31–36
9. Diav-Citrin O et al (2014) Pregnancy outcome following in utero exposure to lithium: a prospective, comparative, observational study. Am J Psychiatry 171(7):785–794
10. Poels EMP et al (2018) Long-term neurodevelopmental consequences of intrauterine exposure to lithium and antipsychotics: a systematic review and meta-analysis. Eur Child Adolesc Psychiatry 27(9):1209–1230
11. Osiro S et al (2013) When lithium hurts: a look at Ebstein anomaly. Cardiol Rev 21(5):257–263

12. Jacobson SJ et al (1992) Prospective multicentre study of pregnancy outcome after lithium exposure during first trimester. Lancet 339(8792):530–533
13. Connoley G, Menahem S (1990) A possible association between neonatal jaundice and long-term maternal lithium ingestion. Med J Aust 152(5):272–273
14. Dorea JG (2015) Exposure to mercury and aluminum in early life: developmental vulnerability as a modifying factor in neurologic and immunologic effects. Int J Environ Res Public Health 12 (2):1295–1313
15. Domingo J, Gomez M, Colomina M (2017) Risks of aluminum exposure during pregnancy. Contrib Sci 1(4):479–487
16. Mountford PJ, Steele HR (1995) Fetal dose estimates and the ICRP abdominal dose limit for occupational exposure of pregnant staff to technetium-99m and iodine-131 patients. Eur J Nucl Med 22(10):1173–1179
17. Maguire C et al (1990) Hepatic uptake of technetium-99m HM-PAO in a fetus. J Nucl Med 31 (2):237–239
18. Heaton B (1979) The build up of technetium in breast milk following the administration of ^{99}Tc (m)O_4 labelled macroaggregated albumin. Br J Radiol 52(614):149–150
19. Owunwanne A et al (1998) Placental binding and transfer of radiopharmaceuticals: technetium-99m d, 1-HMPAO. J Nucl Med 39(10):1810–1813
20. Schaefer C et al (2009) Fetal outcome after technetium scintigraphy in early pregnancy. Reprod Toxicol 28(2):161–166
21. Moynihan M et al (2019) Prenatal cadmium exposure is negatively associated with adiposity in girls not boys during adolescence. Front Public Health 7:61
22. Parodi DA et al (2017) Alteration of mammary gland development and gene expression by in utero exposure to cadmium. Int J Mol Sci 18(9):1939
23. Kippler M et al (2016) Impact of prenatal exposure to cadmium on cognitive development at preschool age and the importance of selenium and iodine. Eur J Epidemiol 31(11):1123–1134
24. Jin S et al (2018) Urinary vanadium concentration in relation to premature rupture of membranes: a birth cohort study. Chemosphere 210:1035–1041
25. Hu X et al (2015) Distributions of heavy metals in maternal and cord blood and the association with infant birth weight in China. J Reprod Med 60(1–2):21–29
26. Rabito FA et al (2014) Changes in low levels of lead over the course of pregnancy and the association with birth outcomes. Reprod Toxicol 50:138–144
27. Rodosthenous RS et al (2017) Prenatal lead exposure and fetal growth: smaller infants have heightened susceptibility. Environ Int 99:228–233
28. Stroustrup A et al (2016) Toddler temperament and prenatal exposure to lead and maternal depression. Environ Health 15(1):71
29. Farzan SF et al (2018) Prenatal lead exposure and elevated blood pressure in children. Environ Int 121(Pt 2):1289–1296
30. Zhou L et al (2017) Prenatal maternal stress in relation to the effects of prenatal lead exposure on toddler cognitive development. Neurotoxicology 59:71–78
31. Dancause KN et al (2010) Chronic radiation exposure in the Rivne-Polissia region of Ukraine: implications for birth defects. Am J Hum Biol 22(5):667–674
32. Lazjuk GI, Nikolaev DL, Novikova IV (1997) Changes in registered congenital anomalies in the Republic of Belarus after the Chernobyl accident. Stem Cells 15(Suppl 2):255–260
33. Racine R et al (2010) Hepatic cholesterol metabolism following a chronic ingestion of cesium-137 starting at fetal stage in rats. J Radiat Res 51(1):37–45
34. Fort M et al (2014) Assessment of exposure to trace metals in a cohort of pregnant women from an urban center by urine analysis in the first and third trimesters of pregnancy. Environ Sci Pollut Res Int 21(15):9234–9241
35. Zhang XQ et al (2011) ZnO, TiO(2), SiO(2,) and Al(2)O(3) nanoparticles-induced toxic effects on human fetal lung fibroblasts. Biomed Environ Sci 24(6):661–669
36. Bar-Ilan O et al (2012) Titanium dioxide nanoparticles produce phototoxicity in the developing zebrafish. Nanotoxicology 6(6):670–679

37. Da Silva GH et al (2018) Toxicity assessment of TiO_2-MWCNT nanohybrid material with enhanced photocatalytic activity on Danio rerio (Zebrafish) embryos. Ecotoxicol Environ Saf 165:136–143
38. Hong F et al (2018) Nano-TiO_2 inhibits development of the central nervous system and its mechanism in offspring mice. J Agric Food Chem 66(44):11767–11774
39. Igra AM et al (2016) Boron exposure through drinking water during pregnancy and birth size. Environ Int 95:54–60
40. Fail PA et al (1998) General, reproductive, developmental, and endocrine toxicity of boronated compounds. Reprod Toxicol 12(1):1–18
41. Navasumrit P et al (2019) Exposure to arsenic in utero is associated with various types of DNA damage and micronuclei in newborns: a birth cohort study. Environ Health 18(1):51
42. Claus Henn B et al (2016) Prenatal arsenic exposure and birth outcomes among a population residing near a mining-related superfund site. Environ Health Perspect 124(8):1308–1315
43. Thomas DJ (2013) The die is cast: arsenic exposure in early life and disease susceptibility. Chem Res Toxicol 26(12):1778–1781
44. Ungvary G et al (2001) The effect of prenatal indium chloride exposure on chondrogenic ossification. J Toxicol Environ Health A 62(5):387–396
45. Badri N et al (2018) Gold and female reproductive organs: an ultrastructural study. Biol Trace Elem Res 183(2):280–287
46. Yang H et al (2018) Murine exposure to gold nanoparticles during early pregnancy promotes abortion by inhibiting ectodermal differentiation. Mol Med 24(1):62
47. Forsberg L et al (2018) Maternal mood disorders and lithium exposure in utero were not associated with poor cognitive development during childhood. Acta Paediatr 107(8):1379–1388
48. Harari F et al (2012) Early-life exposure to lithium and boron from drinking water. Reprod Toxicol 34(4):552–560
49. Liu B et al (2019) Prenatal aluminum exposure is associated with increased newborn mitochondrial DNA copy number. Environ Pollut 252(Pt A):330–335
50. Liu Z et al (2018) The effects of lead and aluminum exposure on congenital heart disease and the mechanism of oxidative stress. Reprod Toxicol 81:93–98
51. Wang Y et al (2016) Effects of prenatal exposure to cadmium on neurodevelopment of infants in Shandong. China Environ Pollut 211:67–73
52. Xu X et al (2015) Associations of cadmium, bisphenol A and polychlorinated biphenyl co-exposure in utero with placental gene expression and neonatal outcomes. Reprod Toxicol 52:62–70
53. Hu J et al (2018) Effects of trimester-specific exposure to vanadium on ultrasound measures of fetal growth and birth size: a longitudinal prospective prenatal cohort study. Lancet Planet Health 2(10):e427–e437
54. Hu J et al (2017) Association of adverse birth outcomes with prenatal exposure to vanadium: a population-based cohort study. Lancet Planet Health 1(6):e230–e241
55. Jiang M et al (2016) A nested case-control study of prenatal vanadium exposure and low birthweight. Hum Reprod 31(9):2135–2141
56. Pi X et al (2018) Concentrations of selected heavy metals in placental tissues and risk for neonatal orofacial clefts. Environ Pollut 242(Pt B):1652–1658
57. Silver MK et al (2016) Low-level prenatal lead exposure and infant sensory function. Environ Health 15(1):65
58. Shah-Kulkarni S et al (2016) Neurodevelopment in early childhood affected by prenatal lead exposure and Iron intake. Medicine (Baltimore) 95(4):e2508
59. Hong YC et al (2014) Postnatal growth following prenatal lead exposure and calcium intake. Pediatrics 134(6):1151–1159
60. Vigeh M et al (2014) Low level prenatal blood lead adversely affects early childhood mental development. J Child Neurol 29(10):1305–1311
61. Wei Y et al (2019) Levels of uranium and thorium in maternal scalp hair and risk of orofacial clefts in offspring. J Environ Radioact 204:125–131

62. Vazquez-Salas RA et al (2014) Prenatal molybdenum exposure and infant neurodevelopment in Mexican children. Nutr Neurosci 17(2):72–80
63. Callan AC et al (2016) Sex specific influence on the relationship between maternal exposures to persistent chemicals and birth outcomes. Int J Hyg Environ Health 219(8):734–741
64. Pi X et al (2019) Association between concentrations of barium and aluminum in placental tissues and risk for orofacial clefts. Sci Total Environ 652:406–412
65. Zhang N et al (2018) Barium exposure increases the risk of congenital heart defects occurrence in offspring. Clin Toxicol (Phila) 56(2):132–139
66. Han BH et al (2011) Pregnancy outcome after 1st-trimester inadvertent exposure to barium sulphate as a contrast media for upper gastrointestinal tract radiography. J Obstet Gynaecol 31 (7):586–588
67. Han BH et al (2010) Conventional barium enema in early pregnancy. J Obstet Gynaecol 30 (6):559–562
68. Barbone F et al (2019) Prenatal mercury exposure and child neurodevelopment outcomes at 18 months: results from the Mediterranean PHIME cohort. Int J Hyg Environ Health 222 (1):9–21
69. Kim Y et al (2018) Prenatal mercury exposure, fish intake and neurocognitive development during first three years of life: prospective cohort mothers and Children's environmental health (MOCEH) study. Sci Total Environ 615:1192–1198
70. Qi J et al (2019) Prenatal thallium exposure and poor growth in early childhood: a prospective birth cohort study. Environ Int 123:224–230
71. Mullin AM et al (2019) Maternal blood arsenic levels and associations with birth weight-for-gestational age. Environ Res 177:108603
72. Suhl J et al (2018) Maternal arsenic exposure and nonsyndromic orofacial clefts. Birth Defects Res 110(19):1455–1467
73. Wang B et al (2018) Prenatal exposure to arsenic and neurobehavioral development of newborns in China. Environ Int 121(Pt 1):421–427
74. Liao CM et al (2008) Arsenic cancer risk posed to human health from tilapia consumption in Taiwan. Ecotoxicol Environ Saf 70(1):27–37
75. Huyck KL et al (2007) Maternal arsenic exposure associated with low birth weight in Bangladesh. J Occup Environ Med 49(10):1097–1104

Prenatal Stress and Offspring Health Outcomes

Guizhen Du and Di Wu

Maternal psychosocial stress during pregnancy has been identified as a robust predictor of offspring health outcomes, especially in neurodevelopmental measures, including behavior and temperament. Thus it is now considered to be a risk factor for the development of childhood behavioral problems.

1 Maternal Stress Measures

Measures to quantify prenatal maternal stress vary widely at present. Unlike the detection of chemical exposures, most studies use questionnaires to assess stress, which have been designed to ascertain perceived stress, life events, depression, anxiety, occupational stress, and trauma. Different standardized questionnaires have been utilized to screen for common mental disorders and measure prenatal affective states, such as the General Health Questionnaire, Self-Reporting Questionnaire, Patient Health Questionnaire, Crisis in Family Systems, Exposure to Violence, Edinburgh Postnatal Depression Scale, Beck Depression Inventory, and State-Trait Anxiety Inventory. It must be emphasized that the results from questionnaires only generally reflect stress and psychosocial health. Great variability and lack of details and validation in some reports make it impossible to compare the stress measured among different studies.

Some researchers analyzed the level of maternal cortisol, which is a hormone whose production is increased when stressed. Usually, multiple measures have been applied to test maternal stress.

G. Du · D. Wu (✉)
State Key Laboratory of Reproductive Medicine, Center for Global Health, School of Public Health, Nanjing Medical University, Nanjing, China
e-mail: diwu@njmu.edu.cn

Y. Xia (ed.), *Early-life Environmental Exposure and Disease*,
https://doi.org/10.1007/978-981-15-3797-4_5

2 Prenatal Stress Exposure and Outcomes in Offspring

2.1 Birth-Related Outcomes in Offspring

Most studies analyzing infant outcomes observed gestational age, birth weight, and Apgar scores at birth. These measures are easily obtained and are usually thought to be basic thus most human studies have included these measure results. The difference in measuring these health indexes among different countries and cultures is small. Studies have shown significant associations between prenatal stress and birth weight, anthropometric measurements, Apgar scores, stillbirth or neonatal death rates, and methylation patterns in newborns (Table 1).

2.1.1 Gestational Age or Preterm Birth

2.1.1.1 Perceived Stress

Perceived stress is a measure of the degree to which situations in one's life are appraised as stressful. Usually, the perceived stress scale is used, which is carefully designed to psychologically determine the perception of stress. The association between perceived stress and gestational age is controversial. Some studies found a significant relationship between perceived stress and preterm birth [1], while others (small-sample-size and case-control studies) indicated that Perceived Stress Scale scores were not related to preterm birth [2]. The discrepancy may be due to the analytical limitations of a small sample size.

2.1.1.2 Life Events

Life events refer to family violence, conflicts among family members, and hospitalization/death of relatives, which can bring stress to the pregnant mothers. Most studies found that life events were significantly related to preterm birth [3]. Negative stressful life events can lead to anxiety or depression [4] and then indirectly relate to decreased gestational age.

2.1.1.3 Cortisol

Cortisol is thought to be a stress hormone. It is the only index which can be measured chemically and thus can be compared among different studies without culture correction. There is a significant relationship between elevated cortisol level, especially during the third trimester [5], and shorter gestational age [1]. In some studies [6], this relationship has been found only in male but not in female infants.

Table 1 Prenatal stress and offspring birth-related health summary

Country	Sample size of pregnant women	Prenatal stress measurement	Outcome measurement	Results (+/–)
Malawi [1]	1391	Perceived Stress Scale, salivary cortisol	Birth weight, birth length, head circumference, arm circumference, WAZ, LAZ, HCAZ	Salivary cortisol: +
				Perceived Stress Scale: –
Brazil [2]	865	Perceived Stress Scale, General Health Quest., State Trait Anxiety Inv.	LBW, preterm birth, intra-uterine growth restriction	LBW, preterm birth: +
				Intra-uterine growth restriction: –
China [3]	2782	Questionnaire: Life events	Preterm birth	+
Iran [4]	550	Depression Anxiety Stress Scales, Stressful Life Events Quest.	Preterm birth	–
Nepal [5]	737	Serum cortisol	Gestational age, LBW, preterm birth	Preterm birth: (OR = 1.04, CI = 1.00, 1.08)
				Birth weight/ LBW: –
Bangladesh [6]	1041	Salivary cortisol	Birth weight, birth length, head circumference, gestational age	+
Iran [7]	600	Spielberger State-Trait Anxiety Inv.	Preterm birth, LBW	Preterm birth, LBW: +
Ghana and Côte d'Ivoire [8]	719	Patient Health Quest., Generalized Anxiety Disorder Scale	Birth weight, LBW, head circumference, gestational age, preterm birth, Apgar score	Apgar: +
				Birth weight/ Gestational age/ Preterm birth: –
Mexico [9]	2623	Karasek's Job Content Quest.	Gestational age, preterm birth, birth weight, SGA	SGA: (OR = 4.93, CI = 2.09, 11.66)
South Africa [10]	544	Childhood Trauma Quest., Mini Int. Neuropsychiatric Interview to assess	WAZ, HCAZ, SGA, preterm birth	SGA, preterm birth, WAZ: –
				HCAZ: +
China [11]	2189	Revised Pregnancy Stress Rating Scale	Preterm birth	High pregnancy specific stress led to preterm birth: +
				Low and medium levels of pregnancy-specific stress: –

(continued)

Table 1 (continued)

Country	Sample size of pregnant women	Prenatal stress measurement	Outcome measurement	Results (+/−)
Romania [12]	474	Perceived Stress Scale	Birth weight, gestational age, SGA, preterm birth	Birth weight (CI = −213, −11)/preterm birth (OR = 2.81, CI = 1.17, 6.76)
Colombia [13]	46	Perceived Stress Scale	Preterm birth, LBW, preterm birth and LBW combined	–
Ethiopia [14]	1065	Self-Reporting Quest. of common mental disorders, List of Threatening Experiences Quest.	Birth weight, stillbirth, neonatal mortality, prolonged labor, time to initiation of breast-feeding	Birth weight, Self-Reporting Quest. stillbirth, or neonatal death: –
				Common mental disorders: low, RR = 1.4, CI = 1.0, 1.9; high, RR = 1.6, CI = 1.0, 2.6
				Delivery: RR = 1.5, CI = 1.0, 2.1
China [15]	1800	19-Item Prenatal Life Events Checklist	Preterm birth, birth weight	Birth weight in the first term: +
				Birth weight in the second and third term: –
Nicaragua [16]	147	Salivary cortisol, intimate partner violence, emotional distress, social resources	LBW, preterm birth, SGA	LBW, SGA: +
				Preterm birth: –
Bangladesh [17]	583	Edinburgh Postnatal Depressive Scale, State Trait Anxiety Inv.	LBW	LBW (OR = 2.24, CI = 1.37, 3.68)
				Anxiety (OR = 2.08, CI = 1.30, 3.25)
South Africa [18]	726	Beck Depression Inv., World Mental Health Life Events Quest.	Birth weight, head circumference, WAZ, HCAZ, SGA	Preterm birth: –
				WAZ (OR = 0.2, CI = 0.02, 0.4) and HCAZ (OR = 0.3, CI = 0.1, 0.6)
Sri Lanka [19]	835	General Health Quest.	SGA	+
China [20]	792	Perceived work stress: single questionnaire item	Birth weight	+

(continued)

Table 1 (continued)

Country	Sample size of pregnant women	Prenatal stress measurement	Outcome measurement	Results (+/−)
China [21]	463	Hospital Anxiety and Depression Scale	Obstetric outcomes	+
Iran [22]	29	Edinburgh Postnatal Depression Scale, Pregnancy-Related Anxiety Quest.	Apgar scores	+
Democratic Republic of Congo [23]	24	Semi-structured ethnographic interviews: Stressful events during pregnancy	Methylation of CRH, CRHBP, NR3C1, and FKBP5, from maternal venous blood, placenta, and umbilical cord blood	+
Democratic Republic of Congo [24]	25	Ethnographic interviews: deprivation, "mundane stressors," war stressors; Peritraumatic Distress Inv.	Methylation of NR3C1 promoter, birth weight	−

+/−:significant positive/negative relationships have been found
WAZ weight for age Z-score, *LAZ* length for age Z-score, *LBW* low birth weight, *PLBW* preterm low birth weight infant, *HCAZ* head circumference for age Z-score, *SGA* small for gestational age, *CRH* corticotropin-releasing hormone, *CRHBP* corticotropin-releasing hormone binding protein, *NR3C1* nuclear receptor subfamily 3 group C member 1, *FKBP5* FK506-binding protein 51, *OR* odds ratio, *CI* confidence interval, *RR* relative risk

2.1.1.4 Anxiety, Depression, and Other Mental Disorders

Researchers have demonstrated that scores from the Depression Anxiety Stress Scale [4] or State-Trait Anxiety Inventory [7] during pregnancy had a negative relationship with gestational age and prenatal maternal mental disorders could lead to preterm birth.

However, other studies [8] showed no significant relationships between anxiety and gestational age. The discrepancy may lie in the fact that these studies only sampled uncomplicated pregnancies. Pregnancy complications may play a key role in the relationship between prenatal maternal mental disorders with birth health outcomes. At the same time, limitations in sample size may also lead to an opposite result.

2.1.1.5 Other Stress Measures

Occupational stress [9], trauma [10], and pregnancy-related stress [11] had been analyzed by a couple of researchers, but the results require further study. They showed that high stress [11], but not occupational stress [9] or trauma [10], had a significant relationship with preterm birth.

2.1.2 Birth Weight

2.1.2.1 Perceived Stress

Studies showed significant relationships between perceived stress and birth weight. High prenatal stress usually leads to reduction in birth weight [12]. Some studies failed [13] to detect this relationship due to small sample size.

2.1.2.2 Life Events

Maternal prenatal life events have not been found [14] to be significantly related to birth weight. However, studies that specified the timing of the life events showed that the occurrence of life events during the first trimester led to low birth weight [15].

2.1.2.3 Cortisol

Studies showed significant negative relationships between third trimester cortisol levels and birth weight in male but not female infants [6]. In fact, high perceived stress had been proved to be related to increased cortisol [16]. Cortisol may play an intermediate role in the relationship.

2.1.2.4 Anxiety, Depression, and Other Mental Disorders

Researchers [7] had demonstrated significant relationships between prenatal maternal common mental disorders (such as anxiety, depression) and low birth weight. Babies of women with high level of anxiety or depression (which could be assessed by the State-Trait Anxiety Inventory [17], Edinburgh Postnatal Depression Scale [18] and State-Trait Anxiety Inventory, Beck Depression Inventory [18], or General Health Questionnaire [2, 19]) tended to have lower birth weight.

2.1.2.5 Other Stress Measures

Occupational stress, trauma, and intimate partner violence had been assessed in some studies. Occupational stress was shown [19] to be significantly related to low birth weight. One study showed [20] that occupational chemical exposure and work stress had interactive decreasing effects on birth weight. Trauma [9, 10] and partner [16] violence had not been found to affect birth weight directly, though these two stress measures could lead to depression.

2.1.3 Anthropometric Measurements (Head Circumference and Birth Length)

Some studies indicated that prenatal depression (Beck Depression Inventory scores) [18] and lifetime trauma [10] had significant relationships with smaller head circumference and birth length, while others found that there was no difference in head circumference [8, 21] and birth length [21] between babies of mothers with or without anxiety and depression during pregnancy.

Interestingly, one study [6] found that there was a negative relationship between cortisol levels during the third trimester and birth length only in male but not in female babies, similar to the results found using gestational age.

2.1.4 Apgar Scores

One case-control study [22] found that women with anxiety or depression during pregnancy but receiving a stress management intervention finally had babies with higher Apgar scores compared to the group with anxiety or depression but without intervention. Apgar scores of offspring have been found [8] to be correlated with the scores from Patient Health Questionnaire and Generalized Anxiety Disorder Scale in pregnant women.

2.1.5 Stillbirth or Neonatal Death

Different from what people usually think, there was no relationship between stillbirth or neonatal death and prenatal maternal mental disorder and negative life events during pregnancy [12].

2.1.6 Methylation Patterns

The measure of methylation patterns is relatively new and has been analyzed only by a few studies with small sample sizes of fewer than 30 participants. Women with chronic stress and trauma during pregnancy showed [23] differences in methylation pattern of placental tissue, umbilical cord blood, and maternal venous blood. Four CpG sites (DNA regions containing cytosine nucleotide-phosphoric acid-guanine nucleotide) have been identified, which could further be linked to other birth measures such as weight. In another study [24], prenatal stress has been found to be related to cord blood methylation of the NR3C1 (Nuclear Receptor Subfamily 3 Group C Member 1) gene, whose function in offspring stress responses is worth researching.

2.2 *Later-Life Outcomes in Offspring*

Prenatal stress has also been related to later-life health problems such as anxiety, attentional deficits, social withdrawal, and helplessness in offspring. Because of follow-up limitations, only a few studies have focused on prenatal stress and later-life outcomes in offspring (Table 2).

2.2.1 Babyhood

Temperament: All the studies measuring temperament found significant results of prenatal maternal stress. Scores of adaptability and approach were higher in babies whose mothers experienced less distress during pregnancy. The scores from Edinburgh Postnatal Depression Scale at second trimester were found to be related to the socioemotional scores from Bayley Scales of Infant Development measured at age of 6 months [25]. Path analyses indicated that prenatal maternal mental disorders led to common postnatal mental disorders and then further affected socioemotional scores of babies. Prenatal maternal negative life events experience could lead to low baby mental development scores and high scores on attention, regularity, and persistence.

2.2.1.1 Motor Development

A study with a small sample size [26] indicated that there was no relationship between maternal negative life events experience and babies' motor development. Other studies [27] had not found a relationship between stress and neuromotor development right after birth, or at the age of 1 and 3 months.

2.2.1.2 Illness

A study among 954 women [28] found that persistent symptoms of common mental disorders during both pregnancy and postpartum (from Self-Reporting Questionnaire scores during third trimester and postpartum) had a relationship with infant diarrhea and illness (maternal-reported) at the age of 2 months. Results on relationships between prenatal stress and other illnesses were inconsistent.

2.2.2 Childhood

2.2.2.1 Behavioral Outcomes

Research has often noted children's behavior as an issue of great concern, but due to the length of time required for a longitudinal study of this nature, there are few

Table 2 Prenatal stress and offspring later-life health summary

Country	Sample size of pregnancy women	Prenatal stress measurement	Outcome measurement	Results (+/−)
Vietnam [25]	378	Edinburgh Postnatal Depression Scale to assess common mental disorder	Bayley Scales of Infant and Toddler Development Social-Emotional Questionnaire	–
China [26]	152	19-Item Prenatal Life Events Checklist	Bayley Mental & Psychomotor Dev. Index, Toddler Temperament Scale	1^{st}T life events: + Life events: −
South Africa [27]	101	Feelings about pregnancy, life events, family relationships	Neuromotor development 3, 32, and 93 days after delivery	Motor scores <3:42.5% in the high-stress group and 15.4% in the low-stress group
Ethiopia [28]	954	Self-Reporting Quest. of common mental disorders	Infant illness episodes since birth	Diarrhea: + Persistent common mental disorders and acute respiratory infection: + In multivariate analyses: –
Brazil [30]	370 (children)	Questionnaire: Mothers were asked "whether the pregnancy was a peaceful time or marked by discord and arguments"	Teacher report form of ADHD symptoms	ADHD: +
South Africa [31]	953	Interviews: Marital, family, economic, and societal stress and violence	Richman Behavior Screening Questionnaire at ages 2 and 4	+
China [33]	216	Hamilton Anxiety Scale, Hamilton Rating Scale for Depression	Resting blood pressure and heart rate at age 7–9 years	+
Brazil [34]	409	Perceived Stress Scale, General Health Quest., State Trait Anxiety Inv.	Body mass index Z-scores at ages 5–8 years	+

(continued)

Table 2 (continued)

Country	Sample size of pregnancy women	Prenatal stress measurement	Outcome measurement	Results (+/−)
Mexico [35]	417	Crisis in Family Systems Revised survey of negative life events	Asthma, wheeze	+

+/−:significant positive/negative relationships have been found
ADHD attention deficit hyperactivity disorder

reports relating prenatal stress with childhood behavior. However, most studies on the matter showed significant relationships between prenatal maternal stress and alterations in child behaviors. One study [29] analyzed second to third trimester maternal salivary cortisol level and scores from Self-Reporting Questionnaire and these pregnant women's children's behavior (Child Behavior Checklist) and cortisol at age of 9. Maternal salivary cortisol level, but not Self-Reporting Questionnaire scores, had a significant relationship with Child Behavior Checklist scores, but not cortisol in children. In another study [30], researchers evaluated the distress of pregnant women using one single retrospective interview question and screened their children (6–13 years old) according to attention deficit hyperactivity disorder (ADHD) symptoms, which had been defined by Teacher Report and the Child Behavior Checklist. Discord during pregnancy was significantly related to reported ADHD. This result was consistent with another study that evaluated prenatal maternal emotional distress using a single retrospective question and compared behavior results in offspring (6–12 years) with and without ADHD. It showed that prenatal maternal stress had a significant relationship with childhood ADHD. One study [31] assessed third trimester stress in pregnant women and their children's behavioral problems using the Behavior Screening Questionnaire when they reached 2–4 years. There was a significant relationship between prenatal maternal stress and children (4 years old) behavioral problems. One study [32] that interviewed women shortly after delivery used a single questionnaire to evaluate mood. Psychological disorders were estimated in their children (6 years old) using the Development and Well-Being Assessment. It showed that maternal mood was significantly related to psychological disorders among children.

2.2.2.2 Other Health Outcomes

Some researchers collected heart rate [33], physical growth [34], and asthma [35] as health outcomes in children after prenatal maternal stress. One study [33] evaluated prenatal maternal depression and anxiety state and these women's children's

(7–9 years old) heart rate and blood pressure before, during, and after a video game (which was thought to bring stress). Children with prenatal anxious mother had high heart rate and blood pressure following the video game stress. Prenatal maternal anxiety had been found to be significantly related to children heart rate and blood pressure. However, another study [33] examined prenatal maternal stress three times during pregnancy according to the data collected from General Health Questionnaire, Perceived Stress Scale, and State-Trait Anxiety Inventory. They also analyzed body mass index Z-scores in their children (5–8 years old). Results indicated that scores from second trimester General Health Questionnaire were significantly related to children's body mass index Z-scores. Further analysis also found that prenatal negative life events were related to wheezing among children.

3 Conclusions

Studies show significant relationships between prenatal maternal stress and health outcomes in offspring at birth, during babyhood, and childhood. It is extremely important to utilize appropriate and well-accepted methods across different studies in order to summarize the discoveries in prenatal stress and offspring health outcomes. Because of the variability in definitions of stress, measures of maternal stress need to be normalized not only by maternal education, age, and household income, etc. but also by the cultures with which both participants and researchers identify. This normalization requires careful collection and analysis of covariates, especially those that might have interactive effects with prenatal maternal stress. Long-term follow-up studies are encouraged since there are only a few at present. One of the main research directions in the near future is the development and validation of brief, simple, well-understood survey measures that can allow fast evaluation of prenatal maternal stress and be integrated into expansive studies on maternal and child health.

References

1. Stewart CP, Oaks BM, Laugero KD, Ashorn U, Harjunmaa U, Kumwenda C et al (2015) Maternal cortisol and stress are associated with birth outcomes, but are not affected by lipid-based nutrient supplements during pregnancy: an analysis of data from a randomized controlled trial in rural Malawi. BMC Pregnancy Childbirth 15(1). https://doi.org/10.1186/s12884-015-0793-8. PMID:26694646
2. Rondo PHC, Ferreira RF, Nogueira F, Ribeiro MCN, Lobert H, Artes R (2003) Maternal psychological stress and distress as predictors of low birth weight, prematurity and intrauterine growth retardation. Eur J Clin Nutr 57(2):266–272
3. Zhang YP, Liu XH, Gao SH, Wang JM, Gu YS, Zhang JY et al (2012) Risk factors for preterm birth in five maternal and child health hospitals in Beijing. PLoS One 7(12):e52780
4. Mirabzadeh A, Dolatian M, Forouzan AS, Sajjadi H, Majd HA, Mahmoodi Z (2013) Path analysis associations between perceived social support, stressful life events and other

psychosocial risk factors during pregnancy and preterm delivery. Iran Red Crescent Med J 15 (6):507–514
5. Christian P, Nanayakkara-Bind A, Schulze K, Wu L, Leclerq SC, Khatry SK (2016) Antenatal micronutrient supplementation and third trimester cortisol and erythropoietin concentrations. Matern Child Nutr 12(1):64–73
6. Frith AL, Naved RT, Persson LA, Frongillo EA (2015) Early prenatal food supplementation ameliorates the negative association of maternal stress with birth size in a randomised trial. Matern Child Nutr 11(4):537–549
7. Nasiri Amiri F, Mohamadpour RA, Salmalian H, Ahmadi AM (2010) The association between prenatal anxiety and spontaneous preterm birth and low birth weight. Iran Red Crescent Med J 12(6):650–654
8. Bindt C, Guo N, Te Bonle M, Appiah-Poku J, Hinz R, Barthel D et al (2013) No association between antenatal common mental disorders in low-obstetric risk women and adverse birth outcomes in their offspring: results from the CDS study in Ghana and Côte D'Ivoire. PLoS One 8(11).
9. Cerón-Mireles P, Harlow SD, Sánchez-Carrillo CI (1996) The risk of prematurity and small-for-gestational-age birth in Mexico City: the effects of working conditions and antenatal leave. Am J Public Health 86(6):825–831
10. Koen N, Brittain K, Donald KA, Barnett W, Koopowitz S, Maré K et al (2016) Psychological trauma and post-traumatic stress disorder: risk factors and associations with birth outcomes in the Drakenstein child health study. Eur J Psychotraumatol 7:28720
11. Qu XL, Zhu WJ, Chen WQ, Cui YY, He P, He ZH et al (2016) Effect of pregnancy-specific stress on spontaneous preterm birth among Chinese people. Clin Exp Obstet Gynecol 43 (1):103–108
12. Meghea CI, Rus IA, Chereches RM, Costin N, Caracostea G, Brinzaniuc A (2014) Maternal smoking during pregnancy and birth outcomes in a sample of Romanian women. Cent Eur J Public Health 22(3):153–158
13. Arteaga-Guerra JJ, Cerón-Souza V, Mafla AC (2010) Dynamic among periodontal disease, stress, and adverse pregnancy outcomes. Rev Salud Publica 12(2):276–286
14. Hanlon C, Medhin G, Alem A, Tesfaye F, Lakew Z, Worku B et al (2009) Impact of antenatal common mental disorders upon perinatal outcomes in Ethiopia: the P-MaMiE population-based cohort study. Tropical Med Int Health 14(2):156–166
15. Zhu P, Tao F, Hao J, Sun Y, Jiang X (2010) Prenatal life events stress: implications for preterm birth and infant birthweight. Am J Obstet Gynecol 203(1):34.e1–34.e8
16. Valladares E, Peña R, Ellsberg M, Persson LÅ, Högberg U (2009) Neuroendocrine response to violence dur-ing pregnancy: impact on duration of pregnancy and fetal growth. Acta Obstet Gynecol Scand 88(7):818–823
17. Nasreen HE, Kabir ZN, Forsell Y, Edhborg M (2010) Low birth weight in offspring of women with depressive and anxiety symptoms during pregnancy: results from a population based study in Bangladesh. BMC Public Health 10:515
18. Brittain K, Myer L, Koen N, Koopowitz S, Donald KA, Barnett W et al (2015) Risk factors for antenatal depression and associations with infant birth outcomes: results from a south African birth cohort study. Paediatr Perinat Epidemiol 29(6):504–514
19. Ruwanpathirana T, Fernando DN (2014) Risk factors for 'small for gestational age babies'. Indian J Pediatr 81(10):1000–1004
20. Chen D, Cho SI, Chen C, Wang X, Damokosh AI, Ryan L et al (2000) Exposure to benzene, occupational stress, and reduced birth weight. Occup Environ Med 57(10):661–667
21. Qiao Y, Li J, Wang J (2012) Effects of depressive and anxiety symptoms during pregnancy on pregnant, obstetric and neonatal outcomes: a follow-up study. J Obstet Gynaecol 32(3):237–240
22. Karamoozian M, Askarizadeh G (2015) Impact of prenatal cognitive-behavioral stress management intervention on maternal anxiety and depression and newborns' Apgar scores. Iran J Neonatol 6(2):14–23

23. Kertes DA, Kamin HS, Hughes DA, Rodney NC, Bhatt S, Mulligan CJ (2016) Prenatal maternal stress predicts methylation of genes regulating the hypothalamic-pituitary-adrenocortical system in mothers and newborns in the Democratic Republic of Congo. Child Dev 87 (1):61–72
24. Mulligan CJ, D'Errico NC, Stees J, Hughes DA (2012) Methylation changes at NR3C1 in newborns associate with maternal prenatal stress exposure and newborn birth weight. Epigenetics 7(8):853–857
25. Tran TD, Biggs BA, Tran T, Simpson JA, De Mello MC, Hanieh S et al (2014) Perinatal common mental disorders among women and the social and emotional development of their infants in rural Vietnam. J Affect Disord 160:104–112
26. Zhu P, Sun MS, Hao JH, Chen YJ, Jiang XM, Tao RX et al (2014) Does prenatal maternal stress impair cognitive development and alter temperament characteristics in toddlers with healthy birth outcomes? Dev Med Child Neurol 56(3):283–289
27. Abramson JH, Singh AR, Mbambo V (1961) Antenatal stress and the baby's development. Arch Dis Child 36(185):42–49
28. Ross J, Hanlon C, Medhin G, Alem A, Tesfaye F, Worku B et al (2011) Perinatal mental distress and infant morbidity in Ethiopia: a cohort study. Arch Dis Child Fetal Neonatal Ed 96(1):F59–F64
29. Isaksson J, Lindblad F, Valladares E, Högberg U (2015) High maternal cortisol levels during pregnancy are associated with more psychiatric symptoms in offspring at age of nine: a prospective study from Nicaragua. J Psychiatr Res 71:97–102
30. Pires TDO, da Silva CMFP, de Assis SG (2013) Association between family environment and attention deficit hyperactivity disorder in children: mothers' and teachers' views. BMC Psychiatry 13:215
31. Ramchandani PG, Richter LM, Norris SA, Stein A (2010) Maternal prenatal stress and later child behavioral problems in an urban South African setting. J Am Acad Child Adolesc Psychiatry 49(3):239–247. PMID: 20410713
32. Santos IS, Matijasevich A, Barros AJD, Barros FC (2014) Antenatal and postnatal maternal mood symptoms and psychiatric disorders in pre-school children from the 2004 Pelotas birth cohort. J Affect Disord 164:112–117
33. Fan F, Zou Y, Tian H, Zhang Y, Zhang J, Ma X et al (2016) Effects of maternal anxiety and depression during pregnancy in Chinese women on children's heart rate and blood pressure response to stress. J Hum Hypertens 30(3):171–176
34. Rondó PHC, Rezende G, Lemos JO, Pereira JA (2013) Maternal stress and distress and child nutritional sta-tus. Eur J Clin Nutr 67(4):348–352
35. Rosa MJ, Just AC, Tamayo y Ortiz M, Schnaas L, Svensson K, Wright RO et al (2016) Prenatal and postnatal stress and wheeze in Mexican children: sex-specific differences. Ann Allergy Asthma Immunol 116(4):306–312.e1

The Unique Vulnerabilities of Children to Environmental Hazards

Karen English, Colleen Lau, and Paul Jagals

1 Introduction

Young children are at extraordinarily high risk of adverse environmental health outcomes because biological and behavioural factors make them more vulnerable to environmental hazards than older children (teens) and adults [1–3]. The most vulnerable times for very young children are the first 1000 days of their lives, from conception up to the end of their second year after birth [4]. The special vulnerabilities of very young children during the first 1000 days are largely due to their environmental settings and their exposures that range widely, depending on their environmental interaction. Their vulnerabilities can be categorised in terms of timing (phases), environmental settings, and the hazards within those settings that characterises their environmental exposures.

The timing categories are (1) of the father and mother and even previous generations up to the point of conception, (2) during pregnancy, and (3) after birth, up to day 1000 [1, 3–6]. Environments range from: (1) environments of the parents-to-be and earlier generations that can influence the young child even before conception and range from domestic, workplace, transport, institutional (healthcare facilities), commercial (shopping), recreational environments (swimming pools, parks), and more—these multiple environments in which we live every day, the potential exposures and hazards vary in intensity and type; (2) in the intra-uterine environment, exposures of the mother determines indirect exposures of the unborn

K. English · P. Jagals (✉)
Children's Health and Environment Program, Child Health Research Centre, The University of Queensland, Brisbane, QLD, Australia
e-mail: p.jagals@uq.edu.au

C. Lau
Department of Global Health, College of Health and Medicine, Australia National University, Canberra, ACT, Australia

Y. Xia (ed.), *Early-life Environmental Exposure and Disease*,
https://doi.org/10.1007/978-981-15-3797-4_6

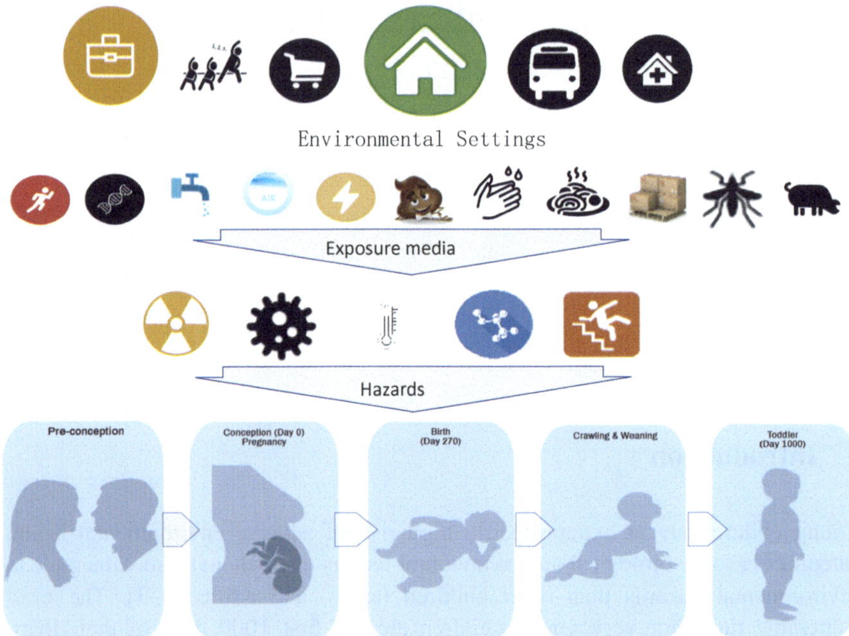

Fig. 1 The outline of the chapter

child; and (3) after birth, the child will be directly exposed to mainly domestic environments but will be interspersed with transport environments, healthcare facilities, and more [1, 4, 7].

We also need to consider the different types of hazards, which can be physical, chemical, or biological, and their specific modes of exposure which are ingestion, sublingual contact, inhalation, and dermal contact [8]. Exposure to hazardous substance found in these environments and during these three timing periods can occur through multiple sources and pathways. These include through the diet (e.g. pesticides and food-borne pathogens entering the food chain at various stages of production and consumption and from contact with chemicals leaching from packaging), particles in dust, natural hazards (e.g. pollens, animals, radiation, infectious agents), air pollution (e.g. traffic-related air pollution), and direct contact with products containing chemicals and microbes [1, 9, 10].

The purpose of this chapter is to inform on phases of exposures to environments and their hazards a child is directly and/or indirectly exposed to in the first 1000 days of life, as conceptualised in Fig. 1.

2 Environmental Hazards

We generally have a good understanding of single and mixtures of exogenous environmental chemical, physical and infectious hazards in the different environments that a child and their parents spend time in [4]. In recent times, rapidly intensifying socio-economic, environmental and technological drivers are exacerbating complex exposures to well-known as well as emerging hazards. Parental behaviour—mostly determined by their socio-economic status and (paradoxically) often in efforts to protect the child—may also lead to increasing early life exposure to environmental hazards. The way we set ourselves up in society—relying on both ecological services (greenness, water, air) and our engineered services (urban environments, healthcare facilities, food and water supply, as well as waste management)—can increase hazard potential if not optimally managed [4, 7, 11–14]. These services are also under pressure from broader regional and global environmental and demographic drivers such as climate change, population growth, urbanisation, antimicrobial resistance, prolific production use of chemicals, emerging infectious diseases, and pollution caused by inadequate waste management. These drivers are rapidly enhancing our environmental hazard potential and thus increasing exogenous pressures on the body's cellular toxicity pathways (internal exposure). Ultimately, these pressures may lead to adverse health outcomes—especially in the window of vulnerability in a child's early life—and could also continue to have negative impacts in later life [1, 12, 15]. More about specific health outcomes can be found in other chapters in this book. This section is about external environmental hazards mostly associated with multiple exposures to multiple hazards over time.

Hazards considered environmental in origin include contaminants that occur naturally, those that occur naturally but are driven to extremes (heat and other environmental disasters), contaminants in goods manufactured for a specific purpose, or by-products and wastes from the way we produce and use those goods to support the way we live. The built environment and social factors may also contribute to the risks and impacts on health in early life [12, 14, 16, 17].

Examples of naturally present hazards include radioactive materials such as rock and soil that emit radon; metals such as arsenic that contaminate drinking water; particulate matter that results from fires, wind, and erosion; pollens and allergens from plants and animals; infectious pathogens from animals (zoonotic diseases) and in water and soil; and dust mites that can be allergenic [9, 13, 18].

Contaminants and products manufactured and transferred through human environments include pesticides used on food crops and chemicals in services such as disinfection by-products in water supplies. More specifically in children, phthalates in toys and specially prepared early-life environments such as baby rooms furnished with goods and textiles that contain flame retardants can be toxic [8, 11].

Hazardous exposures through shortcomings in services and production processes include inadequate safe water supply, airborne particulates and gases from combustion processes derived from generating energy (cooking and heating), inadequate sanitation and waste management [13, 19–21].

Humans are now travelling more than ever before, both in their day-to-day commuting as well as long-distance international travel. Transport environments, such as those that involve cars, trains, buses, planes, ships, as well as their service points such as fuelling and transfer stations and ports, result in exposures to considerably higher levels of emissions from exhaust particles, gases and fuel fumes [14, 20, 22], as well as chemicals used in the manufacturing of vehicles and planes, including plastics and flame retardants [23]. Crowding during transport and at stations also increases the risk of exposure to infectious agents [24]. Very young children are often part of this environment—being taken from and to health care, childcare, and other journeys even at a very young age.

Environmental hazard potential is also increased by low socioeconomic status of the parents. These include the domestic location (distance from the source of pollution), whether the home (domestic) environment is based in an urban, suburban, or rural location, as well as the design, condition, and age of the dwelling, and also the materials of which the goods used in the home are made of [17, 25]. Services such as quality of nutritional and safe food and drinking water supply, condition of indoor air, and efficient waste management all will play a role in moderating environmental exposures in early life [3, 10, 21].

3 Exposure Environments

Why do we differentiate between specific environments? Exposure to chemicals and infectious agents in our environments is ubiquitous and worldwide and especially relevant to vulnerable young children. In the past decades, the manufacture and use of chemicals in our homes, institutions, industries, care facilities, and urban services and utilities have increased substantially [7, 17, 26]. The presence and concentration of these anthropogenic hazards, as well as natural hazards, vary within specific environments. It is important to understand that human exposure to environmental hazards is determined by multiple factors, including time spent in these environments, as well as by physiology and behaviours that modify exposure [27]. Understanding environmental interaction during preconception, pregnancy, and in early infancy is therefore critical to our understanding of how very young children are especially vulnerable to detrimental health outcomes when exposed to hazards in these different environments [28].

3.1 Intrauterine Environment

Preconception and prenatal exposures are especially important because exposure to many and varied synthetic chemicals and infectious agents has now become the norm around the world—not just in the industrialised countries. Maternal exposure to chemicals and infectious agents during pregnancy is known to increase the risk of foetal exposure because of potential transfer across the placenta to the foetus as well as transfer during birth [1, 7]. Maternal exposures during pregnancy can also have multigenerational effects, including direct toxic effects on developing oocytes in female offspring, but also via other mechanisms. Among several proposed mechanisms, epigenetic changes, changes that alter gene function without altering DNA structure, transmitted through generations have been implicated in preconception and multigenerational exposure effects on health [1, 4, 6, 29].

Maternal health status can determine the extent to which chemicals cross the placenta. For example, high blood pressure and maternal drug and alcohol use have been associated with relatively greater concentration of chemicals—notably lead—compared to maternal concentrations, while other factors appear to reduce the degree of transfer [4, 30]. The specific structure, chemical composition, and relative persistence of xenobiotic chemicals also determine the pattern of placental transfer. Persistent chemicals (PBDE and PFC) are lipophilic or are bound to proteins that enter the hepatic bloodstream circulation and directly expose to the foetus. Some chemicals (e.g. methyl mercury) bioaccumulate in the foetus to levels higher than those measured in the mother and can affect the developing brain of the foetus during the first 1000 days and beyond while at the same time having mild adverse effects on the mother [31].

Many infectious diseases during pregnancy are known to adversely affect the foetus [32], and the transmission of many of these diseases is strongly driven by environmental factors. For example, malaria and Zika (both mosquito-borne diseases) are associated with poor health in the pregnant woman as well as a high risk of birth complications and foetal abnormalities [33, 34]. Preconception immunisation is therefore important for protecting the foetus against intrauterine infections, especially pathogens that are strongly associated with congenital abnormalities (e.g. rubella) [35].

3.2 Domestic Environment

Most of us, including pregnant women and young children, spend the majority of our time at home. Yet many households are quite unaware of the high hazard potential of the home environment [4, 14]. Environmental hazards at home will therefore pose the highest risk simply because of the combination of time spent in this environment, and ignorance about how to manage household goods and services that are potentially hazardous.

During pregnancy, an unborn child's exposure to what are in their environments is largely determined by how the mother interacts with the domestic and also other environments. As we have seen with the intra-uterine environment, the modern-day unborn child is not as well protected against the environment as was once thought. After birth, a child generally spends most of the rest of its time during the first 1000 days in its domestic environment [14, 36].

3.3 The Global Environment and Infectious Agents

While environments closer to the very young child are the focus of this chapter, it is worthwhile to consider this much broader context of environment, as it has direct bearing on the condition of the child's direct daily environments. With globalisation, the unprecedented movement of people, animals, and goods around the world has resulted in an increasingly global environment for both infectious and non-infectious diseases [37]. In addition to air, food, water, and soil, exposure to infectious agents can also occur through direct contact with other people and animals (zoonotic diseases) and through insects (e.g. mosquito-borne disease). Globalisation and our increasingly connected world mean that outbreaks and epidemics can spread more rapidly than ever around the world. The emergence and global spread of Zika virus and the devastating consequences of congenital Zika syndrome provide a striking example of the potential impact of infectious disease outbreaks on child health [38].

4 Other Special Vulnerabilities

4.1 Preconception Parental Exposures

The preconception environments of the parents-to-be, and even earlier generations, can influence the very young child. For example, paternal preconception exposures to environmental hazards—which could be encountered in many environments—have been shown to induce epigenetic changes in sperm and are associated with health effects in the child [39]. Similarly, maternal grandmother smoking has been associated with childhood asthma [40]. More about this can be found in other chapters of this book.

4.2 Post-birth Exposures

Infants breathe, drink, and eat more relative to older children, teens, and adults. They are thus subject to proportionally greater exposure to environmental hazards once they are born [4].

In recent years, research has increased our understanding of the reasons environmental contaminants have a different effect on children compared to adults. While children generally have smaller body mass than adults, their exposures (relative to body mass to pollutants) can be much larger, and thus children respond very differently when exposed to environmental hazards than adults [1, 4, 18]..

4.3 Breast Milk

For some chemical hazards, the most significant exposure during early life is through breast milk [31]. Ubiquitous hazardous chemicals include persistent organic pollutants, like organochlorine pesticides, polychlorinated biphenyls, brominated flame retardants, dioxins, and perfluorinated alkyl substances, which are transferable to the young child though breast milk and milk formula [41]. However, at this time, health scientists believe the benefits of breastfeeding far outweigh any risks [4].

4.4 Dermal Exposure

Infants have a higher skin surface area to bodyweight ratio and greater contact with their surroundings than adults. An infant may absorb through the skin a larger dose of a chemical agent on a body weight basis than would an older child or adult. Newborns, especially those who are preterm, experience increased absorption of some compounds through the skin [4, 17].

4.5 Children Have Unique Behaviours

Young children develop rapidly through the first 1000 days. Their activity patterns and behaviours change. Newborns typically spend prolonged periods of time in a single environment such as at home and are thus exposed for relatively longer periods to any hazardous element that might be in the vicinity [17]. They become more mobile and begin to spend more time on the ground as well as in the 'dust' zone of a home, which is approximately up to 1.5 m from the floor level [11]. Behaviours such as pica (tendency to ingest non-dietary substances), crawling, and the tendency to explore items by mouth increase ingestion of contaminants on surfaces. Very young children are also more exposed to pesticide residues from home applications, dust and contaminants carried by dust, volatile organic chemicals from carpets, and chemicals such as chromated copper arsenate from wooden playground equipment [4, 7].

4.6 Children Have Less Mature Immune Systems

Very young children are more susceptible to some infectious diseases (e.g. diarrhoea) and may develop more serious illnesses (e.g. whooping cough) compared to older children and adults. Also some vaccines are not effective in very young children, making it impossible to protect them through immunisation [42, 43].

4.7 *Children Have a Longer Future and Are Generally More Sensitive*

Children are in a rapidly developing stage of their early lives. From birth through the end of the first 1000 days and beyond, children differ from older people in their ability to absorb, metabolise, and excrete contaminants [4]. Detoxifying enzyme systems develop throughout childhood, so the ability to mitigate the effects of chemicals is age dependent and likely to be at its lowest protective capabilities during this phase [2]. Because children are physiologically immature and rapidly developing, environmental hazard exposure can result in long-term irreversible structural changes [44]. Diseases that develop through chronic exposures and/or have long latency periods are likely to have more serious impacts when exposure begins at an early age and continues over long periods of time. For instance, certain cancer outcomes such as melanoma are reported to be primed by exposure to environmental carcinogens early in life rather than total exposure throughout life [45].

5 Conclusions

Children—in the first 1000 days of their lives—are extremely vulnerable to environmental hazards. Their exposures to these hazards are determined by the phase in which the parents, the foetus, newborn, and infant find themselves. Exposures are varied because of the many different chemical, physical and infectious hazards that can be encountered in different environments of the child summarised as preconception, intrauterine, and after birth—predominantly in their domestic environments. This chapter aimed at raising the awareness of this complex exposure matrix of development phase, environmental hazard potential, and various environmental settings.

References

1. Landrigan PJ et al (2019) Pollution and children's health. Sci Total Environ 650:2389–2394
2. Makri A et al (2004) Children's susceptibility to chemicals: a review by developmental stage. J Toxicol Environ Health Part B 7(6):417–435
3. Mattison DR (2010) Environmental exposures and development. Curr Opin Pediatr 22(2):208
4. Landrigan P, Etzel R (2014) Children's environmental health. Oxford University Press, New York
5. Robertson RC et al (2019) The human microbiome and child growth–first 1000 days and beyond. Trends Microbiol 27(2):131–147
6. Soubry A et al (2014) A paternal environmental legacy: evidence for epigenetic inheritance through the male germ line. BioEssays 36(4):359–371
7. Zota AR et al (2017) Reducing chemical exposures at home: opportunities for action. J Epidemiol Community Health 71(9):937–940

8. Healy BF et al (2015) Bisphenol a exposure pathways in early childhood: reviewing the need for improved risk assessment models. J Expo Sci Environ Epidemiol 25(6):544–556
9. Miyake Y et al (2007) Home environment and suspected atopic eczema in Japanese infants: the Osaka maternal and child health study. Pediatr Allergy Immunol 18(5):425–432
10. Gitterman BA, Bearer CF (2001) A developmental approach to pediatric environmental health. Pediatr Clin N Am 48(5):1071–1083
11. English K et al (2015) Assessing exposure of young children to common endocrine-disrupting chemicals in the home environment: a review and commentary of the questionnaire-based approach. Rev Environ Health 30(1):25–49
12. Hystad P et al (2014) Residential greenness and birth outcomes: evaluating the influence of spatially correlated built-environment factors. Environ Health Perspect 122(10):1095–1102
13. Hotez PJ (2013) Pediatric tropical diseases and the World's children living in extreme poverty. J Appl Res Child Inform Pol Child Risk 4(2):10
14. Goldizen FC, Sly PD, Knibbs LD (2016) Respiratory effects of air pollution on children. Pediatr Pulmonol 51(1):94–108
15. Mill J, Petronis A (2008) Pre-and peri-natal environmental risks for attention-deficit hyperactivity disorder (ADHD): the potential role of epigenetic processes in mediating susceptibility. J Child Psychol Psychiatry 49(10):1020–1030
16. Jackson RJ (2011) Designing healthy communities. Wiley, San Francisco
17. Rovira J, Domingo JL (2019) Human health risks due to exposure to inorganic and organic chemicals from textiles: a review. Environ Res 168:62–69
18. Pronczuk-Garbino J (2005) Children's health and the environment: a global perspective: a resource manual for the health sector. World Health Organization, Geneva
19. Kurmi OP, Lam KBH, Ayres JG (2012) Indoor air pollution and the lung in low-and medium-income countries. Eur Respir Soc 4(1):239–254
20. Buonanno G et al (2013) Children exposure assessment to ultrafine particles and black carbon: the role of transport and cooking activities. Atmos Environ 79:53–58
21. Brown J, Cairncross S, Ensink JH (2013) Water, sanitation, hygiene and enteric infections in children. Arch Dis Child 98(8):629–634
22. Shirinde J, Wichmann J, Voyi K (2015) Allergic rhinitis, rhinoconjunctivitis and hay fever symptoms among children are associated with frequency of truck traffic near residences: a cross sectional study. Environ Health 14(1):84
23. English K et al (2017) Polybrominated diphenyl ether flame retardant concentrations in faeces from young children in Queensland, Australia and associations with environmental and behavioural factors. Environ Res 158:669–676
24. Mohr O et al (2012) Evidence for airborne infectious disease transmission in public ground transport–a literature review. Eur Secur 17(35):20255
25. Leventhal T, Newman S (2010) Housing and child development. Child Youth Serv Rev 32 (9):1165–1174
26. World Health Organization (2017) Don't pollute my future! The impact of the environment on children's health. World Health Organization
27. Zartarian V et al (2017) Children's lead exposure: a multimedia modeling analysis to guide public health decision-making. Environ Health Perspect 125(9):097009
28. Tamayo-Uria I et al (2019) The early-life exposome: description and patterns in six European countries. Environ Int 123:189–200
29. Hanson MA, Skinner MK (2016) Developmental origins of epigenetic transgenerational inheritance. Environ Epigenet 2(1)
30. Müller MHB et al (2019) Prenatal exposure to persistent organic pollutants in northern Tanzania and their distribution between breast milk, maternal blood, placenta and cord blood. Environ Res 170:433–442
31. Jacobson JL et al (1984) The transfer of polychlorinated biphenyls (PCBs) and polybrominated biphenyls (PBBs) across the human placenta and into maternal milk. Am J Public Health 74 (4):378–379

32. Zhao J et al (2013) Effect of intrauterine infection on brain development and injury. Int J Dev Neurosci 31(7):543–549
33. Honein MA et al (2017) Birth defects among fetuses and infants of US women with evidence of possible Zika virus infection during pregnancy. JAMA 317(1):59–68
34. Rogerson SJ et al (2018) Burden, pathology, and costs of malaria in pregnancy: new developments for an old problem. Lancet Infect Dis 18(4):e107–e118
35. Yawetz S, Barss V, Weller PF (2015, April) Immunizations during pregnancy. Up to date
36. Gopalan HN, Saksena S (1999) Domestic environment and health of women and children. In: Domestic environment and health of women and children. PNUMA, Delhi
37. De Cock KM et al (2013) The new global health. Emerg Infect Dis 19(8):1192
38. Rasmussen SA et al (2016) Zika virus and birth defects—reviewing the evidence for causality. N Engl J Med 374(20):1981–1987
39. Marcho C, Oluwayiose OA, Pilsner JR (2020) The preconception environment and sperm epigenetics. Andrology
40. Magnus P et al (2006) Cohort profile: the Norwegian mother and child cohort study (MoBa). Int J Epidemiol 35(5):1146–1150
41. Arnold C (2019) Baby steps forward: recommendations for better understanding environmental chemicals in breast milk and infant formula. Environ Health Perspect 127(6):064001
42. Demirjian A, Levy O (2009) Safety and efficacy of neonatal vaccination. Eur J Immunol 39 (1):36–46
43. Simon AK, Hollander GA, McMichael A (2015) Evolution of the immune system in humans from infancy to old age. Proc R Soc B Biol Sci 282(1821):20143085
44. World Health Organization (2005) Children's health and the environment: a global perspective: a resource manual for the health sector
45. Singh K et al (2013) Congenital malignant melanoma: a case report with cytogenetic studies. Am J Dermatopathol 35(8):e135–e138

Early-Life Environmental Influences on Growth

Eva Cecilie Bonefeld-Jorgensen and Manhai Long

1 Introduction

Environmental chemical exposures are ubiquitous; however, they are largely invisible. Human beings are worldwide exposed to thousands of chemicals daily [1, 2], including many known toxicants, as well as numerous potentially hazardous chemicals with more or less well-characterized risks. These chemicals are commonly detected in blood and urine [3–6]. The categorization of these chemicals is based on their uses in commerce (e.g., pesticides), routes of exposure (e.g., inhalation, drinking water, and food), toxicological effects (e.g., neurotoxicity and immune toxicity), or their persistence being hardly metabolized in biological tissues or the environment (e.g., long half-lives).

Exposure to some chemicals may increase the risk of health effects such as obesity, asthma, allergies, neurodevelopmental disorders, and/or reproductive development [7, 8]. Pesticides (e.g., pyrethroids), naturally occurring metals (e.g., lead, mercury), endocrine-disrupting chemicals (EDCs) (e.g., bisphenol A (BPA), and persistent organic pollutants (POPs) are listed chemicals to have health effects to humans.

Endocrine-disrupting chemicals (EDCs) are a class of chemicals which have the potential to alter the homeostasis or action of endogenous hormones or other signaling compounds of the endocrine system and consequently interfere with fetal growth and development, therefore increasing the risk of disease across the lifespan [9]. By altering the production, release, transport, metabolism, binding, action, or elimination of endogenous hormones important for programming and/or maintaining normal growth and development, EDCs might increase the risk of

E. C. Bonefeld-Jorgensen (✉) · M. Long
Centre for Arctic Health & molecular Epidemiology, Aarhus University, Aarhus, Denmark
e-mail: ebj@ph.au.dk

Y. Xia (ed.), *Early-life Environmental Exposure and Disease*,
https://doi.org/10.1007/978-981-15-3797-4_7

diseases. There is a concern that the fetus, infant, or child may have higher exposure to some EDCs or be more vulnerable compared to adults [7].

Epidemiological studies are important to quantify how the risk of diseases in childhood and adult life is influenced by early-life environmental chemical exposures. There are challenges in identifying the signals of associations between chemical exposure and childhood health including accurately estimating chemical exposure, confounding from causes of both exposure and disease, identifying periods of heightened vulnerability to chemical exposures, and determining the effects of chemical mixtures.

Exposure to chemicals during fetal, infant, and child development might be higher than adult due to time-dependent and synchronized nature of rapidly developing organ systems, which makes them to be more sensitive to environmental inputs that disrupt growth and development. Moreover, because of the different in pharmacokinetics compared to adults, a higher chemical body burdens for a given dose of exposure to the fetus, infant, and child may alter the absorption and distribution of chemicals and decrease their capacity to metabolize and excrete chemicals.

To understand the mechanisms behind the exposure and health effects, experimental in vitro and ex vivo studies might help to elucidate which cellular and molecular mechanisms are involved.

Chemical exposures do not occur to single compound alone, and individuals are exposed to multiple chemicals daily during life. A "one chemical at a time" approach that treats exposures as if they occur in isolation from each other has been used by most epidemiological studies to examine these exposures. However, this does not reflect the nature of exposure to a multitude of chemicals that can have cumulative or interactive effects on human health. Thus, identifying signals from chemical mixtures may improve our understanding of risk factors for fetal and childhood diseases.

2 Epidemiological Data on Environmental Exposure and Fetal Growth and Development

2.1 Pyrethroid Pesticides

Pyrethroids are commonly used to control insects around the home and in agricultural production; it is likely for people to come into contact with one or more pyrethroid insecticides. There were dominant metabolites of pyrethroids detected in urine samples collected from the general population. It was suggested that children and adults are widely exposed to one or more pyrethroids. Exposure to pyrethroids in non-occupational (e.g., general population) mainly occurs through ingestion of food, ingestion after household use, or skin contact with contaminated house dust or particles attached to the surface. Although clinical features of acute accidental exposure to pyrethroids are well documented (e.g., respiratory, eye, skin irritation, and paranesthesia), there is limited information on the chronic effects at low concentrations. Recent epidemiological studies address their potential adverse effects on pregnancy outcomes, reproductive hormones, sperm DNA, sperm quality, and early neurobehavioral development [10]. Most epidemiology studies about pyrethroids relied upon a single urinary sample of pyrethroid metabolites, using a poor exposure metric, which could result in misclassification of past exposures. Additionally, cross-sectional studies prevented an evaluation of the exposure–disease association. Moreover, toxicological effects found in the epidemiological studies were inconsistent with the observed effects in parathyroid animal experiments. To provide more reliable evidence on the underlying health effects of low-dose pyrethroid exposure, future epidemiological studies are needed to characterize adverse outcomes, quantify exposure over time, and verify components' exposure [11].

2.2 Bisphenol A

Bisphenol A (BPA) has estrogenic properties that can enter the food and water supply. Researches on exposure-associated health outcomes in humans have revealed the endocrine-disrupting properties of BPA to have the potential effect on children development. An individual may be predisposed to diseases at doses below the prescribed oral reference dose (RfD) by the environmental protection agencies.

A random effects meta-analysis on prenatal exposure to BPA in 3 human studies and 29 rodent studies showed increases in hyperactivity in male rodent, and there is an association between early BPA exposure and hyperactivity in both boys and girls [12]. Several epidemiological studies observed the associations between BPA exposure and altered thyroid function of pregnant women, neonates, or adolescent [7]. Studies found that BPA exposure during prenatal and postnatal periods was related to behavior problems in children, but there were inconsistencies with the greatest vulnerable period to exposure (prenatal vs. infancy vs. childhood) and sex-specific effects. The reason for this heterogeneity could be the variation of urinary BPA concentrations that might result in BPA exposure misclassification [7]. The obesogenic effects of BPA exposure during early life still remain unclear. Both decreases and increases in adiposity with higher early-life BPA exposure were observed [7, 12].

Searhrist et al. have reviewed in vivo literature for the carcinogenic potential of BPA and confirmed from the rodent studies that BPA exposure during early life below the RfD could lead to ascending susceptibility to prostate and mammary cancer [13]. Studies also proposed that BPA may act as a carcinogen in the breast or prostate because of its tumor-promoting properties [13].

2.3 Phthalates

Phthalates, which act as a kind of EDCs, are used in consumer products, including medications, personal care products, and plastics. Biomonitoring studies worldwide indicate that infants, children, and pregnant women are exposed to phthalate universally. Exposure occurs through food, inhalation, or dermal absorption. Moreover, phthalates could pass through the placenta and expose the fetus [7].

Phthalates may disturb the metabolism or action of thyroid hormones, androgens, and glucocorticoids. Potential mechanisms of phthalates are anti-androgenic and reduced testosterone production in testicular and decreases of the expression of genes involved in steroidogenesis and steroid trafficking [7]. Both human and animal studies showed that several phthalates may reduce triiodothyronine concentration and thyroxine in pregnant women and children, antagonize T3 binding to thyroid receptor-β, and reduce cellular T3 uptake, affecting transcription of the sodium-iodine transporter. Phthalates could inhibit 11-β-hydroxysteroid dehydrogenase-2 as well, which deactivates cortisol. Additionally, phthalate exposure may affect offspring health by causing oxidative stress [14] or via epigenetic reprogramming of the fetus and placenta.

There is concern about the health effects of phthalate mixtures since humans are exposed to multiple phthalates simultaneously and rodent studies demonstrated that phthalates have concentration additive effects on fetal androgen production. Thus, the aggregate of individual phthalate exposures may have an additive impact on human health since individual phthalates share a common mechanism of action.

Epidemiological studies suggested that there may be associations between prenatal exposure and child behavioral problems and cognitive decrements. However, the conclusions about the association between early-life phthalate exposure and obesity or adiposity risk of child are inconsistent. The reason for this inconsistency across the studies might be due to the different time windows of exposure, misclassification, for example, using urine samples to assess exposure, child age, and/or neurodevelopment assessment [7].

2.4 Persistent Organic Pollutants

Persistent organic pollutants (POPs) are carbon-based chemicals found ubiquitously in the environment, originating from industrial processes. POPs are transported along sea currents and atmospheric movement and are accumulated in the food chain, especially the arctic marine food chain [15–17]. Humans are exposed to POPs due to their persistence through the diet, including meat, fish, and dairy products [18–22]. Several studies have found that the body burden of lipophilic POPs in the Arctic populations, for example, Greenlandic Inuit, is much higher than that of the people living close to major emission points [3, 23–25].

The POPs include the *amphiphilic perfluoroalkylated substances* (PFASs), the *lipophilic POPs* (e.g., polychlorinated biphenyls (PCBs)), and the organochlorine pesticides (OCPs). Due to their resistance to degradation, they biomagnify and bioaccumulate via the marine food chain [26–28].

Previous studies have shown that POPs, including PFASs, are negatively associated with cognitive development of children [29–31], immune disruption [32–35], cancer, reduced reproductive ability, and metabolic alternations [29, 36, 37]. It has been confirmed by several studies that the endocrine system could be disrupted by POPs and body's defense against oxidative stress could be decreased [3, 29].

Since the 1930s, many organochlorine compounds including PCBs started to be produced. They have been used in an array of products. However, it was prohibited to be used in electrical devices since the late 1970s in most industrialized countries [38–40]. As alternatives to PCBs, polybrominated diphenyl ethers (PBDEs) and polybrominated biphenyls (PBBs) were then introduced as flame retardants. The mixture of PBBs and two types of PBDE (i.e., pentaBDEs and octaBDEs) has been weeded out around the world, and a third type (i.e., decaBDEs) is being regulated [41, 42]. Several OCPs including dichlorodiphenyltrichloroethane (DDT) and hexachlorobenzene (HCB) are banned from use [39, 43]. In the Stockholm Convention, several PCBs, PBDEs, and OCPs are registered as persistent organic pollutants (POPs) [44].

The *amphiphilic PFAAs* have been used as surfactants since the 1940s [45]. The long-chain PFAAs (six or more carbon atoms) are extremely bioaccumulative and persistent with average serum half-life of 4–8 years [46]. Food including fish, meat, and cereals, being among the largest contributors, is the major source of exposure to PFAAs [47–49]. Drinking water, dust, and air could also be other sources [49]. Humans are also under the threat of being exposed to PFAAs and their precursors from consumer products such as food packaging [50, 51], nonstick cookware, dental floss, cosmetics, leather sofa, etc. [52].

2.5 *Prenatal Exposure and Fetal Growth*

Family exposure was expected to be similar because food intake and environmental exposure. A study on PFASs that was carried out in matched parental and cord serum in 369 families from a birth cohort in Shandong, one of the regions seriously polluted by PFASs in China, reported that PFAS levels were positively correlated among family members. Moreover, PFAAs, PFOA levels in particular, were extremely high and had a positive correlation between parents and in cord blood, suggesting that there was a common source of exposure for the family and heavy pollution in this region [53].

Another study on biosamples and data from a prospective birth cohort study in the Shandong province, China, investigated the efficiency of maternal–fetal transfer (369 pairs) of perfluoroalkyl and polyfluoroalkyl substances [54]. The ten PFASs analyzed were nearly detected in all samples including both umbilical cord and maternal serum. There was a close correlation between maternal and cord levels for most PFASs. The transplacental transfer efficiency (TTE) was significantly affected by chain length and functional group carbon. Perfluoroalkylsulfonates (PFSAs) had a lower ratio of maternal to fetal transfer when compared to perfluoroalkylcarboxylates (PFCAs). A U-shaped relationship between carbon chain length and TTE was observed for PFCAs, while a monotonic descending trend was identified between TTE and the increasing carbon chain length for PFSAs. Thus, PFAAs could easily pass through the placenta. Both carbon chain length and functional group are crucial determinants of the TTE of PFASs [54].

Studies have investigated whether prenatal exposure to POPs is associated with fetal growth. Results of meta-analyses including 12 European birth cohorts showed that low-level exposure to PCB (or correlated exposures) had hazardous effects on fetal growth. Evidence from this study confirmed that low-level exposure to PCBs has a negative association with fetal growth [55]. Another European study on pooled analysis of seven birth cohorts showed that prenatal exposure to p,p'-DDE has an increased association with infant growth, and postnatal PCB-153 with decreased growth at European exposure levels [56].

In the Greenlandic birth cohort ACCEPT, POPs had a negative effect on fetal growth. For all lipophilic POPs, an overall trend of negative associations to fetal growth indices was observed. Whereas PFOA affects birth weight and head circumference negatively, a positive association with gestational age (GA) was observed [57].

Similar associations between PFOA and birth weight from previous studies have been observed [58–60], but it is inconsistent with other studies [61, 62]. The reason for this inconsistency could be due to numerous factors not included in the studies which may have impact on the fetal growth. The surprising observation of positive association between PFOA and GA contrasts most observed negative associations of POP exposure and GA [57]. The underlying hypothesis could be that the mother's body is trying to prolong the gestational age to compensate for the lower birth weight caused by PFOA exposure.

For the first time, it was demonstrated that the combined PFAA-induced xenoestrogenic activity in serum of Danish pregnant women was associated with an inverse effect on fetal growth [63]. The actual PFAA mixture was extracted from the serum of 702 pregnant women in Denmark. The PFAA-induced estrogenic receptor transactivation was determined by use of the human stable transfected MVLN cell line [63]. There was an association between higher serum PFAA-induced xenoestrogenic activities with lower birth weight and birth length of the offspring, which suggested that the actual serum PFAA mixtures could have an effect on fetal growth through disruption of the ER function [63].

This study highlights the importance of mixture studies with respect to fetal development and health risk. In the same Danish Birth Cohort studying the "one chemical at a time" approach for 16 PFAAs, PFAAs were not found to be associated with birth weight or other indices of fetal growth consistently [64].

2.6 Prenatal Exposure and Fetal Growth (Metals)

Metals and other elements exist naturally in the Earth's crust. However, there are numerous metal exposures in environment with growing applications of heavy metals in industry, agriculture, technology, and medicine, as well as from domestic settings and workplaces [65–67].

According to the World Health Organization (WHO), mercury (Hg), lead (Pb), arsenic (As), cadmium (Cd), and chromium (Cr) rank among chemicals which are of major public health concerns due to relatively high toxicity [68–70]. Exposure to heavy metals could result in increased risk of diseases, ranging from cancer and allergies to neurological diseases, decreased cognition, and endocrine disorders [24, 71–74]. The exposure may affect the fetal development because of pregnant women being particularly vulnerable [24, 38, 72–75]. Some contaminants are transferred from the mother to fetus through the placental barrier, as well to the newborn through breastfeeding [3, 4, 65, 67, 76–78].

The Greenlandic Birth Cohort ACCEPT study found negative associations between Pb, Cd, and Cu levels and birth outcomes. For females, Pb and Ni were important risk factors for low birth weight, but Cr correlated positively with birth weight. In addition, female head circumference and gestational age were negatively associated with Ni, while not for males [79].

Previous studies also report that lead exposure affects birth outcome with increased prevalence of low birth weight and small for gestation age among term infants [73, 80].

In the ACCEPT study, a higher risk of low birth weight upon exposure to Cd was observed to be similar to the previous findings [73]. Moreover, Bank-Nielsen et al. [79] also found the indication of increased levels of Ni might increase the risk of low birth weight similar to the previous studies, though rarely investigation was documented; the known toxic effects of nickel includes hemolysis, genetic alterations, and oxidative stress [81–83].

2.7 Environmental Exposure and Child Health and Developmental Effects

The timing of the exposure may determine the toxicity of environmental chemicals to some degree. Thalidomide, as one of the most infamous teratogens, was used to treat nausea in pregnant women in the 1950s and 1960s, leading to limb defects in thousands of children [84]. Notably, exposure between 21 and 36 days after conception was necessary to cause these birth defects, demonstrating the presence of limb defects depended on the timing of thalidomide use. Another example was diethylstilbestrol (DES), a pharmaceutical given to women from the 1940s–1970s to prevent spontaneous abortion. The offspring of women who were prescribed DES in the first half of their pregnancy had increased risk of developing vaginal or cervical clear cell adenocarcinoma [85], as well as reproductive problems and some cancers [86, 87]. The question is how could these compounds be available on the market, and the answer might be that the compounds' risk was assessed in rodents but did not respond clearly with adverse outcome upon exposure to thalidomide [84], whereas later studies demonstrated for DES in both rodents and humans [85].

2.8 *Immunological Effects (Autism, Vaccination, Asthma, and Allergy)*

2.8.1 Autism

During pregnancy and after birth, infections played a potential role in the pathophysiology of autism [88]. Children developing autism were more likely to have decreased levels of both T helper-1(Th-1)-like cytokines (i.e., IFN-γ) and Th-2like cytokines (i.e., IL-4, IL-10), suggesting a depressed or hypoactive immune cell activity during neonatal period in autism [89]. The analysis of neonatal inflammatory chemokine levels in amniotic fluid of children diagnosed later in life with autism and controls cautiously suggested an altered cell-mediated immunity during the early neonatal period in autism [90].

2.8.2 Vaccination Response

Prenatal exposure to POPs can influence vaccination response and the immunological protection against infections. Heilmann et al. 2010 [34] reported prenatal exposure to PCBs affect the serum concentrations of antibodies against diphtheria and tetanus vaccines. Examination at 5 and/or 7 years of age showed that the immune system development in early life appears to be particularly vulnerable when exposed to PCBs, whereas Jusko et al. 2016 [91] found little evidence for specific antibody responses at 6 months of age related to maternal or early postnatal PCB exposure.

Another study examined whether PFAA exposure was associated with antibody response to childhood vaccinations similar to PCBs. Higher exposures to PFAAs were associated with reduced humoral immune response to diphtheria and tetanus vaccines in routine childhood immunizations in children aged 5 and 7 years [33]. These findings were consistent with other studies [92–94], though not all [95] experimental studies in rodents, in which adverse effects of PFOS on humoral immune function were observed at serum concentrations similar to those reported in the present study and at levels prevalent in the United States [96].

In a birth cohort study of maternal and infant serum PCB-153 and DDE concentrations on responses to infant tuberculosis vaccination, the results indicated that higher 6-month infant concentrations of PCB-153 and DDE were strongly associated with lower 6-month Bacille Calmette–Guérin (BCG) vaccine-specific antibody levels [91].

These studies link prenatal and child exposure to POP with deficits in immune system functions that might cause less protection against infectious diseases.

2.8.3 Asthma

Exposure to air pollutants during pregnancy and early life is associated with developmental and functional alterations in lung and other negative respiratory conditions in childhood (asthma, wheezing) that may last into adulthood. Plausible mechanisms include changes in maternal physiology such as hypoxia, oxidative stress and maternal systemic inflammation, and DNA methylation in the fetus [97].

POPs existing in maternal serum concentrations have been reported to be linked with increased risk of asthma in the offspring [98], and researches showed that breastfeeding can modify offspring risk of asthma [99].

2.8.4 Allergy

Greenlandic pregnant women have a high frequency of smoking—and it has been related to higher accumulation of serum POPs [[100]]. A preliminary study on the Greenlandic ACCEPT Birth Cohort children at 3–5 years of age observed that the risk of getting allergy among the offspring was higher to maternal smoking exposure and the child being breastfeed <12 months. Furthermore, we found that children with eczema and breastfed >12 months were predisposed to having asthma and allergy [101].

2.8.5 Neurological Effects

Follow-up studies in neurological effects showed conflicting results, indicating associations between neurodevelopmental outcome in children and prenatal exposure to POPs, while other studies observed no associations [102].

Prenatal exposure to PCBs was found to be linked with an increase in attention-deficit/hyperactivity disorder (ADHD)-like behaviors and lower intelligence levels in children and less optimal long-term memory in adolescents [103–107], whereas other findings showed no associations between prenatal exposure to PCBs and attention in adolescents, learning in 12- to 15-year-old adolescents [108–110], and memory in children at school age [111].

Also prenatal exposure to PBDEs was reported to be associated with reduced motor speed and lower intelligence levels [112, 113]. As for PCB exposures, prenatal exposure to DDE was shown to be associated with ADHD-like behaviors in 7- to 11-year-old children [114], while several other studies found no association with intelligence even at a higher level of exposure to DDE [108, 115].

Berghuis et al. 2018 [116] reported for a follow-up of two Dutch birth cohorts on prenatal exposure to POPs that several OH-PCBs were linked to more optimal sustained attention and balance, whereas hexabroomcyclododecane, with lower performance intelligence, and PCB-183 were linked to lower total intelligence. PCBs, PBDEs, and OH-PCBs were negatively linked to verbal memory.

Numerous studies have indicated that PFASs may interfere with thyroid hormone homeostasis in pregnant women. A recent systematic review reported that three PFASs were negatively correlated with free thyroxine and positively correlated with thyroid-stimulating hormone [117–120]. Thyroid hormones transferred from the mother to the embryo and fetus might be essential for normal brain development of the offspring [121]. Subclinical maternal hypothyroxinemia has been associated with adverse neurodevelopmental outcomes. Deficiency of severe thyroid hormone during gestation might cause cretinism and cognitive and/or mental disorders [122–126]. Research has also observed that even a slight reduction of circulating free thyroid hormone in mothers might cause a loss of 4–7 IQ points in children [127].

We conducted a review on "Exposure to perfluoroalkyl acids and fetal and maternal thyroid status." Including 13 studies, the results indicated a mainly positive relationship between maternal PFAA exposure and TSH levels, and a suggestion of an inverse association with T4 and/or T3 levels. Associations of infant TH upon PFAA exposure were less consistent (Boesen et al. submitted).

A study on the Danish National Birth Cohort showed gestational-week-specific associations between high exposure to several PFAAs and TSH level in early gestations [128]. Further researches within the biology and the adverse clinical outcome regarding thyroid hormones disruptions in early pregnancy are needed.

Few data have been reported on PFAA exposure and child IQ. A study on the Danish National Birth Cohort found no strong associations between a natural-log unit increase in each of the seven PFASs and child IQ scores, while a few positive and negative associations were found in the sex-stratified PFAS quartile analyses, but the patterns were inconsistent [129].

3 Possible Molecular Mechanisms

In vitro and ex vivo cell systems have been introduced for the assessment of EDCs such as the integrated level of xenobiotic cellular effects in human beings. In this section, the in vitro and ex vivo studies of EDCs mainly using cell-based reporter gene bioassays are described. In addition, some in vivo animal studies about the development effect are also elaborated.

3.1 *In Vitro (and In Vivo)*

3.1.1 Pesticides

Previous in vitro studies showed that pesticides (methiocarb, endosulfan, dieldrin, and fenarimol) acted as both estrogen receptor (ER) agonists and androgen receptor (AR) antagonists. Prochloraz reacted as both an estrogen and an androgen antagonist. Furthermore, fenarimol and prochloraz were potent aromatase inhibitors, while endosulfan was a weak inhibitor. Hence, there are at least three different ways in which pesticides potentially disturb sex hormone actions. Chlorpyrifos, deltamethrin, tolclofos-methyl, and tribenuron-methyl induced weak estrogenic responses, while endosulfan and pirimicarb, propamocarb, and daminozide potentiated the estrogenic response of natural ER ligand 17-estradiol. Methomyl, pirimicarb, propamocarb, and iprodione weakly stimulated activity of aromatase, an enzyme converting testosterone to estrogen. Although the potencies of the pesticides were low compared to the natural ligands, the integrated response in the organism might be amplified by the ability of the pesticides to act via several mechanisms and the frequent simultaneous exposure to several pesticides [43].

Furthermore, studies showed that the pesticides endosulfan, prochloraz, tolclofos-methyl, and propamocarb elicited the estrogenic potential in both stable and transient transfected cell lines [130] and demonstrated organochlorine and organophosphorus pesticides such as prochloraz, fenarimol, and chlorpyrifos possess the ability to interfere with the ERα and ERβ mRNA steady-state levels [131, 132].

Different receptor conformations induce diverse effects of different natural and synthetic ER ligands, allowing differential interactions with other transcription factors. It was reported that the peptide recognition pattern induced by a group of chlorinated pesticides including 2, 4-dichlorodiphenyl-dichloroethylene (DDE) is different from the classical ER ligand [133].

A recent in vitro study showed a weakly induced ER transactivity by the pesticides propiconazole, terbuthylazine, cypermethrin, prothioconazole, and malathion [134], while bitertanol, propiconazole, and mancozeb antagonized the AR activity in a concentration-dependent manner. The mixture consisting of five pesticides (bitertanol, terbuthylazine, cypermethrin, malathion, propiconazole) induced the aromatase activity and the ER transactivity while additively antagonized the AR transactivity [134].

A study on the fungicide fenarimol indicated estrogenic effects both in vitro and in vivo and a dual effect being estrogenic at higher concentrations and aromatase inhibitor at low concentrations [135].

Studies have reported that prochloraz, an imidazole fungicide, elicits multiple mechanisms of action in vitro, antagonizing the androgen and the estrogen receptor and inhibiting activity of aromatase [43] while agonizing the aryl hydrocarbon receptor (AhR) [136]. The in vivo Hershberger assay using castrate-immature male rats showed that prochloraz as an antiandrogen might reduce weights of reproductive organs, affects androgen-regulated gene expressions in the prostate, and increases luteinizing hormone (LH) levels [137]. A study investigating the developmental effects of prochloraz, upon exposure of pregnant Wistar rat dams, observed that plasma and testicular testosterone levels in gestational day 21 male fetuses were significantly reduced, whereas testicular progesterone was increased by prochloraz, indicating that the male offspring might be feminized by perinatal prochloraz exposure and these effects are due to diminished fetal steroidogenesis. Thus prochloraz acts as an antiandrogen eliciting dual mechanisms of action both by blocking the androgen receptor and by inhibiting fetal steroidogenesis [138].

The potential endocrine activity was studied on pesticides bitertanol, propiconazole, cypermethrin, malathion, and terbuthylazine alone and as mixtures in vitro and in vivo. It was shown that the pesticides alone and as mixtures affected steroidogenesis in adrenal cells in vitro and caused the increases in progesterone and decreases in testosterone. The mixture of five pesticides elicited an increase in estradiol, indicating increased aromatase activity [139]. Furthermore, the in vivo animal study showed a decreased estradiol and reduced placental testosterone for dams exposed to pesticide mixture and a significant increase in aromatase mRNA-levels in female adrenal glands [139]. This study indicated the potential aromatase induction of the mixture of the five pesticides both in vitro and in vivo. However, the hormonal responses in vitro were only partly reflected in vivo, probably due to some toxicokinetic issues, since the amount of compound mixtures affect pesticide levels negatively in the amniotic fluid [139].

The aryl hydrocarbon receptor (AhR) acts as a ligand-activated transcription factor mediating many of the biologic and toxicological effects of 2,3,7,8-tetrachlorodibenzo-p-dioxin (TCDD) and related compounds. The cross-talks between AhR and ER, AR have been reported [140]. AhR is involved in syntheses of steroids and metabolism of steroids and xenobiotic compounds [141]. Studies showed that the pesticides iprodione, chlorpyrifos, prochloraz, terbuthylazine, propiconazole, mancozeb, cypermethrin, and tau-fluvalinate elicited dose-dependent AhR agonistic effects [136, 142]. The mixture of bitertanol, propiconazole, cypermethrin, malathion, and terbuthylazine induced as well AhR transactivity [142].

The actions of thyroid hormones (THs) are mediated by the thyroid hormone receptor (TR). Agonistic effects on cell growth (cell proliferation) may be caused by interaction of compounds with the TRs, whereas interference with the triiodothyronine (T3)-TR association or binding of antagonists to the TRs may result in inhibiting effects on T3-mediated cell growth. Studies showed that the pesticides prochloraz, chlorpyrifos, prothioconazole, malathion, tau-fluvalinate, cypermethrin, terbuthylazine, and mancozeb significantly stimulated rat pituitary GH3 cell proliferation and bitertanol and propiconazole slightly reduced the GH3 cell proliferation [142, 143]. In the presence of triiodothyronine (T3), prochloraz, iprodione, prothioconazole, tau-fluvalinate, propiconazole, cypermethrin, and bitertanol significantly antagonized the T3-induced GH3 cell proliferation [142, 143]. Moreover, an additive combined effect on TH-dependent cell proliferation of pesticide mixture composed of terbuthylazine, propiconazole, cypermethrin, and malathion was observed [142].

3.1.2 Plasticizers/Phthalates

In vitro studies showed that widely used phenols and plasticizers including bisphenol A (BPA) and bisphenol A dimethacrylate (BPA-DM), 4-n-nonylphenol (nNP), and 4-n-octylphenol (nOP) have endocrine-disrupting potentials and the effects can be mediated via several cellular pathways, including the two sex steroid hormone receptors (ER and AR), aromatase activity, and AhR [144]. Moreover, BPA and BPA-DM elicited an inhibitory effect on thyroid hormone (TH)-dependent cell growth [143]. In addition, benzyl butyl phthalate (BBP), 4-chloro-3-methylphenol (CMP), 2,4-dichlorophenol (2,4-DCP), and resorcinol affected AR and AhR transactivity, whereas bis(2-ethylhexyl) phthalate (DEHP), diisodecyl phthalate (DIDP), and dibutyl phthalate (DBP) affected only the AhR and 4-tert-octylphenol (tOP), and 2-phenylphenol (2-PP) antagonized the AR activity in vitro [145].

The mixture composed of six plasticizers, of which one weakly induced the AhR but all others antagonized the AR-elicited additive effects for both AR and AhR. This in vitro data indicate that when assessing the risk to human health, the effect of a mixture depends on the character, potency, concentration, and composition of the single mixture compounds and also the combined effects of the compounds should be taken into account [145].

Furthermore, in vitro study showed that BBP, DBP, dioctyl phthalate (DOP), DIDP, diisononyl phthalate (DINP), DEHP, bis(2-ethylhexyl) adipate (DEHA), tOP, CMP, 2,4-DCP, and resorcinol significantly affected the thyroid hormone-dependent GH3 cell proliferation: tOP, BBP, and DBP activated ER transactivity, whereas DEHP antagonized the 17-estradiol-induced ER function. The mixture of six plasticizers significantly induced ER transactivity in an additive manner, whereas elicited antagonized effect for the thyroid hormone-dependent GH3 cell proliferation [146].

3.1.3 Persistent Organic Pollutants

3.1.3.1 Lipophilic POPs

There are many interactions in the bloodstream of mammals connected with the transport of lipophilic xenobiotic compounds. POPs including DDT, and especially its metabolite DDE would cause a range of deleterious health effects by interacting with nuclear hormone receptors and resulting in malfunction. A study of lipoprotein receptors in mouse embryonic fibroblast cells in conjunction with uptake of DDT–lipoprotein compounds from supplemented media in vitro showed that DDT uptake decreased with increased low-density lipoprotein (LDL) concentration. However, there was no strong evidence for a receptor-mediated uptake of the DDT–lipoprotein complex, suggesting DDT might be transported as a DDT–lipoprotein complex without receptors to cross cell membranes, since passive diffusion constitutes a major passageway [147].

Among the lipophilic POPs, PCBs are ubiquitous environmental POPs giving rise to potential health hazard. Dioxin-like PCBs such as PCB 105, PCB 118, PCB126, PCB 156, exert dioxin-like activities mediated through AhR. The di-ortho, multiple-chloro-substituted biphenyls (PCB138, PCB153, and PCB180) were shown to have pleiotropic effects on the estrogen receptor (ER) and androgen receptor (AR). They can compete with the binding of the natural ligand to ER and AR and thus possess the ability to interfere with sexual hormone-regulated processes [148].

The PCB metabolites (OH-PCB 106, OH-PCB 121, OH-PCB 69) and brominated flame retardants (tetrabromobisphenol A) were shown to interfere with the TH-dependent GH3 cell proliferation alone or upon co-treatment with T3 [143].

Several rodent researches reported behavioral alterations after developmental, neonatal, or adult exposure to PBDEs, among which subtle structural and functional changes in brains were observed. In the brain, functional effects have been found on synaptic plasticity and the glutamate–nitric oxide–cyclic guanosine monophosphate pathway. Furthermore, some studies reported expression changes of genes and proteins involved in synapse and axon formation, neuronal morphology, cell migration, synaptic plasticity, ion channels, and vesicular neurotransmitter release. Cellular and molecular mechanisms include effects on neuronal differentiation and migration, neuronal viability (via apoptosis and oxidative stress), neurotransmitter release/uptake, neurotransmitter receptors and ion channels, calcium (Ca^{2+}) homeostasis, and intracellular signaling pathways [149–151].

3.1.3.2 Amphiphilic POPs (PFAAs)

An in vitro study analyzed seven PFAA congeners [perfluorooctanoate (PFOA), perfluorooctane sulfonate (PFOS), perfluorodecanoate (PFDA), perfluorononanoate (PFNA), perfluorohexane sulfonate (PFHxS), perfluorododecanoate (PFDoA), and perfluoroundecanoate (PFUnA)] for their potential to affect estrogen receptor (ER) and androgen receptor (AR) transactivity as well as aromatase enzyme activity in individual and in an equimolar mixture. The results showed that PFHxS, PFOS, and PFOA and a mixture of the seven PFAAS significantly induced the ER transactivity [152], while PFHxS, PFOS, PFOA, PFNA, and PFDA significantly antagonized the AR activity in a concentration-dependent manner. A synergistic mixture effect on AR function was observed for the equimolar mixture of the seven PFAAs. Moreover, PFDA weakly decreased the aromatase activity at a high test concentration [152].

Furthermore, the above seven PFAAs were shown to elicit a dose-dependent inhibition of GH3 cell growth and PFOS, PFHxS, PFNA, and PFUnA antagonized the T3-induced GH3 cell proliferation [153], while only PFDoA and PFDA elicited an activating effect on the AhR [153].

PFAAs were shown to affect oxidative stress biomarkers in vitro. Wielsøe M et al. [154] reported that PFHxS, PFOA, PFOS, and PFNA showed a dose-dependent increase in DNA damage; except for PFDoA, all the other PFAAs increased the generation of reactive oxygen species (ROS) significantly with PFHxS and PFUnA dose-dependently. PFOA decreased the total antioxidant capacity (TAC) level in human liver cells [154].

3.1.4 Phytoestrogens

Phytoestrogens (PEs) can mimic or modulate the production or action of endogenous hormones resulting in biologic responses in vertebrates. PEs are produced in a large range of plants as naturally occurring plant components.

An in vitro study examined the mixtures of 12 foods relevant PEs including coumestrol, isoflavonoids and lignans for the effects on estrogenic and aromatase activity, steroid hormone production, and for the interaction with the androgen receptor. The results indicated an induced aromatase activity by the mixture of all tested PEs causing increased estradiol production and decreased testosterone production of adrenal corticocarcinoma cells in human. Furthermore, various mixtures of PEs significantly stimulated human breast adenocarcinoma cell growth and induced aromatase activity in human choriocarcinoma cells. It was reported that isoflavonoid may cause reduction of testosterone, and isoflavonoid mixture and coumestrol might decrease ERα expression while increase progesterone receptor protein expression [155].

Among the 12 PEs mentioned above, most PEs and their mixtures showed effects on both the TH and AhR cell system. Single isoflavonoid metabolites and their mixture and coumestrol induced T3-dependent GH3 cell growth and AhR transactivity dose-dependently. Furthermore, isoflavonoid metabolites may also affect T3-dependent GH3 cell growth and cause a synergistic effect on the AhR transactivity [156]. Therefore, nutrition-relevant PEs, alone and in mixture, may possess endocrine-disrupting potential through various modes of actions.

3.1.5 Other Compounds

Based on previous studies, polyhalogenated carbazoles (PHCZs) are a general class of contaminants characterized by persistence and bioaccumulation property. It was shown that nine PHCZs significantly activated AhR in a concentration-dependent manner, with 1000–100,000-fold less potential than that of the most potent AhR ligand TCDD. The AhR activation was partly consistent with the induction of AhR-mediated CYP1A1 expression. In in silico analysis, the nine PHCZs could be docked into the same pocket as TCDD, owing to their high structural similarity. However, the shrunk size of the heterocyclic moieties in PHCZs compared with that in TCDD dramatically contributed to a lower compound stability provided by intermolecular interactions. Moreover, two distinguished docking poses adopted by the nine PHCZs were found. Thus PHCZ may possess the toxicity via interaction with AhR [157].

Dehydroepiandrosterone sulfate (DHEAS) and estrone sulfate (E1S) are two of the most abundant steroids existing in the human circulation. The enzyme steroid sulfatase (STS) cracks the sulfate group of DHEAS and E1S resulting in biosynthesis of endogenous hormones such as testosterone and estrone. In vitro study showed both E1S and DHEAS dose-dependently transactivated the ER and the AR in dose-dependent manners [158].

3.2 *Ex Vivo Studies (as Exposure Biomarker)*

The toxicological assessment of EDCs in human is complicated. The adverse health effects of environment contaminants are probably due to disruption of various hormonal systems, e.g., ER, AR, TR, and/or AhR. Toxicological studies have shown that the individual POPs possess very different biological effects and potentials; many of the bioaccumulated POPs are estrogenic while others are antiestrogenic, as well as anti-androgenic, and some have dioxin-like potentials. Additive enhancement of hormone actions has been reported in vitro and in vivo. Therefore, it is of great significance to evaluate the integrated biological effect of the actual chemical mixture in human body. Extractions followed by cell culture system analyses have recently been introduced to assess the ex vivo integrated effect on hormone receptor activities of xenobiotic compounds such as POPs in human adipose tissue and in human serum [29].

Extracting the compounds from human tissues, such as human serum, is one way to study the effects of the actual mixture of compounds related to the human body [29]. A method of extracting lipophilic POPs from human serum, including PCBs and organochlorine pesticides (OCPs) but free of endogenous hormones, was established and validated, making the extraction method as a valuable tool to assess the combined effects such as additive/synergistic and agonistic/antagonistic effects of ER and AR of serum lipophilic POPs and may give an overall estimate of exposure and bioactivity [159]. Recently, a method of extracting in parallel the lipophilic POPs and the amphiphilic PFAAs, free of endogenous hormones, separated from the same serum sample, was developed and validated [160]. This method can be used for studying the effects of the actual serum lipophilic POPs mixture as well as PFAA mixture on both steroid hormones and other hormonal systems, e.g., thyroid hormone function, and possibly elucidate the relationship between exposure to lipophilic POPs and PFAAs and related biological effects and health outcomes [161].

The lipophilic POPs were extracted from Greenland Inuit serum, and the extract elicited in cell culture ex vivo xenoestrogenic and xenoandrogenic transactivities and AhR transactivity which were related to age, marine food intake, and smoking years and negatively correlated to the serum levels of lipophilic POPs. These data indicate that the POP mixture induced xenohormone and AhR transactivities can serve as a comprehensive biomarker of POP exposure and lifestyle characteristics. The data clearly showed the hormone-disruptive potentials of serum POPs [162–164].

A study measured the xenoestrogenic activity in human serum extracts consisting of mixtures of PFAAs of 397 Danish nulliparous pregnant women. Fifty-two percent of the PFAA serum extracts agonized the ER transactivation, and 46% further enhanced the 17β estradiol-induced ER transactivation. The serum PFAA extracts induced the ER in a non-monotonic concentration-dependent manner. The serum extract containing the actual mixtures of PFAAs induced the estrogenic activity corresponding to the effect of 0.5 pg 17β estradiol per milliliter serum. Thus, nearly all of the serum extracts containing the PFAA mixtures from pregnant women's serum elicited estrogenic potentials, agonizing the ER, and further promoted the E2-induced effects in non-monotonic concentration-dependent manners [165].

The lipophilic POPs induced AhR transactivity were analyzed in serum samples from Danish schoolchildren and their mothers living in urban and rural areas. The serum lipophilic POP-induced AhR transactivities were dramatically higher in schoolchildren living in the urban area compared with the rural. A high correlation between the AhR transactivity of mothers and children was observed. The results also showed that AhR transactivity can be measured as a biomarker of exposure and effects in blood samples from children and women and indicated that people living in urban areas may be exposed to higher concentrations of PCBs, dioxins, and dioxin-like chemicals, which may result in a greater risk of adverse effects for urban populations [166].

3.2.1 POP-Induced Receptor Transactivity and Health Outcome (as Effect Biomarker)

3.2.1.1 Fetal Growth

A newly published ex vivo study showed that the maternal serum extract of PFAAs in cell culture-induced xenoestrogenic receptor transactivation (XER) was related to a decrease in birth weight and birth length [63]. The associations of maternal serum dioxin-like compounds measured as ex vivo AhR transactivity and birth outcomes are inconsistent [167, 168]. An international study showed the cord blood AhR transactivity was inversely associated with gestational age but found a tendency of a positive, non-significant association between maternal serum AhR transactivity and birth weight and gestational age [169].

3.2.1.2 Autism (Molecular Mechanisms)

Several studies support the hypothesis that the pathogenesis of autism is most likely to be polygenic [170], and environmental factors may interact with genetic factors to increase the risk of autism [171, 172]. Although the genetic risk factors remain difficult to identify, several chromosomal disorders and single gene disorders are associated with an increased risk for autism. Furthermore, evidence has indicated that some non-inherited factors such as exposure to environmental pollutants bear upon autism [173]. The epigenetic mechanisms play an important role in the gene–environment interactions in autism [174]. In addition, prenatal stress and maternal immune dysregulation are also associated with autism [175].

A Danish case-control study measured the amniotic fluid (AF) levels of EDCs and metals as well as the receptor transactivity induced by AF and also investigated the possible connection between prenatal exposure to EDCs and heavy metals and risk of autism [176]. The biomarkers of effect such as ER-, AR-, AhR-, and TH-like transactivity were determined in the AF samples, which indicated the presence of EDCs in amniotic fluid. This study suggested that EDCs might alter the risk of autism by affecting the hormone receptor function. The observed inverse correlation between PFAAs and autism risk might be associated with the weak estrogenic activities and anti-androgenic activities of PFAAs. As autism is a typical male trait, regardless of whether EDCs together with endogenous hormones play a role in the development of autism, the observed tendency of positive association between the ratio of combined androgenic effect to the combined estrogenic effect and autism risk needs further studies to explore [176].

4 Summary

Humans are exposed to complicated mixtures of chemicals, which have individually significant differences in biological potentials and effects. Endocrine disruptors (EDCs) can mimic or block endogenous hormones, thereby disrupting normal hormone homeostasis. EDCs include compounds with long half-life such as POPs and non-accumulating compounds such as certain pesticides, BPA, and phthalates.

In particular, prenatal and children's exposure to chemicals in surrounding environment are of great concern that may have the potential to influence the risk of diseases in childhood and adult life.

Epidemiological researches play a critical part in quantifying how environmental chemical exposures prenatally and postnatally contribute to diseases in childhood and adult life. Although there are some challenges for estimating accurately exposure and the period of exposure sensitivity that needs further exploration.

In epidemiological studies, pesticides such as pyrethroids effects were reported for acute accidental exposure to pyrethroids such as paranesthesia; respiratory, eye, and skin irritation; and so on, whereas information on their chronic effects at low concentrations is not only limited but also controversial. The effects observed in the epidemiological literature were inconsistent with toxicological effects observed in extensive testing of pyrethroids in animals.

Considerable research on BPA exposure-associated health risks in humans has elucidated BPA's endocrine-disrupting properties, suggesting BPA's potential impact on development during early life. This may make individuals more susceptible to diseases, including neurological and carcinogenic potential, below the oral reference dose (RfD) determined by the environmental protection agencies.

Epidemiological studies on exposure to phthalates during pregnancy suggest behavioral and cognitive effects in children as well as child obesity.

POPs, including lipophilic POPs and amphiphilic PFASs and some metals, were relevant to negative influence on development of fetal, child cognitive, immune, and reproductive disruption. POPs can disrupt the endocrine system and decrease the defense against oxidative stress. A new method to study the actual serum mixture of POPs has suggested that the mixtures exposure approach reflect more precisely the real daily exposure to multiple chemicals instead of "one chemical at a time" approach.

POP exposures were also associated with decreased vaccination response and immunological protection to tetanus, diphtheria, and tuberculosis.

Prenatal environmental exposures were also associated with the risk of autism/ADHD, asthma, and allergy.

5 Mechanisms

EDCs such as pesticides, PCBs, PFAAs, plasticizers/phthalates, phenols, and phytoestrogens are shown to work as an estrogen receptor (ER) agonist/antagonist, androgen receptor (AR), and aryl hydrocarbon receptor (AhR), to interfere with thyroid hormone (TH) function and to interfere with the steroid enzymes such as aromatase enzyme that convert testosterone to E2 (17b-estradiol) and can work through a variety of mechanisms. In addition, due to the cross interaction of the AhR with the ER, AR, and TH, the effects of EDCs on AhR can help to elucidate the cellular mechanisms behind hormone disorders. The final response may be determined by the interaction of all pathways implicated. Moreover, the mixture analyses showed that the combined effect of all the compounds present in the human body must be taken into consideration for risk assessment.

Ex vivo studies have shown comprehensive biomarker effect of complex mixture extracted from human serum to reflect the regional differences in serum levels of bioaccumulated POPs, e.g., in the Arctic region. Xenobiotic receptor activity can be used as an in vitro biomarker of POP exposure and effects. The potential impact of the comprehensive effect of EDCs on human health has been supported by epidemiological and in vitro/ex vivo studies.

Other mechanisms such as oxidative stress and DNA alterations and inflammation also play important roles in effects of the early exposure to environmental contaminants on growth and development (Fig. 1).

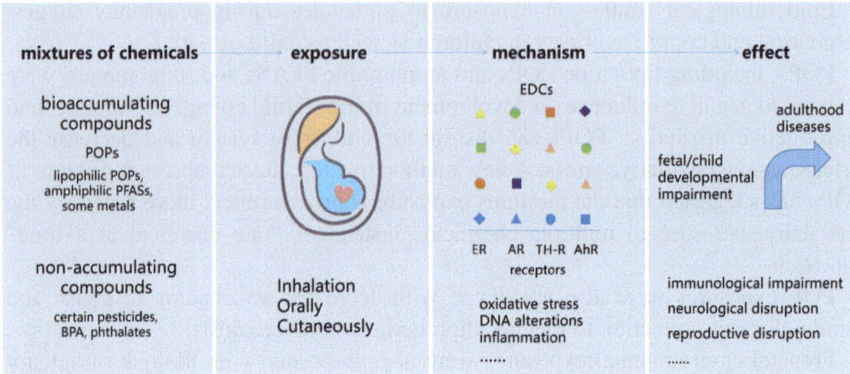

Fig. 1 The outline of the chapter (*POPs* persistent organic pollutants, *PFAS* per- and polyfluoroalkyl substances, *BPA* bisphenol A, *EDCs* endocrine-disrupting chemicals, *ER* estrogen receptor, *AR* androgen receptor, *TH-R* thyroid receptor, *AhR* aryl hydrocarbon receptor)

References

1. Agency, E.C. Available from: https://echa.europa.eu/information-on-chemicals
2. EP, A (2017) How to access the TSCA inventory 2017 [cited 2017 June 22]. Available from: https://www.epa.gov/tsca-inventory/how-access-tsca-inventory#download
3. AMAP (2015) AMAP assessment 2015: human health in the Arctic. Arctic Monitoring and Assessment Programme (AMAP), Oslo, vii + 165 pp. https://www.amap.no/documents/download/2594
4. AMAP (2017) AMAP assessment 2015 chemicals of emerging arctic concern. 2015, Arctic Monitoring and Assessment Programme (AMAP): Oslo, Norway
5. CDC CfDCaP, U.T Fourth national report on human exposure to environmental chemicals, Updated Tables 2012. Available from: http://www.cdc.gov/exposurereport/pdf/FourthReport_UpdatedTables_Feb2012.pdf
6. OECD (2019) Environmental performance reviews: Denmark 2019, Chapter 5, Chemical management. Available from: https://books.google.dk/books?id=bT6DwAAQBAJ&pg=PA202&lpg=PA202&dq=biomonitorering+in+Denmark&source=bl&ots=tUaRkEStZ&sig=ACfU3U19a2IHP7IGnaYy7SxkaNFAvz_soQ&hl=da&sa=X&ved=2ahUKEwiPm5L6_PmAhVO_qQKHVFhBKIQ6AEwBXoECAoQAQ#v=onepage&q=biomonitorering%20in%20Denmark&f=false
7. Braun JM (2017) Early-life exposure to EDCs: role in childhood obesity and neurodevelopment. Nat Rev Endocrinol 13(3):161–173
8. Grandjean P, Landrigan PJ (2014) Neurobehavioural effects of developmental toxicity. Lancet Neurol 13(3):330–338
9. Zoeller RT et al (2012) Endocrine-disrupting chemicals and public health protection: a statement of principles from The Endocrine Society. Endocrinology 153(9):4097–4110
10. Saillenfait AM, Ndiaye D, Sabate JP (2015) Pyrethroids: exposure and health effects – an update. Int J Hyg Environ Health 218(3):281–292
11. Burns CJ, Pastoor TP (2018) Pyrethroid epidemiology: a quality-based review. Crit Rev Toxicol 48(4):297–311
12. Rochester JR, Bolden AL, Kwiatkowski CF (2018) Prenatal exposure to bisphenol A and hyperactivity in children: a systematic review and meta-analysis. Environ Int 114:343–356
13. Seachrist DD et al (2016) A review of the carcinogenic potential of bisphenol A. Reprod Toxicol 59:167–182

14. Ferguson KK et al (2015) Urinary phthalate metabolites and biomarkers of oxidative stress in pregnant women: a repeated measures analysis. Environ Health Perspect 123(3):210–216
15. Barrie LA et al (1992) Arctic contaminants: sources, occurrence and pathways. Sci Total Environ 122(1–2):1–74
16. Burkow IC, Kallenborn R (2000) Sources and transport of persistent pollutants to the Arctic. Toxicol Lett 112–113:87–92
17. Hung H et al (2016) Temporal trends of Persistent Organic Pollutants (POPs) in arctic air: 20 years of monitoring under the Arctic Monitoring and Assessment Programme (AMAP). Environ Pollut 217:52–61
18. Diamanti-Kandarakis E et al (2009) Endocrine-disrupting chemicals: an Endocrine Society scientific statement. Endocr Rev 30(4):293–342
19. Thomsen C, Liane VH, Becher G (2007) Automated solid-phase extraction for the determination of polybrominated diphenyl ethers and polychlorinated biphenyls in serum – application on archived Norwegian samples from 1977 to 2003. J Chromatogr B Anal Technol Biomed Life Sci 846(1–2):252–263
20. Brauner EV et al (2011) Predictors of polychlorinated biphenyl concentrations in adipose tissue in a general Danish population. Environ Sci Technol 45(2):679–685
21. Brauner EV et al (2012) Predictors of adipose tissue concentrations of organochlorine pesticides in a general Danish population. J Expo Sci Environ Epidemiol 22(1):52–59
22. Halldorsson TI et al (2008) Linking exposure to polychlorinated biphenyls with fatty fish consumption and reduced fetal growth among Danish pregnant women: a cause for concern? Am J Epidemiol 168(8):958–965
23. Bonefeld-Jorgensen EC (2010) Biomonitoring in Greenland: human biomarkers of exposure and effects – a short review. Rural Remote Health 10(2):1362
24. Long M et al (2015) Food intake and serum persistent organic pollutants in the Greenlandic pregnant women: the ACCEPT sub-study. Sci Total Environ 529:198–212
25. Frank W, Mackay D (1993) Global fractionation and cold condensation of low volatility organochlorine compounds in polar regions. Ambio 22(1):10–18
26. Borga K et al (2004) Biological and chemical factors of importance in the bioaccumulation and trophic transfer of persistent organochlorine contaminants in Arctic marine food webs. Environ Toxicol Chem 23(10):2367–2385
27. Corsolini S, Sara G (2017) The trophic transfer of persistent pollutants (HCB, DDTs, PCBs) within polar marine food webs. Chemosphere 177:189–199
28. Krafft MP, Riess JG (2015) Per- and polyfluorinated substances (PFASs): Environmental challenges. Curr Opin Colloid Interface Sci 20(3):192–212
29. Bonefeld-Jorgensen EC et al (2014) Biomonitoring and hormone-disrupting effect biomarkers of persistent organic pollutants in vitro and ex vivo. Basic Clin Pharmacol Toxicol 115 (1):118–128
30. Boucher O et al (2012) Response inhibition and error monitoring during a visual go/no-go task in Inuit children exposed to lead, polychlorinated biphenyls, and methylmercury. Environ Health Perspect 120(4):608–615
31. Lam J et al (2017) Developmental PBDE exposure and IQ/ADHD in childhood: a systematic review and meta-analysis. Environ Health Perspect 125(8):086001
32. Dallaire F et al (2006) Effect of prenatal exposure to polychlorinated biphenyls on incidence of acute respiratory infections in preschool Inuit children. Environ Health Perspect 114 (8):1301–1305
33. Grandjean P et al (2012) Serum vaccine antibody concentrations in children exposed to perfluorinated compounds. JAMA 307(4):391–397
34. Heilmann C et al (2010) Serum concentrations of antibodies against vaccine toxoids in children exposed perinatally to immunotoxicants. Environ Health Perspect 118 (10):1434–1438
35. Schaebel LK et al (2017) The influence of persistent organic pollutants in the traditional Inuit diet on markers of inflammation. PLoS One 12(5):e0177781

36. Ghisari M et al (2014) Polymorphisms in phase I and phase II genes and breast cancer risk and relations to persistent organic pollutant exposure: a case-control study in Inuit women. Environ Health 13(1):19
37. Weihe P et al (2016) Health effects associated with measured levels of contaminants in the Arctic. Int J Circumpolar Health 75:33805
38. Takeuchi S et al (2011) Characterization of steroid hormone receptor activities in 100 hydroxylated polychlorinated biphenyls, including congeners identified in humans. Toxicology 289 (2–3):112–121
39. Noren K, Meironyte D (2000) Certain organochlorine and organobromine contaminants in Swedish human milk in perspective of past 20–30 years. Chemosphere 40(9–11):1111–1123
40. Medehouenou TC et al (2011) Polychlorinated biphenyls and organochlorine pesticides in plasma of older Canadians. Environ Res 111(8):1313–1320
41. Wu JP et al (2011) Several current-use, non-PBDE brominated flame retardants are highly bioaccumulative: Evidence from field determined bioaccumulation factors. Environ Int 37 (1):210–215
42. Sjodin A et al (2004) Retrospective time-trend study of polybrominated diphenyl ether and polybrominated and polychlorinated biphenyl levels in human serum from the United States. Environ Health Perspect 112(6):654–658
43. Andersen HR et al (2002) Effects of currently used pesticides in assays for estrogenicity, androgenicity, and aromatase activity in vitro. Toxicol Appl Pharmacol 179(1):1–12
44. Stockholm_Convention (2009) Listing of POPs in Stockholm convention [cited 2014 July 24th]. Available from: http://chm.pops.int/Convention/ThePOPs/ListingofPOPs/tabid/2509/Default.aspx
45. Schultz MM, Barofsky DF, Field JA (2003) Fluorinated alkyl surfactants. Environ Eng Sci 20 (5):487–501
46. Olsen GW et al (2007) Half-life of serum elimination of perfluorooctanesulfonate, perfluorohexanesulfonate, and perfluorooctanoate in retired fluorochemical production workers. Environ Health Perspect 115(9):1298–1305
47. Haug LS et al (2011) Characterisation of human exposure pathways to perfluorinated compounds – comparing exposure estimates with biomarkers of exposure. Environ Int 37 (4):687–693
48. Haug LS et al (2010) Diet and particularly seafood are major sources of perfluorinated compounds in humans. Environ Int 36(7):772–778
49. Trudel D et al (2008) Estimating consumer exposure to PFOS and PFOA. Risk Anal 28 (2):251–269
50. D'Eon JC et al (2009) Observation of a commercial fluorinated material, the polyfluoroalkyl phosphoric acid diesters, in human sera, wastewater treatment plant sludge, and paper fibers. Environ Sci Technol 43(12):4589–4594
51. Trier X, Granby K, Christensen JH (2011) Polyfluorinated surfactants (PFS) in paper and board coatings for food packaging. Environ Sci Pollut Res Int 18(7):1108–1120
52. Ramli MR et al (2020) Level and determinants of serum perfluoroalkyl acids (PFAAs) in a population in Klang Valley, Malaysia. Int J Hyg Environ Health 223(1):179–186
53. Han W et al (2018) Perfluoroalkyl and polyfluoroalkyl substances in matched parental and cord serum in Shandong, China. Environ Int 116:206–213
54. Wang Y et al (2019) Efficiency of maternal-fetal transfer of perfluoroalkyl and polyfluoroalkyl substances. Environ Sci Pollut Res Int 26(3):2691–2698
55. Govarts E et al (2012) Birth weight and prenatal exposure to polychlorinated biphenyls (PCBs) and dichlorodiphenyldichloroethylene (DDE): a meta-analysis within 12 European Birth Cohorts. Environ Health Perspect 120(2):162–170
56. Iszatt N et al (2015) Prenatal and postnatal exposure to persistent organic pollutants and infant growth: a pooled analysis of seven European birth cohorts. Environ Health Perspect 123 (7):730–736

57. Hjermitslev MH et al (2020) Persistent organic pollutants in Greenlandic pregnant women and indices of foetal growth: The ACCEPT study. Sci Total Environ 698:134118
58. Apelberg BJ et al (2007) Cord serum concentrations of perfluorooctane sulfonate (PFOS) and perfluorooctanoate (PFOA) in relation to weight and size at birth. Environ Health Perspect 115 (11):1670–1676
59. Chen MH et al (2012) Perfluorinated compounds in umbilical cord blood and adverse birth outcomes. PLoS One 7(8):e42474
60. Cao W et al (2018) Perfluoroalkyl substances in umbilical cord serum and gestational and postnatal growth in a Chinese birth cohort. Environ Int 116:197–205
61. Bach CC et al (2016) Perfluoroalkyl acids in maternal serum and indices of fetal growth: the Aarhus Birth Cohort. Environ Health Perspect 124(6):848–854
62. Darrow LA, Stein CR, Steenland K (2013) Serum perfluorooctanoic acid and perfluorooctane sulfonate concentrations in relation to birth outcomes in the Mid-Ohio Valley, 2005–2010. Environ Health Perspect 121(10):1207–1213
63. Bjerregaard-Olesen C et al (2019) Associations of fetal growth outcomes with measures of the combined xenoestrogenic activity of maternal serum perfluorinated alkyl acids in Danish pregnant women. Environ Health Perspect 127(1):17006
64. Bach CC et al (2015) Perfluoroalkyl acids and time to pregnancy revisited: An update from the Danish National Birth Cohort. Environ Health 14:59
65. Adal A, Wiener S, Louden M. Heavy metal toxicity: back ground, pathophysiology, epidemiology [cited 2018 February 14]. Available from: https://emedicine.medscape.com/article/814960-overview#a5
66. Jaishankar M et al (2014) Toxicity, mechanism and health effects of some heavy metals. Interdiscip Toxicol 7(2):60–72
67. Tchounwou PB et al (2012) Heavy metal toxicity and the environment. Exp Suppl 101:133–164
68. Gavidia T et al (2011) Children's environmental health – from knowledge to action. Lancet 377(9772):1134–1136
69. WHO (2010) World Health Organization: Action is needed on chemicals of major public health concern. World Health Organization, Geneva. http://www.who.int/ipcs/features/10chemicals_en.pdf
70. WHO (2011) World Health Organization: adverse health effects of heavy metals in children. Children's Health and the Environment WHO Training Package for the Health Sector World Health Organization, pp 1–77. https://www.who.int/ce
71. Boucher O et al (2014) Domain-specific effects of prenatal exposure to PCBs, mercury, and lead on infant cognition: results from the Environmental Contaminants and Child Development Study in Nunavik. Environ Health Perspect 122(3):310–316
72. Knudsen AS et al (2018) Persistent organic pollutants and haematological markers in Greenlandic pregnant women: the ACCEPT sub-study. Int J Circumpolar Health 77(1):1456303
73. Luo Y et al (2017) Maternal blood cadmium, lead and arsenic levels, nutrient combinations, and offspring birthweight. BMC Public Health 17(1):354
74. Vrijheid M et al (2016) Environmental pollutants and child health-A review of recent concerns. Int J Hyg Environ Health 219(4–5):331–342
75. Veyhe AS et al (2015) The Northern Norway Mother-and-Child Contaminant Cohort (MISA) Study: PCA analyses of environmental contaminants in maternal sera and dietary intake in early pregnancy. Int J Hyg Environ Health 218(2):254–264
76. Caserta D et al (2013) Heavy metals and placental fetal-maternal barrier: a mini-review on the major concerns. Eur Rev Med Pharmacol Sci 17(16):2198–2206
77. Odland JO, Nieboer E (2012) Human biomonitoring in the Arctic. Special challenges in a sparsely populated area. Int J Hyg Environ Health 215(2):159–167
78. Zietz BP et al (2008) Long-term biomonitoring of polychlorinated biphenyls and organochlorine pesticides in human milk from mothers living in northern Germany. Int J Hyg Environ Health 211(5–6):624–638

79. Bank-Nielsen PI, Long M, Bonefeld-Jorgensen EC (2019) Pregnant Inuit women's exposure to metals and association with fetal growth outcomes: ACCEPT 2010–2015. Int J Environ Res Public Health 16(7):1171
80. Berkowitz Z et al (2006) Lead exposure and birth outcomes in five communities in Shoshone County, Idaho. Int J Hyg Environ Health 209(2):123–132
81. Brocato J, Costa M (2015) 10th NTES conference: Nickel and arsenic compounds Alter the epigenome of peripheral blood mononuclear cells. J Trace Elem Med Biol 31:209–213
82. McDermott S et al (2015) Systematic review of chromium and nickel exposure during pregnancy and impact on child outcomes. J Toxicol Environ Health A 78(21–22):1348–1368
83. Zhang Y et al (2015) Toxicity of nickel ions and comprehensive analysis of nickel ion-associated gene expression profiles in THP-1 cells. Mol Med Rep 12(3):3273–3278
84. Kim JH, Scialli AR (2011) Thalidomide: the tragedy of birth defects and the effective treatment of disease. Toxicol Sci 122(1):1–6
85. Swan SH (2000) Intrauterine exposure to diethylstilbestrol: long-term effects in humans. APMIS 108(12):793–804
86. Hoover RN et al (2011) Adverse health outcomes in women exposed in utero to diethylstilbestrol. N Engl J Med 365(14):1304–1314
87. Braun JM, Gray K (2017) Challenges to studying the health effects of early life environmental chemical exposures on children's health. PLoS Biol 15(12):e2002800
88. Abdallah MW et al (2012) Infections during pregnancy and after birth, and the risk of autism spectrum disorders: a register-based study utilizing a Danish historic birth cohort. Turk Psikiyatri Derg 23(4):229–235
89. Abdallah MW et al (2012) Neonatal levels of cytokines and risk of autism spectrum disorders: an exploratory register-based historic birth cohort study utilizing the Danish Newborn Screening Biobank. J Neuroimmunol 252(1–2):75–82
90. Abdallah MW et al (2013) Neonatal chemokine levels and risk of autism spectrum disorders: findings from a Danish historic birth cohort follow-up study. Cytokine 61(2):370–376
91. Jusko TA et al (2016) A birth cohort study of maternal and infant serum PCB-153 and DDE concentrations and responses to infant tuberculosis vaccination. Environ Health Perspect 124 (6):813–821
92. Fair PA et al (2011) Effects of environmentally-relevant levels of perfluorooctane sulfonate on clinical parameters and immunological functions in B6C3F1 mice. J Immunotoxicol 8 (1):17–29
93. Keil DE et al (2008) Gestational exposure to perfluorooctane sulfonate suppresses immune function in B6C3F1 mice. Toxicol Sci 103(1):77–85
94. Peden-Adams MM et al (2008) Suppression of humoral immunity in mice following exposure to perfluorooctane sulfonate. Toxicol Sci 104(1):144–154
95. Qazi MR et al (2010) Dietary exposure to perfluorooctanoate or perfluorooctane sulfonate induces hypertrophy in centrilobular hepatocytes and alters the hepatic immune status in mice. Int Immunopharmacol 10(11):1420–1427
96. Kato K et al (2009) Polyfluoroalkyl compounds in pooled sera from children participating in the National Health and Nutrition Examination Survey 2001-2002. Environ Sci Technol 43 (7):2641–2647
97. Veras MM et al (2017) Before the first breath: prenatal exposures to air pollution and lung development. Cell Tissue Res 367(3):445–455
98. Hansen S et al (2013) Maternal concentrations of persistent organochlorine pollutants and the risk of asthma in offspring: results from a prospective cohort with 20 years of follow-up. Environ Health Perspect 122(1):93–99
99. Silvers KM et al (2012) Breastfeeding protects against current asthma up to 6 years of age. J Pediatr **160**(6):991–996. e1
100. Deutch B et al (2003) Smoking as a determinant of high organochlorine levels in Greenland. Arch Environ Health 58(1):30–36

101. Haugaard Rasmussen IM, Bonefeld-Jorgensen EC, Long M (2019) Greenlandic women s lifestyle and diet during pregnancy and child risk for asthma, eczema and allergy: an ACCEPT-substudy. Int J Circumpolar Health **78**(1):1682421
102. Berghuis SA et al (2015) Developmental neurotoxicity of persistent organic pollutants: an update on childhood outcome. Arch Toxicol 89(5):687–709
103. Neugebauer J et al (2015) The influence of low level pre- and perinatal exposure to PCDD/Fs, PCBs, and lead on attention performance and attention-related behavior among German school-aged children: results from the Duisburg Birth Cohort Study. Int J Hyg Environ Health 218(1):153–162
104. Polanska K, Jurewicz J, Hanke W (2013) Review of current evidence on the impact of pesticides, polychlorinated biphenyls and selected metals on attention deficit/hyperactivity disorder in children. Int J Occup Med Environ Health 26(1):16–38
105. Newman J et al (2009) Analysis of PCB congeners related to cognitive functioning in adolescents. Neurotoxicology 30(4):686–696
106. Chen YC, Guo YL, Hsu CC (1992) Cognitive development of children prenatally exposed to polychlorinated biphenyls (Yu-Cheng children) and their siblings. J Formos Med Assoc 91 (7):704–707
107. Lai TJ et al (2002) A cohort study of behavioral problems and intelligence in children with high prenatal polychlorinated biphenyl exposure. Arch Gen Psychiatry 59(11):1061–1066
108. Lee DH, Jacobs DR, Porta M (2007) Association of serum concentrations of persistent organic pollutants with the prevalence of learning disability and attention deficit disorder. J Epidemiol Community Health 61(7):591–596
109. Newman J et al (2014) PCBs and ADHD in Mohawk adolescents. Neurotoxicol Teratol 42:25–34
110. Strom M et al (2014) Persistent organic pollutants measured in maternal serum and offspring neurodevelopmental outcomes – a prospective study with long-term follow-up. Environ Int 68:41–48
111. Orenstein ST et al (2014) Prenatal organochlorine and methylmercury exposure and memory and learning in school-age children in communities near the New Bedford Harbor Superfund site, Massachusetts. Environ Health Perspect 122(11):1253–1259
112. Zhang H et al (2017) Prenatal PBDE and PCB exposures and reading, cognition, and externalizing behavior in children. Environ Health Perspect 125(4):746–752
113. Kicinski M et al (2012) Neurobehavioral function and low-level exposure to brominated flame retardants in adolescents: a cross-sectional study. Environ Health 11:86
114. Sagiv SK et al (2010) Prenatal organochlorine exposure and behaviors associated with attention deficit hyperactivity disorder in school-aged children. Am J Epidemiol 171 (5):593–601
115. Gaspar FW et al (2015) Prenatal DDT and DDE exposure and child IQ in the CHAMACOS cohort. Environ Int 85:206–212
116. Berghuis SA et al (2018) Prenatal exposure to persistent organic pollutants and cognition and motor performance in adolescence. Environ Int 121(Pt 1):13–22
117. Wang Y et al (2014) Association between maternal serum perfluoroalkyl substances during pregnancy and maternal and cord thyroid hormones: Taiwan maternal and infant cohort study. Environ Health Perspect 122(5):529–534
118. Wang Y et al (2013) Association between perfluoroalkyl substances and thyroid stimulating hormone among pregnant women: a cross-sectional study. Environ Health 12(1):76
119. Webster GM et al (2014) Associations between perfluoroalkyl acids (PFASs) and maternal thyroid hormones in early pregnancy: a population-based cohort study. Environ Res 133:338–347
120. Ballesteros V et al (2017) Exposure to perfluoroalkyl substances and thyroid function in pregnant women and children: a systematic review of epidemiologic studies. Environ Int 99:15–28

121. Lazarus JH (1999) Thyroid hormone and intellectual development: a clinician's view. Thyroid 9(7):659–660
122. Hong T, Paneth N (2008) Maternal and infant thyroid disorders and cerebral palsy. Semin Perinatol 32(6):438–445
123. Modesto T et al (2015) Maternal mild thyroid hormone insufficiency in early pregnancy and attention-deficit/hyperactivity disorder symptoms in children. JAMA Pediatr 169(9):838–845
124. Oppenheimer JH, Schwartz HL (1997) Molecular basis of thyroid hormone-dependent brain development. Endocr Rev 18(4):462–475
125. Andersen SL et al (2014) Attention deficit hyperactivity disorder and autism spectrum disorder in children born to mothers with thyroid dysfunction: a Danish nationwide cohort study. BJOG 121(11):1365–1374
126. Andersen SL et al (2018) Maternal thyroid function in early pregnancy and neuropsychological performance of the child at 5 years of age. J Clin Endocrinol Metab 103(2):660–670
127. Haddow JE et al (1999) Maternal thyroid deficiency during pregnancy and subsequent neuropsychological development of the child. N Engl J Med 341(8):549–555
128. Inoue K et al (2019) Perfluoroalkyl substances and maternal thyroid hormones in early pregnancy; findings in the Danish national birth cohort. Environ Health Perspect 127 (11):117002
129. Liew Z et al (2018) Prenatal exposure to perfluoroalkyl substances and IQ scores at age 5; A Study in the Danish National Birth Cohort. Environ Health Perspect 126(6):067004
130. Bonefeld-Jorgensen EC, Grunfeld HT, Gjermandsen IM (2005) Effect of pesticides on estrogen receptor transactivation in vitro: a comparison of stable transfected MVLN and transient transfected MCF-7 cells. Mol Cell Endocrinol 244(1–2):20–30
131. Grunfeld HT, Bonefeld-Jorgensen EC (2004) Effect of in vitro estrogenic pesticides on human oestrogen receptor alpha and beta mRNA levels. Toxicol Lett 151(3):467–480
132. Hofmeister MV, Bonefeld-Jorgensen EC (2004) Effects of the pesticides prochloraz and methiocarb on human estrogen receptor alpha and beta mRNA levels analyzed by on-line RT-PCR. Toxicol in Vitro 18(4):427–433
133. Sumbayev VV et al (2005) A novel pesticide-induced conformational state of the oestrogen receptor ligand-binding domain, detected by conformation-specific peptide binding. FEBS Lett 579(2):541–548
134. Kjeldsen LS, Ghisari M, Bonefeld-Jorgensen EC (2013) Currently used pesticides and their mixtures affect the function of sex hormone receptors and aromatase enzyme activity. Toxicol Appl Pharmacol 272:453
135. Andersen HR et al (2006) Estrogenic effects in vitro and in vivo of the fungicide fenarimol. Toxicol Lett 163(2):142–152
136. Long M et al (2003) Effects of currently used pesticides in the AhR-CALUX assay: comparison between the human TV101L and the rat H4IIE cell line. Toxicology 194(1–2):77–93
137. Vinggaard AM et al (2002) Antiandrogenic effects in vitro and in vivo of the fungicide prochloraz. Toxicol Sci 69(2):344–353
138. Vinggaard AM et al (2006) Prochloraz: an imidazole fungicide with multiple mechanisms of action. Int J Androl 29(1):186–192
139. Taxvig C et al (2013) In vitro-in vivo correlations for endocrine activity of a mixture of currently used pesticides. Toxicol Appl Pharmacol 272(3):757–766
140. Pocar P et al (2005) Molecular interactions of the aryl hydrocarbon receptor and its biological and toxicological relevance for reproduction. Reproduction 129(4):379–389
141. Baba T et al (2005) Intrinsic function of the aryl hydrocarbon (dioxin) receptor as a key factor in female reproduction. Mol Cell Biol 25(22):10040–10051
142. Ghisari M et al (2015) Effects of currently used pesticides and their mixtures on the function of thyroid hormone and aryl hydrocarbon receptor in cell culture. Toxicol Appl Pharmacol 284 (3):292–303
143. Ghisari M, Bonefeld-Jorgensen EC (2005) Impact of environmental chemicals on the thyroid hormone function in pituitary rat GH3 cells. Mol Cell Endocrinol 244(1–2):31–41

144. Bonefeld-Jorgensen EC et al (2007) Endocrine-disrupting potential of bisphenol A, bisphenol A dimethacrylate, 4-n-nonylphenol, and 4-n-octylphenol in vitro: new data and a brief review. Environ Health Perspect 115(Suppl 1):69–76
145. Kruger T, Long M, Bonefeld-Jorgensen EC (2008) Plastic components affect the activation of the aryl hydrocarbon and the androgen receptor. Toxicology 246(2–3):112–123
146. Ghisari M, Bonefeld-Jorgensen EC (2009) Effects of plasticizers and their mixtures on estrogen receptor and thyroid hormone functions. Toxicol Lett 189(1):67–77
147. Hjelmborg PS, Andreassen TK, Bonefeld-Jorgensen EC (2008) Cellular uptake of lipoproteins and persistent organic compounds – an update and new data. Environ Res 108(2):192–198
148. Bonefeld-Jorgensen EC et al (2001) Effect of highly bioaccumulated polychlorinated biphenyl congeners on estrogen and androgen receptor activity. Toxicology 158(3):141–153
149. Dingemans MM et al (2007) Neonatal exposure to brominated flame retardant BDE-47 reduces long-term potentiation and postsynaptic protein levels in mouse hippocampus. Environ Health Perspect 115(6):865–870
150. Llansola M et al (2007) Prenatal exposure to polybrominated diphenylether 99 enhances the function of the glutamate-nitric oxide-cGMP pathway in brain in vivo and in cultured neurons. Eur J Neurosci 25(2):373–379
151. Dingemans MM, van den Berg M, Westerink RH (2011) Neurotoxicity of brominated flame retardants: (in)direct effects of parent and hydroxylated polybrominated diphenyl ethers on the (developing) nervous system. Environ Health Perspect 119(7):900–907
152. Kjeldsen LS, Bonefeld-Jorgensen EC (2013) Perfluorinated compounds affect the function of sex hormone receptors. Environ Sci Pollut Res Int 20:8031
153. Long M, Ghisari M, Bonefeld-Jorgensen EC (2013) Effects of perfluoroalkyl acids on the function of the thyroid hormone and the aryl hydrocarbon receptor. Environ Sci Pollut Res Int 20:8045
154. Wielsoe M et al (2015) Perfluoroalkylated substances (PFAS) affect oxidative stress biomarkers in vitro. Chemosphere 129:239–245
155. Taxvig C et al (2010) Effects of nutrition relevant mixtures of phytoestrogens on steroidogenesis, aromatase, estrogen, and androgen activity. Nutr Cancer 62(1):122–131
156. Long M et al (2012) Effects of selected phytoestrogens and their mixtures on the function of the thyroid hormone and the aryl hydrocarbon receptor. Nutr Cancer 64(7):1008–1019
157. Ma D et al (2019) Aryl hydrocarbon receptor activity of polyhalogenated carbazoles and the molecular mechanism. Sci Total Environ 687:516–526
158. Bjerregaard-Olesen C et al (2016) Estrone sulfate and dehydroepiandrosterone sulfate: transactivation of the estrogen and androgen receptor. Steroids 105:50–58
159. Hjelmborg PS, Ghisari M, Bonefeld-Jorgensen EC (2006) SPE-HPLC purification of endocrine-disrupting compounds from human serum for assessment of xenoestrogenic activity. Anal Bioanal Chem 385(5):875–887
160. Bjerregaard-Olesen C et al (2015) Extraction of perfluorinated alkyl acids from human serum for determination of the combined xenoestrogenic transactivity: a method development. Chemosphere 129:232–238
161. Bjerregaard-Olesen C, Bonefeld-Jørgensen E (2015) Receptor research on xenohormone effects of human serum extracts containing the actual mixture of perfluorinated alkyl acids: a short review. Receptor Clin Invest 2:e702
162. Kruger T et al (2008) Xenohormone transactivities are inversely associated to serum POPs in Inuit. Environ Health 7:38
163. Long M, Deutch B, Bonefeld-Jorgensen EC (2007) AhR transcriptional activity in serum of Inuits across Greenlandic districts. Environ Health 6:32
164. Kruger T et al (2012) The combined effect of persistent organic pollutants in the serum POP mixture in Greenlandic Inuit: xenoestrogenic, xenoandrogenic and dioxin-like transactivities. Biomarkers 17(8):692–705

165. Bjerregaard-Olesen C, Ghisari M, Bonefeld-Jorgensen EC (2016) Activation of the estrogen receptor by human serum extracts containing mixtures of perfluorinated alkyl acids from pregnant women. Environ Res 151:71–79
166. Morck TA et al (2014) PCB concentrations and dioxin-like activity in blood samples from Danish school children and their mothers living in urban and rural areas. Basic Clin Pharmacol Toxicol 115(1):134–144
167. Halldorsson TI et al (2009) Dioxin-like activity in plasma among Danish pregnant women: dietary predictors, birth weight and infant development. Environ Res 109(1):22–28
168. Konishi K et al (2009) Prenatal exposure to PCDDs/PCDFs and dioxin-like PCBs in relation to birth weight. Environ Res 109(7):906–913
169. Vafeiadi M et al (2014) In utero exposure to compounds with dioxin-like activity and birth outcomes. Epidemiology 25(2):215–224
170. Bill BR, Geschwind DH (2009) Genetic advances in autism: heterogeneity and convergence on shared pathways. Curr Opin Genet Dev 19(3):271–278
171. Gardener H, Spiegelman D, Buka SL (2011) Perinatal and neonatal risk factors for autism: a comprehensive meta-analysis. Pediatrics 128(2):344–355
172. Hallmayer J et al (2011) Genetic heritability and shared environmental factors among twin pairs with autism. Arch Gen Psychiatry 68(11):1095–1102
173. Windham GC et al (2006) Autism spectrum disorders in relation to distribution of hazardous air pollutants in the San Francisco bay area. Environ Health Perspect 114(9):1438–1444
174. Tordjman S et al (2014) Gene x environment interactions in autism spectrum disorders: role of epigenetic mechanisms. Front Psychiatry 5:53
175. Beversdorf DQ, Stevens HE, Jones KL (2018) Prenatal stress, maternal immune dysregulation, and their association with autism spectrum disorders. Curr Psychiatry Rep 20(9):76
176. Long M et al (2019) Autism spectrum disorders, endocrine disrupting compounds, and heavy metals in amniotic fluid: a case-control study. Mol Autism 10:1

Early-Life Environmental Toxic Influences on Neural Development

Gro D. Villanger, Johan Øvrevik, Heidi Aase, and Oddvar Myhre

1 Background

Exposure to environmental toxicants has gradually become a growing concern. We are daily exposed to multiple chemicals through several ways, such as inhalation, diet, and dermal contact. Environmental pollution is reported to cause 9 million annual deaths worldwide, 3 times more than the combined number of deaths from AIDS, malaria, and tuberculosis and 15 times more than from all wars and other forms of violence [1]. Pollution is among the top risk factors for noncommunicable diseases (NCDs), even in high-income countries. The likelihood of being exposed to pollution is affected by socioeconomic status with low-income neighborhoods and countries taking its heaviest toll [1–3]. Pollution was responsible for 940,000 deaths in 2016 among children, two-thirds of whom were under 5 years old. Exposure to environmental pollution is related to multiple NCDs in children such as neurodevelopmental disorders which are on the increase [4].

The Developmental Origins of Health and Disease (DOHaD) paradigm (evolved from the Barker's hypothesis [5]) posits that there are windows during development, in particular related to cell differentiation and tissue formation, of particular sensitivity toward environmental factors such as nutrients, environmental toxicants,

G. D. Villanger · H. Aase
Department of Child Health and Development, Norwegian Institute of Public Health, Oslo, Norway

J. Øvrevik
Section of Air Pollution and Noise, Norwegian Institute of Public Health, Oslo, Norway

Department of Biosciences, University of Oslo, Oslo, Norway

O. Myhre (✉)
Section of Toxicology and Risk Assessment, Norwegian Institute of Public Health, Oslo, Norway
e-mail: Oddvar.Myhre@fhi.no

Y. Xia (ed.), *Early-life Environmental Exposure and Disease*,
https://doi.org/10.1007/978-981-15-3797-4_8

drugs, and other stressors. These sensitive windows are primarily related to the in utero period and first years of postnatal life, but may also encompass exposure of parents prior to conception and for some outcomes extend into puberty. As such, the DOHaD paradigm suggests that research and prevention strategies should focus more on these early developmental stages of life [6, 7].

In line with the DOHaD paradigm, there has been an increase in the prevalence of learning disabilities, attention deficit hyperactivity disorder (ADHD), and autism spectrum disorders (ASD) in children over the last decades [8, 9]. Early-life (pre- and early postnatal) exposure to environmental pollution (toxicants and air pollution) has been linked to neuropsychological disorders and may also adversely affect the development of motor, cognitive, and behavioral functions.

Despite decades of research, only 12 of the more than 10,000 chemicals present on the market today have been verified to cause adverse neurodevelopment in humans, whereas 218 chemicals are identified as neurotoxic [10, 11]. A concern for the newborn child is that human breast milk contains chemicals regulated as pesticides, cosmetics, and persistent organic pollutants (POPs) [12]. This clearly illustrates that the present knowledge on environmental toxicants as potential causative factors for adverse neurodevelopment is inadequate. The aim of this chapter is to summarize existing knowledge on the influence of environmental toxicants on adverse neurodevelopment, mainly focusing on knowledge gaps and how to combine recent developments in different research areas to prevent adverse health outcomes.

2 Neurodevelopmental and Neurological Disorders in Children

Neurodevelopmental and neurological disorders (NDDs) are frequent causes of long-term disability in children. *Attention deficit hyperactivity disorder (ADHD)*, which is the most common, affects 5% of children all around the world [13]. The disorder's characteristics are inattention, hyperactivity, and impulsivity, with common additional dysfunctions like compromised motor skills and cognitive functions [13]. *Autism spectrum disorders (ASD)* constitute a heterogeneous group of disorders characterized by persistent deficits in social communication and social interaction, as well as restricted, repetitive patterns of interests, behavior, or activities [14]. Children with ASD display a large scale of cognitive skills, from high intelligence to severe intellectual disability [15]. Recent studies from the Nordic countries have found the current ASD prevalence in children to be just over 1% [16, 17]. *Epilepsy*, the most common serious neurological disorder in childhood, is characterized by an enduring predisposition to generate epileptic seizures in the brain [18]. The overall prevalence of childhood epilepsy is 0.5–1% [19]. Children with epilepsy often have other cognitive, behavioral, and emotional problems, and they are at increased risk of comorbid NNDs such as ASD and ADHD [20]. *Cerebral palsy*

(CP) is a disorder of movement and posture due to a permanent, nonprogressive insult to the developing fetal or infant brain [21]. CP has a prevalence of 0.15–0.35% and is the most common cause of childhood physical disability [22]. Children with CP often have learning and language difficulties, hearing and vision impairments, and epilepsy [18]. The etiologies of these various disorders are multifactorial as well as complex. Genetic predisposition is a major determinant of risk, but heritability is not 100%, and genetic factors are likely to interact with environmental and psychosocial and socioeconomic factors [23–28]. Since the 1980s, the incidence of diagnosed ADHD and ASD has increased rapidly in developed countries, and this increase has led to concerns that environmental toxicants may be one of the causes [11, 29–31].

There are considerable comorbidities among NDDs [32] as well as several phenotypic similarities such as problems with language and communication, cognitive functions, social interaction, motor skills, attention, affect, and sleep. Together with shared genetic and environmental risk factors, there could be overlapping similarities in the multifactorial etiologies of NDDs and related behavioral problems or cognitive deficits. The NDDs can be viewed as the extreme end of a continuum of neurodevelopmental phenotypes involving interaction between genetic and environmental risk and protective factors acting on the developmental trajectories – from neurotypical to aberrant neurodevelopment, where the latter can result in adaptive or maladaptive outcomes (e.g., cognitive deficits, NDDs) in the child. This complex and interdisciplinary interpretation is conceptualized in developmental psychopathology as the reflection of the probabilistic, bidirectional, and transactional nature of genetic, neurobiological, social, psychological, and pre- and postnatal environmental influences in the course of life [33]. This also means that there is not just one single pathway to a given outcome or disorder, but also that similar pathways may lead to different outcomes [33], thus establishing the causality of early exposure to toxicants in the environment as risk factors for adverse neurodevelopment in later childhood, and thus susceptibility for a specific disorder need studies that investigate general and differential effects. It also questions the use of standard animal models in chemical testing to predict potential human developmental neurotoxicity.

3 Adverse Neurodevelopment and Environmental Toxicants

The developing brain seems particularly sensitive to toxic insults [9, 34], because of the numerous precisely timed and complex processes that occur during fetal and postnatal growth. Additionally, the fetus has a limited ability to detoxify and eliminate contaminants, as well as an immature blood-brain barrier, together conferring little protection from the effects of toxic chemicals [29, 35]. From animal studies, we acknowledge that during critical periods of brain development, even low exposures that would have little to no negative effect in adults can cause permanent disruptions in brain development and maturation [29, 36], potentially leading to adverse effects on functioning in the offspring. Epidemiological studies report that various toxic metals or POPs are present in maternal blood, cord blood, placenta as well as in breast milk, and in child's blood [37–41]. Toxicants may reach the growing nervous system of the fetus because of the absence of a fully formed blood-brain barrier [42, 43]. Therefore, vulnerability of the growing nervous system raises concern regarding the impact of environmental toxicants on brain development and their potential contribution to the recently observed higher prevalence of neurodevelopmental disorders (NDDs).

Human exposure to toxic metals is a global challenge, and the World Health Organization (WHO) ranks these among the priority metals that are of great public health concerns [44]. Mercury (Hg), arsenic (As), and lead (Pb) are examples of metals that may seriously harm the unborn child.

Pb is a toxic metal where extensive use has resulted in health problems in various parts of the world. Children are especially vulnerable to the neurotoxic effects of Pb and even relatively low levels of exposure can lead to acute and irreversible neurotoxicity [45, 46]. For instance, it has been shown that early-life Pb exposure leads to changes in brain volume [47]. Subtle negative effects on IQ can be expected when blood lead levels rise as a result of daily life exposure in polluted areas, and the effects aggravate with increasing levels of lead in blood [45]. A previous review concluded that there are no indications of a threshold for key adverse effects (including adverse neurodevelopment) of lead [48]. Lead exposure has also been linked epidemiologically to attention deficit disorder and aggression, in addition to cognitive deficits [49]. Experimental data have illustrated mechanistic relationships between exposure to Pb and inhibition of the brain NMDA receptor (molecular initiating event) leading, through a cascade of key events, to disability of learning and memory in children (AOP-Wiki; https://aopwiki.org/wiki/index.php/Aop:13). Due to its intrinsic toxic properties, it is urgent that we take action to reduce the use and releases of Pb in order to lower exposures, especially for children and women of childbearing age.

Arsenic exposure is another major health concern, specifically during early-life exposure where the developing brain is a susceptible target. Intake of inorganic arsenic over a long period can lead to chronic arsenic poisoning (arsenicosis). Organic As compounds, which are abundant in seafood, have less adverse effects on health, and are rapidly eliminated by the body. Human exposure to elevated levels of inorganic As occurs mainly through the consumption of groundwater containing naturally high levels of inorganic As and food prepared and food crops irrigated with this water. In one estimate, As-contaminated drinking water in Bangladesh alone was attributed 9100 deaths and 125,000 disability-adjusted life years (DALYs) in 2001 [44]. As is reported to pass the placenta as well as the blood-brain barrier, and its lipophilic nature implies lactational transfer to offspring [41]. Although some studies show a relationship between As exposure and neurodevelopmental outcomes, a systematic review reports that the overall evidence does not consistently support a causal dose-response relationship at low doses [50]. A more recent review concluded that an increased risk for neurotoxic effects due to As, Pb, and Hg exposure among breastfed infants in most regions of the world cannot be excluded [41]. Therefore, more data on relevant effect biomarkers of As exposure and developmental neurotoxicity data are needed to improve human risk assessment of pre- and postnatal exposure.

The central nervous system is the primary target of methyl mercury (MeHg) in neonates, children, adolescents, and adults [51]. The brain has high affinity for MeHg, with its concentrations 3–6 times higher than in blood [52]. MeHg can cross the blood-brain barrier via the neutral amino acid transport system L as a complex with L-cysteine [53] and finally distribute to all brain areas, exposing the fetus during critical windows of development. In the brain, Hg can affect critical neurodevelopmental processes like cell proliferation, migration, differentiation, synaptogenesis, myelination, as well as apoptosis [54, 55]. Mild or severe mental retardation, decreased IQ, in addition to impaired movements, visuospatial perception, and speech have been reported in children exposed to MeHg [56–58]. Exposure of MeHg is mainly via seafood. Thus, dietary advice, particularly to pregnant women, should balance information of the positive nutritional health benefits from eating seafood versus potential health-damaging effects of co-exposure to MeHg and other toxicants (e.g. POPs).

Although exposure levels of toxic metals in the general population are generally low, safe threshold levels of exposure during fetal brain development are yet to be determined [11, 29]. Growing evidence of neurotoxicity and other health effects demands further research in the area of cumulative risk assessment of these metals.

Halogenated POPs are of concern to human health and wildlife because of their potential toxicity. Many of them are structurally closely connected and share common characteristics, most notably their ubiquitous distribution in the environment and their potential ability for bioaccumulation in living organisms. This has led to some POPs being banned from production via the Stockholm Convention or regulated through REACH (Registration, Evaluation, Authorisation and Restriction of Chemicals), but a huge number of compounds are not even tested for toxic properties. As such, POPs continue to be of considerable human and environmental concern. In children prenatally exposed to organochlorine compounds including pesticides, adverse neurodevelopmental effects like delayed neurodevelopment, memory loss, poorer verbal ability, behavioral impairment, lowered IQ, inattention, and hyperactivity are reported [59–68]. Cohort studies show that children prenatally exposed to different brominated diphenyl ethers (BDEs) were more at risk of suffering from symptoms of attention deficit disorders, poorer social competence, lower intelligence [69–71]. This is supported by animal studies, where mice or rats pre- or postnatally exposed to brominated POPs exhibited cognitive deficits, in addition to disturbed attention [72–77]. Perfluorinated alkylated substances (PFASs) are among the most prominent pollutant groups found in human blood including pregnant women, and the intake of fish and shellfish are the major determinants of blood levels [78, 79]. Some studies indicate health effects in the child from prenatal exposure to PFASs [80–84]. Several animal and human studies indicate that PFASs act as thyroid-disrupting chemicals [84–88], and they are suspected developmental neurotoxicants based on behavioral effects in animal studies [89]. However, the epidemiological data are scarce and the results are inconclusive [11, 89, 90]. For example, a recent Danish study reported increased risk of cerebral palsy (CP) in girls with elevated maternal PFAS levels [91], but similar findings were not reported for ASD and ADHD [92].

In contrast to persistent toxicants with long biological half-lives and biomagnifying properties, exposure levels for non-persistent toxicants with a short half-life (e.g. phthalates) often vary in a single day or between days for an individual. Phthalates are high production volume chemicals, found in a wide array of consumer products, and there is also substantial dietary exposure [93]. Women have higher phthalate concentrations than men [94]. Increasing evidence points to associations with reproductive toxicity/function [93], hormone regulation [95–97], and neurodevelopment [98–104]. In a recent study of prenatal phthalate exposure, a 47% increase in risk of ADHD diagnoses associated with every 1-log unit increase in $\sum$DEHP exposure [105] was reported, demonstrating associations with a clinically diagnosed developmental disability. Although some phthalates have been regulated in consumer products in the United States, European Union, and other countries [106, 107], there are few regulations that apply to products used by the general population (all existing US regulations pertain to childcare products). Therefore, efforts should be made to exclude phthalate exposure during pregnancy as a precautionary act to protect the unborn child.

Particulate matter (PM) air pollution is the main urban-related environmental problem and a significant contributor to the global burden of disease based on its cardiovascular effects [108]. However, due to the inadequacy of the available evidence, the potential influence of air pollution on brain development (and cognitive decline) has not been considered when estimating the burden associated with air pollution [109]. Still, some studies of children provide support for the importance of PM exposure during the prenatal period. Examples are children in New York, who showed structural brain alterations after exposure to high air pollution levels in the womb, while postnatal exposure was little related to structural alterations [110]. Similar findings are also reported from Mexico City [111]. Air pollution has also been linked to ADHD and ASD; however, recent reviews report that the epidemiological evidence of the influence of air pollution on NDDs is still inadequate [109, 112], and mechanistic data are needed to support causalities.

4 Adverse Neurodevelopment: Genes or Environment?

4.1 Susceptibilities

There are many critical stages during prenatal, neonatal, and early childhood where perturbations and deviation from normal brain development can occur. Neurotoxicants can have particular negative effects on neurodevelopment during the sensitive developmental windows, especially at fetal and newborn stages, and even within these periods, there are specific developmental events (windows) of

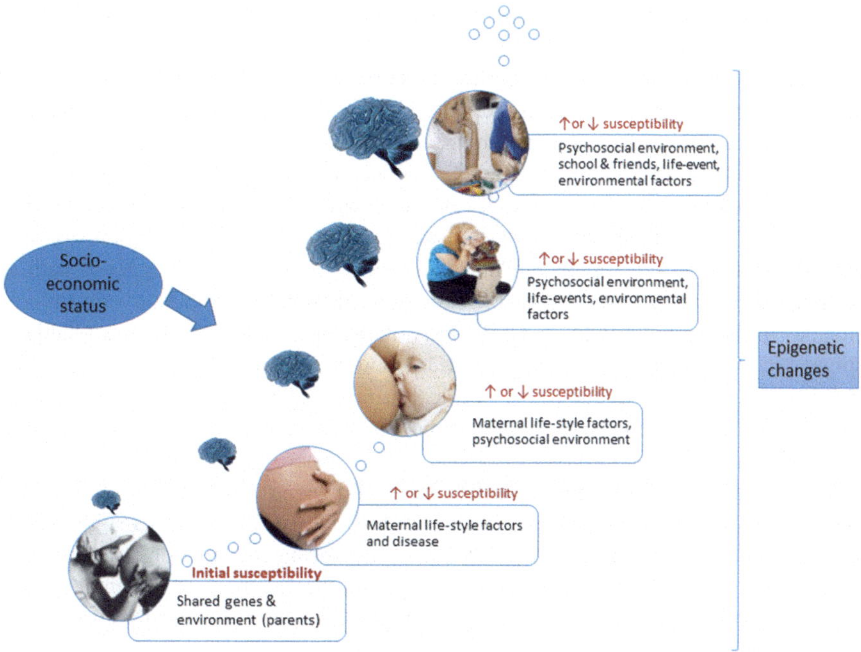

Fig. 1 Accumulated susceptibility for adverse neurodevelopment

heightened sensitivity to specific neurotoxicants [9]. Identification of the true risk or susceptibility of environmental toxicants for child adverse behavioral phenotypes and NDDs will ultimately require consideration of interactions between genetic (and epigenetic), environmental, psychosocial, and socioeconomic factors on the developmental trajectory [33]. This can be conceptualized as the accumulated susceptibility of all factors contributing to the developmental trajectory, many of which can be considered as either risk or protective factors depending on the direction of impact (negative or positive), see illustration in Fig. 1.

4.2 *Genetic Susceptibility*

Family, twin, and molecular genetic studies have documented that neurodevelopmental disorders are, to a large extent, of heritable origin [28, 113, 114]. Recent multi-cohort genome-wide association studies (GWAS) and genome-wide DNA methylation studies of particularly ASD and ADHD have identified genetic variations in multiple different gene loci [115]. Additional studies have shown shared genetic risks across psychiatric disorders and in phenotypic characteristics (below "threshold" of clinical diagnosis) [27, 28]. The GWAS have directed most attention from individual genes to genetically and/or environmentally impaired gene regulatory networks and associated alterations in neuronal function during development [115, 116].

Environmental factors (e.g., nutrition, smoking, and toxicants) during early development can influence the epigenome [117–119], and such gene-environment interactions are linked to many human diseases in childhood or later-life stages, such as cancer, asthma, and neuropsychological deficits or NDDs [120, 121]. The effects of environmental factors on neurodevelopment are suggested to be mediated by epigenetic changes in specific neuronal sites [120]. Within environmental toxicology, the importance of epigenetic mechanisms is increasingly recognized with a heightened focus on the ability of endocrine-disruptive compounds to induce changes in the epigenome [117, 122]. DNA methylation is among the most studied epigenetic biomarkers and is an important part of the maintenance of genomic stability [120, 123]. Perinatal life is a critical time for establishing DNA methylation patterns and for susceptibility to environmental factors, and early-life environment might play a role in the etiology of NNDs [123–125] as indicated by recent studies [126–128]. Human and animal studies have shown associations between DNA methylation and environmental toxicants such as POPs, toxic metals, phthalates, and air pollution [119, 122, 129–132]. Thus, measuring methylation patterns may explain how toxicants change gene expression and thus neurodevelopmental events (e.g., neuronal migration) and even phenotypes dependent on the proteins these genes encode.

A possible causal role of perturbed epigenetic and transcriptional processes in ASD has been supported by both human and animal studies [116]. Several recent sequencing studies of families with children with ASD led to the identification of genes conferring risk for the disorder [133–135]. The disturbed transcriptional regulation in ASD may lead to erroneous timing of gene expression during the tightly regulated developmental trajectories of neurons in the developing brain. Data support that the convergence of the varied ASD risk genes onto the same behavioral outcome may reflect the defective timing of neuronal subtype specification and associated circuit formation during prenatal and postnatal brain development. Genetic lesions acting on multiple pathways during the differentiation processes in the fetal brain have an effect on the stability of neuronal networks. Consequently, the social challenges after birth confront a neuronal network with impaired robustness and hence increased susceptibility to activity-driven changes that may lead to the establishment of the disease phenotype [116]. The described scenario views attenuated brain robustness instead of defects in specific genes or cell types, as an underlying mechanism for ASD pathophysiology.

It is tempting to speculate that the diverse genetic susceptibilities as well as environmental factors contributing to NDD risk, i.e. targeting various sets of genes during the critical phase of fetal and early postnatal brain development, may converge to disease phenotype characteristics. Therefore, NDDs can be viewed as a pathological state where slight variations in the input factors drive the severity of the clinical phenotypic manifestations.

Genetic susceptibility and environmental interactions can also be linked to polymorphism in specific genomic areas that code for proteins that are involved in toxicokinetics (i.e., uptake, metabolism, and excretion) of a chemical. For example, polymorphism of the PON1 gene in mother and/or fetus can lead to altered metabolism, resulting in more toxic metabolites. Other examples are polymorphism in enzymes involved in metabolism of As [136] or manganese and genes coding for proteins serving as transporters over cell membranes [137]. In fact, element/metal dysregulation has been proposed as a risk factor for ASD and ADHD [138, 139]. This would ultimately mean that even normal, population level exposures can be associated with increased risk of adverse neurodevelopment or NDDs with the existence of polymorphism of such genes.

4.3 Prenatal Environmental Factors

What are the environmental factors affecting neurodevelopment? These can be all kinds of exposures during pre- and postnatal life. Prenatal factors will often be of biological nature. Maternal lifestyle factors during pregnancy that may affect the fetus include intake of medicines, drugs, alcohol and tobacco, macro- and micronutrients, and BMI, but also diseases and infections, hormonal dysfunction, stress, depression or other psychiatric illnesses, and exposure to toxicants via air, food, drinking water, and skin. Although exposure to neurotoxicants can perturb normal brain development, and thus is a negative risk factor, many environmental factors can also be considered both risk and protective factors, depending on how they influence brain development.

4.4 Psychosocial Factors

During infancy and childhood, brain development will be influenced by a host of psychosocial factors, like parenting style and care, social interaction with other children and adults, but also exposure to maltreatment and traumatic events. Nutrition may also play an important role. These factors act bidirectionally, as brain development is shaped by behavioral and environmental factors and vice versa [140]. In addition, these factors can be either protective, and thus counteract the negative influence of toxicants and genetics, or they can be adding to the accumulated susceptibility (Fig. 1).

4.5 Socioeconomic Position

Socioeconomic position is a principal characteristic of most environmental factors as well as an important determinant of exposure to toxicants. The sociodemographics of sub-populations are related to educational level, work, income, nutritional quality, habitation, housing situation, and more. Negative sociodemographic and environmental factors are known risks to brain development globally, but research linking cognitive and behavioral outcomes with early childhood inequalities – in particular unequal exposures to environmental toxicants (e.g., air pollution, food contaminants, industrial byproducts, etc.) – is just emerging. Socioeconomic status (SES) of the child is most often shared with parents. While most environmental epidemiologic studies tend to incorporate variables reflecting SES, e.g., maternal educational level, by adjusting for SES as a potential confounder, studies now point to SES being a possible effect modifier [141–143]; the toxicant-neurodevelopmental outcome relationships are different in low versus higher SES strata. Fish or seafood intake is among the most important routes of exposure for POPs and metals in human populations; however, the simultaneous dietary intake of nutritional factors (omega-3 fatty acids, iodine, selenium, etc.) is beneficial for brain development and may counterbalance negative effects of environmental toxicants. Fish intake is additionally associated with SES status. To unravel the true impact of toxicants on brain developmental outcomes in children, both SES status and the relationship with maternal/child nutritional quality (especially fish intake) must be characterized.

5 Toxicity Testing

The purpose of toxicity testing is to produce data that can ensure appropriate protection of public health and the environment from negative influence of exposure to environmental agents [144]. As such, there is a clear overlap with the goals of environmental epidemiology, but toxicity testing also enables prediction of toxicity from new chemicals before adverse effects are manifested in the population. Animal studies are both time- and resource-intensive, hampering the possibility of testing complex mixtures, which may require a multitude of combinations of chemicals. In vitro models may be more suited to detect low-dose effects and to elucidate mechanistic pathways after toxicants exposure. The US National Academy of Sciences report *Toxicity Testing in the 21st Century: A Vision and a Strategy* therefore suggested the implementation of a new testing strategy firmly based on human biology by a combination of human cell-based tissue models, advanced analytical methods, and computational systems biology. The report emphasizes the importance of utilizing human exposure and biomonitoring data to identify compounds of interest and setting dose ranges for testing, as well as the need of pharmacokinetic models for extrapolation from in vitro results to human tissue concentrations in vivo and back [144].

6 The Need of an Integrative Approach Unifying Epidemiology and Mechanistic Studies

Casual relations cannot be reduced to biochemical reactions, nor can they be solved by more "fine-grained" statistical associations among macro-variables (external factors). The solution is therefore a unifying framework where epidemiological associations ("difference making") and evidence of the underlying biological mechanisms ("productive causality") are combined to produce causal evidence [145]. However, a systematic procedure to bridge the data as well as the analysis of epidemiology and mechanistic studies (toxicology) in a way that provides a unified view on the adverse causal relationship between exposure and diseases has been lacking [146, 147]. The ultimate aim is that experimental and mechanistic data can give support as well as biological plausibility for the human epidemiological observations and vice versa, and that epidemiological observations can confirm or negate adverse effects predicted from toxicological studies. However, this relies on establishment of mechanistic models that are sufficiently representative (of the human body and its organs/compartments) and suitable for the high-throughput screening required to cope with the large number of environmental exposure factors included in exposome research. Human in vitro neuronal cultures derived from neural progenitor cells are now making this possible, as they are primarily of human origin and expandable [148, 149] (Fig. 2). Neural progenitor cells can be differentiated into different types of postmitotic neurons, astrocytes, and oligodendrocytes. Currently, the differentiation of human-induced pluripotent stem cells (hiPSCs) into microglia-like cells has been achieved by exposure to defined factors and co-culture with astrocytes [150]. It is supposed that mixed neuronal/glial (preferably organotypic, 3D brain organoids) cultures of human origin are the most relevant test systems for the evaluation of human developmental neurotoxicity, as they provide a higher level of functional integration between different neuronal and glial cell types, which is hampered in monolayer cultures. Except the neural progenitor cells from healthy subjects, somatic cells can also be reprogrammed into PSCs from patient biopsies [151, 152]. As a result, this technology allows the delivery of human neurons in vitro derived from patients with, e.g., ASD and ADHD. This may be an attractive technology because it allows to recapitulate in a culture dish precisely those developmental events that are putatively abnormal and thus involved in the pathology of the disorders [153–155]. It is therefore an attractive approach to combine toxicological screening studies of environmental toxicants in hiPSCs from healthy individuals, with targeted mechanistic studies in hiPSCs and brain organoids from patients with NDD diagnosis to reveal possible gene-environment interactions.

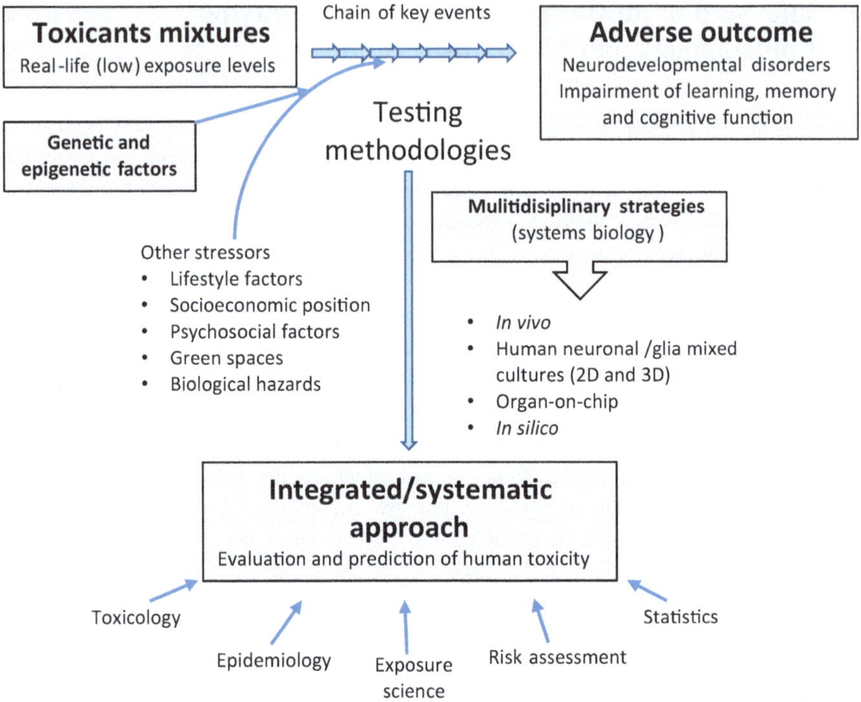

Fig. 2 Suggested approach for hazard assessment of neurodevelopmental adverse health outcomes from long-term exposure to multiple stressors and integration of multiple lines of evidence from toxicity testing. (Modified from [156])

References

1. Landrigan PJ et al (2018) The lancet commission on pollution and health. Lancet 391:462–512
2. Hajat A et al (2013) Air pollution and individual and neighborhood socioeconomic status: evidence from the Multi-Ethnic Study of Atherosclerosis (MESA). Environ Health Perspect 121:1325–1333
3. Said S, Hernandez GT (2015) Environmental exposures, socioeconomics, disparities, and the kidneys. Adv Chronic Kidney Dis 22:39–45
4. Landrigan PJ et al (2019) Pollution and children's health. Sci Total Environ 650:2389–2394
5. Barker DJ (1998) In utero programming of chronic disease. Clin Sci (Lond) 95:115–128
6. Barouki R, Gluckman PD, Grandjean P, Hanson M, Heindel JJ (2012) Developmental origins of non-communicable disease: implications for research and public health. Environ Health 11:42
7. Heindel JJ, Vandenberg LN (2015) Developmental origins of health and disease: a paradigm for understanding disease cause and prevention. Curr Opin Pediatr 27:248–253
8. Bennett D et al (2016) Project TENDR: targeting environmental neuro-developmental risks the TENDR consensus statement. Environ Health Perspect 124:A118–A122
9. Grandjean P, Kishi R, Kogevinas M, International Society for Environmental, E (2017) Prevention of developmental neurotoxicity. Epidemiology 28:157–158

10. Evans RM, Martin OV, Faust M, Kortenkamp A (2016) Should the scope of human mixture risk assessment span legislative/regulatory silos for chemicals? Sci Total Environ 543:757–764
11. Grandjean P, Landrigan PJ (2014) Neurobehavioural effects of developmental toxicity. Lancet Neurol 13:330–338
12. Schlumpf M et al (2010) Exposure patterns of UV filters, fragrances, parabens, phthalates, organochlor pesticides, PBDEs, and PCBs in human milk correlation of UV filters with use of cosmetics. Chemosphere 81:1171–1183
13. Polanczyk G, de Lima MS, Horta BL, Biederman J, Rohde LA (2007) The worldwide prevalence of ADHD: a systematic review and metaregression analysis. Am J Psychiatry 164:942–948
14. American Psychiatric Association (2013) Diagnostic and Statistical Manual of Mental Disorders, 5th edn. American Psychiatric Association, Arlington
15. Johnson CP, Myers SM (2007) Identification and evaluation of children with autism spectrum disorders. Pediatrics 120:1183–1215
16. Idring S et al (2015) Changes in prevalence of autism spectrum disorders in 2001-2011: findings from the Stockholm youth cohort. J Autism Dev Disord 45:1766–1773
17. Hansen SN, Schendel DE, Parner ET (2015) Explaining the increase in the prevalence of autism spectrum disorders: the proportion attributable to changes in reporting practices. JAMA Pediatr 169:56–62
18. Saunders (2004) Nelson textbook of pediatrics, 17th edn
19. Shinnar S, Pellock JM (2002) Update on the epidemiology and prognosis of pediatric epilepsy. J Child Neurol 17:S4–S17
20. Lin JJ, Mula M, Hermann BP (2012) Uncovering the neurobehavioural comorbidities of epilepsy over the lifespan. Lancet 380:1180–1192
21. Baxter P, Morris C, Rosenbaum P, Paneth N, Leviton A, Goldstein M, Bax M, Colver A, Damiano D, Graham HK, Brien GO (2007) The definition and classification of cerebral palsy. Dev Med Child Neurol 49:1–44
22. Nelson KB, Blair E (2015) Prenatal factors in singletons with cerebral palsy born at or near term. N Engl J Med 373:946–953
23. Aguiar A, Eubig PA, Schantz SL (2010) Attention deficit/hyperactivity disorder: a focused overview for children's environmental health researchers. Environ Health Perspect 118:1646–1653
24. Sandin S, Lichtenstein P, Kuja-Halkola R, Larsson H, Hultman CM, Reichenberg A (2014) The familial risk of autism. JAMA 311:1770–1777
25. Guerrini R (2006) Epilepsy in children. Lancet 367:499–524
26. Tollanes MC, Wilcox AJ, Lie RT, Moster D (2014) Familial risk of cerebral palsy: population based cohort study. BMJ 349:g4294
27. Martin J, Taylor MJ, Lichtenstein P (2018) Assessing the evidence for shared genetic risks across psychiatric disorders and traits. Psychol Med 48:1759–1774
28. Anttila V et al (2018) Analysis of shared heritability in common disorders of the brain. Science 360:eaap8757
29. Grandjean P, Landrigan PJ (2006) Developmental neurotoxicity of industrial chemicals. Lancet 368:2167–2178
30. Mendola P, Selevan SG, Gutter S, Rice D (2002) Environmental factors associated with a spectrum of neurodevelopmental deficits. Ment Retard Dev Disabil Res Rev 8:188–197
31. de Cock M, Maas YGH, van de Bor M (2012) Does perinatal exposure to endocrine disruptors induce autism spectrum and attention deficit hyperactivity disorders? Rev Acta Paediatr 101:811–818
32. Suren P et al (2012) Autism spectrum disorder, ADHD, epilepsy, and cerebral palsy in Norwegian children. Pediatrics 130:e152–e158
33. Cicchetti D, Toth SL (2009) The past achievements and future promises of developmental psychopathology: the coming of age of a discipline. J Child Psychol Psychiatry 50:16–25

34. Moog NK et al (2017) Influence of maternal thyroid hormones during gestation on fetal brain development. Neuroscience 342:68–100
35. Ek CJ, Dziegielewska KM, Habgood MD, Saunders NR (2012) Barriers in the developing brain and Neurotoxicology. Neurotoxicology 33:586–604
36. Rice D, Barone S Jr (2000) Critical periods of vulnerability for the developing nervous system: evidence from humans and animal models. Environ Health Perspect 108(Suppl 3):511–533
37. Huang R et al (2019) The human body burden of polychlorinated dibenzo-p-dioxins/furans (PCDD/Fs) and dioxin-like polychlorinated biphenyls (DL-PCBs) in residents' human milk from Guangdong Province, China. Toxicol Res UK 8:552–559
38. Muller MHB et al (2019) Prenatal exposure to persistent organic pollutants in Northern Tanzania and their distribution between breast milk, maternal blood, placenta and cord blood. Environ Res 170:433–442
39. Caspersen IH et al (2016) Determinants of plasma PCB, brominated flame retardants, and organochlorine pesticides in pregnant women and 3 year old children in The Norwegian Mother and Child Cohort Study. Environ Res 146:136–144
40. Lenters V et al (2019) Early-life exposure to persistent organic pollutants (OCPs, PBDEs, PCBs, PFASs) and attention-deficit/hyperactivity disorder: a multi-pollutant analysis of a Norwegian birth cohort. Environ Int 125:33–42
41. Rebelo FM, Caldas ED (2016) Arsenic, lead, mercury and cadmium: Toxicity, levels in breast milk and the risks for breastfed infants. Environ Res 151:671–688
42. Rodier PM (1995) Developing brain as a target of toxicity. Environ Health Perspect 103(Suppl 6):73–76
43. Adinolfi M (1985) The development of the human blood-CSF-brain barrier. Dev Med Child Neurol 27:532–537
44. WHO (2010) Preventing disease through healthy environments. Action is needed on chemicals of major public health concern. https://www.who.int/ipcs/features/10chemicals_en.pdf?ua=1. Accessed 8 Nov 2019
45. Fewtrell L, Kaufman R, Prüss-Üstün A (2003) Lead: assessing the environmental burden of disease at national and local levels, Environmental burden of disease series, No. 2.; http://www.who.int/quantifying_ehimpacts/publications/en/leadebd2.pdf, 2. World Health Organization, Geneva
46. IPCS (1995) Inorganic Lead, Environmental Health Criteria 165.; http://www.inchem.org/documents/ehc/ehc/ehc165.htm. World Health Organization, International Programme on Chemical Safety, Geneva
47. Cecil KM et al (2008) Decreased brain volume in adults with childhood lead exposure. PLoS Med 5:e112
48. FAO/WHO (2010) Summary and conclusions of the seventy-third meeting of the Joint FAO/WHO Expert Committee on Food Additives, Geneva, 8–17 June 2010. Rome, Food and Agriculture Organization of the United Nations; Geneva, World Health Organization (JECFA/73/SC; http://www.who.int/entity/foodsafety/publications/chem/summary73.pdf)
49. IARC (2006) Summaries & evaluations: inorganic and organic lead compounds, IARC monographs for the evaluation of carcinogenic risks to humans, vol 87.; http://www.inchem.org/documents/iarc/vol87/volume87.pdf. International Agency for Research on Cancer, Lyon
50. Tsuji JS, Garry MR, Perez V, Chang ET (2015) Low-level arsenic exposure and developmental neurotoxicity in children: a systematic review and risk assessment. Toxicology 337:91–107
51. dos Santos AA et al (2016) Methylmercury and brain development: a review of recent literature. J Trace Elem Med Biol 38:99–107
52. Syversen T, Kaur P (2012) The toxicology of mercury and its compounds. J Trace Elem Med Biol 26:215–226
53. Aschner M, Clarkson TW (1988) Uptake of methylmercury in the rat brain: effects of amino acids. Brain Res 462:31–39
54. Choi BH, Lapham LW, Amin-Zaki L, Saleem T (1978) Abnormal neuronal migration, deranged cerebral cortical organization, and diffuse white matter astrocytosis of human fetal

brain: a major effect of methylmercury poisoning in utero. J Neuropathol Exp Neurol 37:719–733
55. Choi BH (1986) Methylmercury poisoning of the developing nervous system: I. Pattern of neuronal migration in the cerebral cortex. Neurotoxicology 7:591–600
56. Castoldi AF et al (2008) Human developmental neurotoxicity of methylmercury: impact of variables and risk modifiers. Regul Toxicol Pharmacol 51:201–214
57. Grandjean P et al (1997) Cognitive deficit in 7-year-old children with prenatal exposure to methylmercury. Neurotoxicol Teratol 19:417–428
58. Harada M (1995) Minamata disease: methylmercury poisoning in Japan caused by environmental pollution. Crit Rev Toxicol 25:1–24
59. Eskenazi B et al (2006) In utero exposure to dichlorodiphenyltrichloroethane (DDT) and dichlorodiphenyldichloroethylene (DDE) and neurodevelopment among young Mexican American children. Pediatrics 118:233–241
60. Urabe H, Koda H, Asahi M (1979) Present state of yusho patients. Ann N Y Acad Sci 320:273–276
61. Schantz SL (1996) Developmental neurotoxicity of PCBs in humans: what do we know and where do we go from here? Neurotoxicol Teratol 18:217–227.; Discussion 229–276
62. Park HY et al (2010) Neurodevelopmental toxicity of prenatal polychlorinated biphenyls (PCBs) by chemical structure and activity: a birth cohort study. Environ Health 9:51
63. Winneke G et al (1998) Developmental neurotoxicity of polychlorinated biphenyls (PCBS): cognitive and psychomotor functions in 7-month old children. Toxicol Lett 102-103:423–428
64. Korrick SA, Sagiv SK (2008) Polychlorinated biphenyls, organochlorine pesticides and neurodevelopment. Curr Opin Pediatr 20:198–204
65. Ribas-Fito N et al (2003) Breastfeeding, exposure to organochlorine compounds, and neurodevelopment in infants. Pediatrics 111:e580–e585
66. Torres-Sanchez L et al (2013) Prenatal p,p -DDE exposure and neurodevelopment among children 3.5–5 years of age. Environ Health Perspect 121:263–268
67. Ribas-Fito N et al (2007) Exposure to hexachlorobenzene during pregnancy and children's social behavior at 4 years of age. Environ Health Perspect 115:447–450
68. Kilburn KH, Thornton JC (1995) Protracted neurotoxicity from chlordane sprayed to kill termites. Environ Health Perspect 103:690–694
69. Gascon M et al (2011) Effects of pre and postnatal exposure to low levels of polybromodiphenyl ethers on neurodevelopment and thyroid hormone levels at 4 years of age. Environ Int 37:605–611
70. Herbstman JB et al (2010) Prenatal exposure to PBDEs and neurodevelopment. Environ Health Perspect 118:712–719
71. Cowell WJ et al (2015) Prenatal exposure to polybrominated diphenyl ethers and child attention problems at 3-7 years. Neurotoxicol Teratol 52:143–150
72. Koenig CM, Lango J, Pessah IN, Berman RF (2012) Maternal transfer of BDE-47 to offspring and neurobehavioral development in C57BL/6J mice. Neurotoxicol Teratol 34:571–580
73. Sun W et al (2017) PBDE-209 exposure damages learning and memory ability in rats potentially through increased autophagy and apoptosis in the hippocampus neuron. Environ Toxicol Pharmacol 50:151–158
74. Dingemans MM et al (2007) Neonatal exposure to brominated flame retardant BDE-47 reduces long-term potentiation and postsynaptic protein levels in mouse hippocampus. Environ Health Perspect 115:865–870
75. Viberg H, Fredriksson A, Eriksson P (2004) Investigations of strain and/or gender differences in developmental neurotoxic effects of polybrominated diphenyl ethers in mice. Toxicol Sci 81:344–353
76. Eriksson P, Fischer C, Wallin M, Jakobsson E, Fredriksson A (2006) Impaired behaviour, learning and memory, in adult mice neonatally exposed to hexabromocyclododecane (HBCDD). Environ Toxicol Pharmacol 21:317–322

77. Miller-Rhodes P et al (2014) Prenatal exposure to the brominated flame retardant hexabromocyclododecane (HBCD) impairs measures of sustained attention and increases age-related morbidity in the Long-Evans rat. Neurotoxicol Teratol 45:34–43
78. Haug LS et al (2010) Diet and particularly seafood are major sources of perfluorinated compounds in humans. Environ Int 36:772–778
79. Brantsaeter AL et al (2013) Determinants of plasma concentrations of perfluoroalkyl substances in pregnant Norwegian women. Environ Int 54:74–84
80. Saikat S, Kreis I, Davies B, Bridgman S, Kamanyire R (2013) The impact of PFOS on health in the general population: a review. Environ Sci Process Impacts 15:329–335
81. Whitworth KW et al (2012) Perfluorinated compounds in relation to birth weight in the Norwegian Mother and Child Cohort Study. Am J Epidemiol 175:1209–1216
82. Granum B et al (2013) Pre-natal exposure to perfluoroalkyl substances may be associated with altered vaccine antibody levels and immune-related health outcomes in early childhood. J Immunotoxicol 10:373–379
83. Starling AP et al (2014) Perfluoroalkyl substances and lipid concentrations in plasma during pregnancy among women in the Norwegian Mother and Child Cohort Study. Environ Int 62:104–112
84. Kim S et al (2011) Trans-placental transfer of thirteen perfluorinated compounds and relations with fetal thyroid hormones. Environ Sci Technol 45:7465–7472
85. Wang Y et al (2013) Association between perfluoroalkyl substances and thyroid stimulating hormone among pregnant women: a cross-sectional study. Environ Health 12:7
86. Lau C et al (2003) Exposure to perfluorooctane sulfonate during pregnancy in rat and mouse. II: Postnatal evaluation. Toxicol Sci 74:382–392
87. Thibodeaux JR et al (2003) Exposure to perfluorooctane sulfonate during pregnancy in rat and mouse. I: Maternal and prenatal evaluations. Toxicol Sci 74:369–381
88. Berg V et al (2015) Assessing the relationship between perfluoroalkyl substances, thyroid hormones and binding proteins in pregnant women; a longitudinal mixed effects approach. Environ Int 77:63–69
89. Mariussen E (2012) Neurotoxic effects of perfluoroalkylated compounds: mechanisms of action and environmental relevance. Arch Toxicol 86:1349–1367
90. Miodovnik A (2011) Environmental neurotoxicants and developing brain. Mt Sinai J Med 78:58–77
91. Liew Z et al (2014) Prenatal exposure to perfluoroalkyl substances and the risk of congenital cerebral palsy in children. Am J Epidemiol 180:574–581
92. Liew Z et al (2015) Attention deficit/hyperactivity disorder and childhood autism in association with prenatal exposure to perfluoroalkyl substances: a nested case–control study in the Danish National Birth Cohort. Environ Health Perspect 123:367
93. CPSC (2014) Chronic Hazard Advisory Panel on Phthalates and Phthalate Alternatives. U.S. Consumer Product Safety Commission, Bethesda
94. Centers for Disease, Control and Prevention (2005) Third National Report on Human Exposure to Environmental Chemicals. CDC, Atlanta
95. Johns LE, Ferguson KK, McElrath TF, Mukherjee B, Meeker JD (2016) Associations between repeated measures of maternal urinary phthalate metabolites and thyroid hormone parameters during pregnancy. Environ Health Perspect 124:1808–1815
96. Johns LE et al (2015) Urinary phthalate metabolites in relation to maternal serum thyroid and sex hormone levels during pregnancy: a longitudinal analysis. Reprod Biol Endocrinol 13:4
97. Villanger GD, Drover SSM, Nethery RC, Thomsen C, Sakhi AK, Overgaard KR, Zeiner P, Hoppin JA, Reichborn-Kjennerud T, Aase H, Engel SM (2020) Associations between urine phthalate metabolites and thyroid function in pregnant women and the influence of iodine status. Environ Int 137:105509
98. Lien YJ et al (2015) Prenatal exposure to phthalate esters and behavioral syndromes in children at 8 years of age: Taiwan Maternal and Infant Cohort Study. Environ Health Perspect 123:95–100

99. Kobrosly RW et al (2014) Prenatal phthalate exposures and neurobehavioral development scores in boys and girls at 6-10 years of age. Environ Health Perspect 122:521–528
100. Philippat C et al (2015) Phthalate concentrations in house dust in relation to autism spectrum disorder and developmental delay in the CHildhood Autism Risks from Genetics and the Environment (CHARGE) study. Environ Health 14:56.
101. Philippat C et al (2017) Prenatal exposure to nonpersistent endocrine disruptors and behavior in boys at 3 and 5 years. Environ Health Perspect 125:097014
102. Engel SM et al (2010) Prenatal phthalate exposure is associated with childhood behavior and executive functioning. Environ Health Perspect 118:565–571
103. Factor-Litvak P et al (2014) Persistent associations between maternal prenatal exposure to phthalates on child IQ at age 7 years. PLoS One 9:e114003
104. Tellez-Rojo MM et al (2013) Prenatal urinary phthalate metabolites levels and neurodevelopment in children at two and three years of age. Sci Total Environ 461-462:386–390
105. Engel SM et al (2018) Prenatal phthalates, maternal thyroid function, and risk of attention-deficit hyperactivity disorder in the Norwegian Mother and Child Cohort. Environ Health Perspect 126:Artn 057004
106. California Safe Cosmetics Act of 2005. p. p. Chapter 729
107. Consumer Product Safety Improvement Act of 2008, in STAT. 3016-122 STAT. 3077. 2008 United States of America, p 122
108. Cohen AJ, Brauer M, Burnett R (2018) Estimates and 25-year trends of the global burden of disease attributable to ambient air pollution: an analysis of data from the global burden of diseases study 2015 (vol 389, pg 1907, 2017). Lancet 391:1576–1576
109. Sunyer J, Dadvand P (2019) Pre-natal brain development as a target for urban air pollution. Basic Clin Pharmacol Toxicol 125(Suppl 3):81–88
110. Peterson BS et al (2015) Effects of prenatal exposure to air pollutants (polycyclic aromatic hydrocarbons) on the development of brain white matter, cognition, and behavior in later childhood. JAMA Psychiat 72:531–540
111. Calderon-Garciduenas L et al (2011) Exposure to severe urban air pollution influences cognitive outcomes, brain volume and systemic inflammation in clinically healthy children. Brain Cogn 77:345–355
112. Myhre O et al (2018) Early life exposure to air pollution particulate matter (PM) as risk factor for attention deficit/hyperactivity disorder (ADHD): need for novel strategies for mechanisms and causalities. Toxicol Appl Pharmacol 354:196–214
113. Thapar A, Cooper M (2016) Attention deficit hyperactivity disorder. Lancet 387:1240–1250
114. Thapar A, Cooper M, Rutter M (2017) Neurodevelopmental disorders. Lancet Psychiatry 4:339–246
115. Faraone SV, Larsson H (2019) Genetics of attention deficit hyperactivity disorder. Mol Psychiatry 24:562–575
116. Sullivan JM, De Rubeis S, Schaefer A (2019) Convergence of spectrums: neuronal gene network states in autism spectrum disorder. Curr Opin Neurobiol 59:102–111
117. Jirtle RL, Skinner MK (2007) Environmental epigenomics and disease susceptibility. Nat Rev Genet 8:253–262
118. Skinner MK, Manikkam M, Guerrero-Bosagna C (2011) Epigenetic transgenerational actions of endocrine disruptors. Reprod Toxicol 31:337–343
119. Alvarado-Cruz I, Alegria-Torres JA, Montes-Castro N, Jimenez-Garza O, Quintanilla-Vega B (2018) Environmental epigenetic changes, as risk factors for the development of diseases in children: a systematic review. Ann Glob Health 84:212–224
120. Latham KE, Sapienza C, Engel N (2012) The epigenetic lorax: gene-environment interactions in human health. Epigenomics 4:383–402
121. Banik A et al (2017) Maternal factors that induce epigenetic changes contribute to neurological disorders in offspring. Genes (Basel) 8.
122. Bollati V, Baccarelli A (2010) Environmental epigenetics. Heredity 105:105–112

123. Mill J, Petronis A (2008) Pre- and peri-natal environmental risks for attention-deficit hyperactivity disorder (ADHD): the potential role of epigenetic processes in mediating susceptibility. J Child Psychol Psychiatry 49:1020–1030
124. LaSalle JM (2013) Epigenomic strategies at the interface of genetic and environmental risk factors for autism. J Hum Genet 58:396–401
125. Henshall DC, Kobow K (2015) Epigenetics and Epilepsy. Cold Spring Harb Perspect Med 5. https://doi.org/10.1101/cshperspect.a022731
126. van Mil NH et al (2014) DNA methylation profiles at birth and child ADHD symptoms. J Psychiatr Res 49:51–59
127. Wong CC et al (2014) Methylomic analysis of monozygotic twins discordant for autism spectrum disorder and related behavioural traits. Mol Psychiatry 19:495–503
128. Schoendorfer NC et al (2012) Methylation capacity in children with severe cerebral palsy. Eur J Clin Investig 42:768–776
129. Wright RO et al (2010) Biomarkers of Lead exposure and DNA methylation within Retrotransposons. Environ Health Perspect 118:790–795
130. Pilsner JR et al (2010) Mercury-associated DNA hypomethylation in polar bear brains via the LUminometric Methylation Assay: a sensitive method to study epigenetics in wildlife. Mol Ecol 19:307–314., MEC4452 [pii]
131. Cardenas A et al (2015) Differential DNA methylation in umbilical cord blood of infants exposed to mercury and arsenic in utero. Epigenetics 10:508–515
132. Rusiecki J, Baccarelli A, Bollati V, Moore L, Bonefeld-Jorgensen E (2007) DNA methylation among Greenlandic Inuit with varying levels of exposures to specific persistent organic pollutants. Epidemiology 18:S151–S152
133. De Rubeis S et al (2014) Synaptic, transcriptional and chromatin genes disrupted in autism. Nature 515:209–215
134. Iossifov I et al (2014) The contribution of de novo coding mutations to autism spectrum disorder. Nature 515:216–221
135. Sanders SJ et al (2015) Insights into autism spectrum disorder genomic architecture and biology from 71 risk loci. Neuron 87:1215–1233
136. Steinmaus C et al (2007) Genetic polymorphisms in MTHFR 677 and 1298, GSTM1 and T1, and metabolism of arsenic. J Toxicol Environ Health A 70:159–170
137. Broberg K et al (2019) Manganese transporter genetics and sex modify the association between environmental manganese exposure and neurobehavioral outcomes in children. Environ Int 130:104908
138. Austin C et al (2019) Dynamical properties of elemental metabolism distinguish attention deficit hyperactivity disorder from autism spectrum disorder. Transl Psychiatry 9:238
139. Arora M et al (2017) Fetal and postnatal metal dysregulation in autism. Nat Commun 8:15493
140. Dórea JG (2019) Environmental exposure to low-level lead (Pb) co-occurring with other neurotoxicants in early life and neurodevelopment of children. Environ Res 177:108641
141. Hendriks AM et al (2019) Comparing the genetic architecture of childhood behavioral problems across socioeconomic strata in the Netherlands and the United Kingdom. Eur Child Adolesc Psychiatry. https://doi.org/10.1007/s00787-019-01357-x
142. Rice DC (2008) Overview of modifiers of methylmercury neurotoxicity: chemicals, nutrients, and the social environment. NeuroToxicology 29:761–766
143. Bellinger DC (2008) Lead neurotoxicity and socioeconomic status: conceptual and analytical issues. NeuroToxicology 29:828–832
144. Krewski D et al (2010) Toxicity testing in the 21st century: a vision and a strategy. J Toxicol Environ Health B Crit Rev 13:51–138
145. Vineis P, Illari P, Russo F (2017) Causality in cancer research: a journey through models in molecular epidemiology and their philosophical interpretation. Emerg Themes Epidemiol 14:7
146. Adami HO et al (2011) Toxicology and epidemiology: improving the science with a framework for combining toxicological and epidemiological evidence to establish causal inference. Toxicol Sci 122:223–234

147. Teeguarden JG et al (2016) Completing the link between exposure science and toxicology for improved environmental health decision making: the aggregate exposure pathway framework. Environ Sci Technol 50:4579–4586.
148. Moors M, Cline JE, Abel J, Fritsche E (2007) ERK-dependent and -independent pathways trigger human neural progenitor cell migration. Toxicol Appl Pharmacol 221:57–67
149. Breier JM et al (2010) Neural progenitor cells as models for high-throughput screens of developmental neurotoxicity: state of the science. Neurotoxicol Teratol 32:4–15
150. Pandya H et al (2017) Differentiation of human and murine induced pluripotent stem cells to microglia-like cells. Nat Neurosci 20:753
151. Takahashi K, Yamanaka S (2006) Induction of pluripotent stem cells from mouse embryonic and adult fibroblast cultures by defined factors. Cell 126:663–676
152. Takahashi K et al (2007) Induction of pluripotent stem cells from adult human fibroblasts by defined factors. Cell 131:861–872
153. Vaccarino FM et al (2011) Annual research review: the promise of stem cell research for neuropsychiatric disorders. J Child Psychol Psychiatry 52:504–516
154. Kathuria A, Sala C, Verpelli C, Price J (2017) Modelling autistic neurons with induced pluripotent stem cells. Adv Anat Embryol Cell Biol 224:49–64
155. Adegbola A, Bury LA, Fu C, Zhang M, Wynshaw-Boris A (2017) Concise review: induced pluripotent stem cell models for neuropsychiatric diseases. Stem Cells Transl Med 6:2062–2070
156. Hernandez AF, Tsatsakis AM (2017) Human exposure to chemical mixtures: challenges for the integration of toxicology with epidemiology data in risk assessment. Food Chem Toxicol 103:188–193

Early-Life Environmental Influences on Allergic Diseases

Yu Ait Bamai, Chihiro Miyashita, Atsuko Araki, and Reiko Kishi

1 Introduction

An allergy is a chronic condition involving an abnormal reaction to an ordinarily harmless substance (i.e., an allergen). The resultant response can lead to conditions such as asthma, food allergies, atopic dermatitis (eczema), allergic rhinitis or hay fever, and anaphylaxis. Allergens can include aeroallergens such as dust mites, mold, and plants pollen, as well as food allergens such as milk, eggs, wheat, nuts, or fish proteins. Responses to allergens result in allergic symptoms, including increased levels of immunoglobulin-E (IgE). Allergies first present in early childhood. Interestingly, the severity of symptoms of allergic asthma in childhood predicts disease persistence into adulthood. Type 2 immune responses are the basis of an allergic response. However, increasing allergies in early childhood cannot be simply explained by type 2 immune responses only. It is clear that the genetic component certainly contributes to allergy susceptibility. In fact, various gene variants associated with Th2 cell differentiation are noted as risk factors for allergy [15]. For example, loss-of-function mutation(s) in the *filaggrin* gene is a risk factor of atopic dermatitis. However, *filaggrin* gene mutations can explain only 40% of the cases of atopic dermatitis [67], and the remaining 60% are thought to occur due to environmental risk factors. Furthermore, epigenetic modifications play a key role in the differentiation of allergy-related T-cell lineages as well as influence the balance between distinct Th cell populations such as Th1, Th2, and regulatory T cells. Epigenetic regulation also mediates the effect of various environmental exposures resulting in both allergy protection and conferring susceptibility to allergic diseases [65]. Many environmental factors have been identified and investigated as "environmental influences of allergic diseases." These include various toxic and harmful

Y. Ait Bamai · C. Miyashita · A. Araki · R. Kishi (✉)
Center for Environmental and Health Sciences, Hokkaido University, Sapporo, Japan
e-mail: rkishi@med.hokudai.ac.jp

Y. Xia (ed.), *Early-life Environmental Exposure and Disease*,
https://doi.org/10.1007/978-981-15-3797-4_9

physical, chemical, biological, and sociopsychological factors. Such factors are introduced into people's lives through their environment (e.g., via air), water source, soil, indoor public spaces, food, etc. In regard to chemical factors, the prevalence of asthma has increased since the 1970s, which coincides with an increased use of numerous new chemicals in manufacturing processes, with increased exposure of the general population during the same period. Asthma and allergy have not only a genetic but also an environmental component, and, because of the increases in incidence, prevalence cannot be due solely to genetics. These newly produced synthetic chemicals have shown endocrine-disrupting effects on humans, which interfere in some way with hormone action and can alter endocrine function such as immune, reproductive, endocrine, cardiopulmonary, and brain systems [84]. In this section, we provide up-to-date evidence based on epidemiological findings, specifically focused on the influence of prenatal and postnatal environmental chemical exposures, such as persistent organic pollutants (POPs) and short half-life compounds, on early childhood allergic diseases outcomes. We also investigate the possible pathophysiological mechanisms involved based on experimental data.

2 Persistent Organic Pollutants (POPs)

2.1 Perfluoroalkyl Substances (PFAS)

Perfluoroalkyl substances (PFAS) are persistent bioaccumulative chemicals which are widely used in industry including textiles, non-stick housewares, food packaging, furnishings, fire-fighting formulations, and more. The main exposure routes of PFAS for people are through the intake of contaminated food and water [28], although inhalation and ingestion of indoor dust are also contributing factors [40]. Since perfluorooctane sulfonate (PFOS) and perfluorooctanoate (PFOA) were included in the Stockholm Convention on Persistent Organic Pollutants, both substances have been replaced by shorter or longer carbon-chain PFAS. In human biomonitoring, results have shown that the exposure levels of PFOS and PFOA have decreased in recent years, while the levels of shorter and longer carbon-chain have increased [31, 61, 78]. Despite the introduction of the shorter or longer carbon-chain PFAS, epidemiological studies have reported that these substances are immunotoxic and immunomodulating (Table 1). Data from a birth cohort from the "Hokkaido Study" showed that prenatal exposure to PFOS was linked to decreased cord blood IgE levels among female infants [63] and reduced risk of eczema among 2-year-old girls [62]. In the same population, prenatal exposure to longer chain PFAS, such as perfluorohexane sulfonate (PFHxS), perfluorododecanoic acid (PFDoDA), and perfluorotridecanoic acid (PFTrDA), was linked to reduced risk of eczema at 4 years old [34]. Similar results have been reported from other birth cohorts. The Norwegian Mother and Child (MoBA) cohort has reported that prenatal exposure to longer carbon-chain PFAS and perfluoroundecanoic acid (PFUnDA) was inversely linked to a risk of atopic eczema [44]. Furthermore, a study conducted

Table 1 Early-life exposure to PFAS and associations with allergies or infectious disease

Author, year	No. of participants and age	Exposure	Outcome	Results
Stain et al. (2016) USA	1191 (12–19 years)	PFOS, PFOA, PFHxS, PFNA in maternal blood	Measles, mumps, rubella	PFOS was associated with decrease in rubella and mumps antibody. No adverse association between exposure and current allergies
			Asthma, wheeze, rhinitis, allergy	
Granum et al. (2013) Norway	640 (3 years)	PFOS, PFOA, PFHxS, PFNA in maternal blood	Vaccine antibody levels, common infectious diseases, and allergy- and asthma-related health outcomes	Inverse association between the level of anti-rubella antibodies at 3 years and PFAS. A positive association between the maternal PFOA and PFNA levels and the number of episodes of common cold. No associations were found between maternal PFAS and the allergy- and asthma-related health outcomes
Smit et al. (2015) Greenland and Ukraine	1024 (5–9 years)	PFHxS, PFHpA, PFOS, PFOA, PFNA, PFDA, PFUnDA, and PFDoDA in maternal blood	Wheeze, rhino-conjunctivitis, eczema (ISAAC)	PFAS in maternal blood was inversely associated with wheeze
Impinen et al. (2019) Norway	1270 (3 years), 972 (7 years)	PFOS, PFOA, PFHxS, PFNA, PFUnDA, and PFHpS in maternal blood	Asthma	Prenatal exposure to lPFAS and PFUnDA was inversely associated with risk of atopic eczema. Significant positive associations were seen between PFASs and airway infections
			Atopic eczema	
			Food allergy, infectious diseases	
Okada et al. (2012) Japan	343 (at birth)	PFOS, PFOA in maternal blood	Cord blood IgE	Prenatal exposure to PFOS was associated with decreased cord blood IgE levels among girl infants, but not associated with any allergic symptoms at 1.5 years of age

(continued)

Table 1 (continued)

Author, year	No. of participants and age	Exposure	Outcome	Results
Okada et al. (2014) Japan	2063 (2 years)	PFHxS, PFHxA, PFHpA, PFOS, PFOA, PFNA, PFDA, PFUnDA, PFDoDA, PFTrDA, PFTeDA in maternal blood	Wheeze, rhino-conjunctivitis, eczema (ISAAC)	Prenatal exposure to PFOS was associated with reduced risk of eczema among girls at 2 years of age
Goudarzi et al. (2016) Japan	1558 (4 years)			Prenatal exposure to PFHxS, PFDoDA, and PFTrDA was associated with reduced risk of eczema
Goudarzi et al. (2017) Japan			Otitis media, pneumonia, RS virus, varicella, total infectious diseases	Prenatal exposure to PFHxS, PFDoDA, and PFTrDA was associated with increased risk of infectious diseases
Dalsager et al. (2016) Denmark	346 (1–4 years)	PFOS, PFOA, PFHxS, PFNA, PFDA in maternal blood	Fever, stuffed or runny nose, cough, diarrhea, and vomiting	Prenatal exposure to PFOS and PFOA and the prevalence of fever at 1–4 years of age
Grandjean et al. (2012) Denmark	587 (5 years, 7 years)	PFOS, PFOA in maternal blood	Tetanus and diphtheria antibody	A twofold increase levels of PFAS was associated with a decline in the diphtheria antibody levels
Zeng et al. (2019) China	201 (3 months old)	PFOA, PFOS, PFDA PFDoDA PFHxS PFNA PFUnDA in maternal blood	Hand-foot-mouth disease antibody	Cord blood PFAS in 3 month-old-infants was associated with significant increase in the risk of hand-foot-mouth disease antibody concentration below clinical protection level

in Greenland and Ukraine showed that a principal component of PFAS in maternal blood, dominated by PFOS, was inversely linked to wheeze at 5–9 years old [68]. On the other hand, some studies are incongruent with those results. A study from Taiwanese asthmatic case-control study reported that positive dose-response associations were found between PFAS concentrations and risk of asthma at 15 years old [25]. National Health and Nutrition Examination Survey, a cross-sectional study, reported that the levels of PFOS were linked to higher odds of diagnosed asthma at 12–15 years old [43].

Data from the same population as Goudarzi et al. showed that prenatal exposure to PFHxS, PFDoDA, and PFTrDA was linked to an increasing risk of infectious diseases at 4 years old [33]. The Denmark Odense Child Cohort has reported that exposure to PFOS and PFOA during the prenatal period increases the prevalence of fever at 1–4 years of age [22]. This inverse association of allergic symptoms and infectious diseases is thought to be plausible due to the immunosuppressive effects of PFAS. Grandjean et al. first reported the possibilities of the immunosuppressive effects of PFAS when they showed that a twofold increase in PFAS levels was linked to a decline in diphtheria antibody levels [35]. Similar associations have been found between prenatal or postnatal exposure to PFAS and childhood vaccination antibodies, such as mumps and rubella [36, 71]. Moreover, the Guangzhou Birth Cohort Study has reported that cord blood PFAS was linked to a significant increase in the risk of hand-food-mouth-disease antibody concentration below the level of clinical protection among 3-month-old infants [86]. These findings are in line with animal studies. It has been demonstrated that in PFOS-exposed mice, IgM, which was suppressed, responses to T-cell-dependent and T-cell-independent antigens and natural killer (NK)-cell function [24, 37]. However, the experimental conditions employed used higher doses than the general exposure levels seen in humans. Evidence from experimental studies cannot be directly related to human health outcomes. Moreover, epidemiological findings are not fully consistent; this may be due to study designs, the age to which the health outcomes are related, confounding factors, and varied definitions of outcomes. Evidence regarding the immunosuppressive effects of PFAS, especially longer carbon-chain of PFAS in early childhood, is still under consideration.

2.2 *PCBs/PCDDs/PCDFs*

Polychlorinated biphenyls (PCBs), polychlorinated dibenzo-p-dioxins, and polychlorinated dibezofurans (PCDDs/PCDFs) have a long half-life and are categorized as POPs. PCBs, PCDDs, and PCDFs exist persistently not only in the food chain but also in the environment. Primary sources of exposure to these compounds are food items such as fish, seafood, meat, and eggs. PCBs, PCDDs. For many years, it has been shown that PCDFs accumulate mainly in adipose tissue due to the high lipophilicity and resistance to biodegradation. In bodies, they traverse the placenta and are transferred to fetal tissues and cord blood. The most toxic congener of

Table 2 Prenatal exposure to PCBs and dioxins at high levels and association with allergies or infectious diseases

Authors (year), place	No. of participants and age	Exposure	Results
Dallaire et al. (2004[a], 2006[b]) Nunavik in Canada	a: 199 (1 years)	PCB 153 in cord blood	a: GI infections/PCB: RR = 1.7 (1.0–2.8), otitis media/PCB: RR = 1.6 (1.0–2.5)
	b: 343 (5–7 years)		b: Acute otitis/PCB: RR=1.1 (1.1-1.1), lower respiratory infections/PCB: RR = 1.1 (1.0–1.2)
Heilmann et al. (2006) Faroe Island	a: 129 (7 years)	PCBs in maternal serum	a: Decreased antibody response to diphtheria toxoid/PCB:24% (p = 0.04)
	b: 119 (18mo.)		b: Decreased antibody response to tetanus toxoid/PCB: 17% (p = 0.03)
Park et al. (2008)	982 (3–4 days)	PCBs in maternal serum	Small thymus size/PCBs: $\beta = -36 (p = 0.047)$
Yu et al. 1998 Taiwan	105Yuchengs / 101Controls (born between 1978 and 1987)	PCBs/PCDFs by maternal infestation of contaminated rice oil	Bronchitis/PCDFs (6 months)
			Respiratory tract infections/ PCDFs (6 years)
			Ear infection/PCDFs (6 years) (significant higher frequency in Yuchengs than unexposed controls)

PCDDs/PCDFs is 2,3,7,8-tetrachlorodibenzo-p-dioxin (TCDD). The offspring of maternal rats treated with TCDD during pregnancy are more sensitive to immune toxicity caused by TCDD compared to adult rats and the negative influence that occurs at crucial windows of maturation persists later in life. Besides, the aforementioned toxic susceptibility appears to be sex-dependent. The offspring of male rats is more sensitive to TCDD-mediated inhibition of T cell activity than that of female rats [83].

There have been reports of exposure of high levels of PCBs/PCDDs/PCDFs, accidental poisoning, or contaminated food intake of PCBs/PCDDs/PCDFs in humans (Table 2). In one such incident in Taiwan Yucheng, pregnant women were exposed to high levels of PCDFs, and their children were more frequent to have bronchitis and reduced serum levels of immunoglobulins at 6 months of age and more likely to develop diseases of influenza and otitis media at 6 years of age. In Japan, pregnant women exposed to contaminated food were exposed to high levels of PCB. The children that these women bore were more likely to catch colds and gastrointestinal symptoms [30]. In Inuit infants born to mothers who were exposed to contaminated marine mammals, higher levels of prenatal PCB caused an apparent increased incidence of infections (e.g., acute otitis) and respiratory problems [20, 21]. On the Faroe Islands, PCB levels in maternal serum were inversely linked

Table 3 Prenatal exposure to PCBs and dioxins at environmental levels and association with allergies or infectious diseases

Authors (year), Place	No. of participants and age	Exposure	Results
Weisglas-Kupherus et al. (2000) Rotterdam in Netherland	193 mother-infant pairs (42 months)	PCBs (118, 128, 153, 18) Dioxins (PCDD, PCDF, Mono-ortho PCB) in maternal blood and breast milk	Asthma/∑PCB (maternal blood): (OR: 0.44; 95 % CI: 0.18–0.99)
			Otitis media/mono-ortho PCB TEQ (breast milk): (OR: 1.2; 95% CI: 1.0–1.3)
			Cough
			Chest congestion
			Phlegm/dioxin TEQ (breast milk): (OR: 1.1; 95% CI: 1.0–1.1)
Sunyer et al. (2005) Menorca in Spain	482 mother-infant pairs (4 years)	PCBs (28,52,101,118,153,138,180) in cord blood	Asthma/PCBs: No association
ten Tusscher et al. (2003) Amsterdam in Netherland	27 mother–infant pairs (8 years)	17 PCDDs /PCDFs in breast milk	Allergies/dioxins: Slope = −0.14 ($p = 0.023$)
			Infections/dioxins: No association
Miyashita et al. (2011) Hokkaido in Japan	364 mother-infant pairs (1.5 years)	Dioxin-like PCBs, PCDDs, PCDFs in maternal blood	Otitis media (male)/PCDFs (OR: 2.5, 95% CI: 1.1–5.9)
			Otitis media (male)/2,3,4,7,8-pentachlorodibenzo-furan (OR: 5.3; 95% CI: 1.5–19)
Hansen et al. (2014[a], 2016[b]) [38, 39] Aarhus in Denmark	421 mother-infant pairs (20 years)	PCBs, PCDDs, PCDFs in maternal blood	a: Asthma medical intake/PCB118 (OR: 1.90; 95% CI: 1.12–3.23)
			b: Allergic sensitization/PCBs, PCDDs, PCDFs: No association
			c: Airway obstruction/PCBs (OR: 2.96; 95% CI: 1.14–7.70)
Miyashita et al. (2018) Hokkaido in Japan	264 mother-infant pairs (7 years)	Dioxin-like PCBs, PCDDs, PCDFs in maternal blood	Wheezing/PCBs, PCDDs, PCDFs (OR: 7.8; 95% CI: 1.4–42.9)

to an antibody response to diphtheria toxoid in 18-month-old children and tetanus toxoid in 7-year-old children [41]. According to a study in Eastern Slovakia, higher PCB levels in maternal serum were linked to newborns with a smaller thymus, the organ associated with lymphocyte maturation [64].

The associations between prenatal exposure to PCBs and dioxins at environmental levels and allergies or infectious diseases among general population have been also reported (Table 3). In the Rotterdam study, children's otitis media and chicken pox were more prevalent due to maternal exposure to PCBs during pregnancy. Moreover, these implications were associated with a decrease in measles, mumps, and rubella reactivity after primary vaccination and a growing number of T lymphocytes in 42-month-old children [79, 80]. In contrast, in the Amsterdam study, children's allergies were found to have decreased at 8 years of age due to increased maternal dioxin levels [73]. PCB levels in cord blood have no associations with the prevalence of asthma in 4-year-old children in Spain [72]. In Japan, PCBs/PCDDs/PCDF levels in breast milk were notably linked to an increase of lymphocyte subset ratio in the peripheral blood of breast-fed infants at 10 months of age [60]; however, there was no observation in another cohort of Japanese infants at 12 months of age [47]. A systematic review published by Gascon et al. included several studies demonstrating a higher risk of respiratory infections, including acute otitis media, among infants [16, 20, 32, 58] with regard to in utero exposure to PCBs and/or dioxins. The majority of the current knowledge surrounding in utero exposure to PCBs/PCDDs/PCDFs in the context of downregulation of immune response and higher incidences of infectious symptoms in early infancy has been relatively consistent.

Regarding long-term effects, in a Danish cohort, the number of children with asthma was higher during a follow-up period lasting for 20 years according to higher maternal PCBs during pregnancy. Airway obstruction in children but not allergic sensitization, at age 20, was associated with maternal PCB levels during pregnancy in that cohort [39]. The Hokkaido Study in Japan reported that exposure to PCBs/PCDDs/PCDFs in utero may modify immune responses in offspring, resulting in a growing risk of allergy among school-age children. Besides, male infants may be more susceptible to maternal exposure to PCBs/PCDDs/PCDFs [57]. In summary, excluding accidental poisoning and contaminated food intake, the general population is continually exposed to PCBs/PCDDs/PCDF at relatively low levels. Even at low-level exposure, prenatal PCB/PCDD/PCDF exposure may modify the immune responses of the offspring of exposed individuals, resulting in an increased risk of allergy and infection during childhood and adolescence. There is insufficient evidence detailing the long-term effects of exposure to PCBs/PCDDs/PCDFs. Therefore, further studies targeted at the general population are vital to elucidate the long-term influence of such exposure.

2.3 Brominated Flame Retardants (BFRs)

Brominated flame retardants (BFRs) consist of different groups of chemicals with a range of physiochemical properties. BFRs are widely used in industrial applications such as production of polybrominated diphenyl ethers (PBDEs), hexabromocyclododecane (HBCD), tetrabromobisphenol A (TBBPA), as well as other brominated compounds. PBDEs contain up to 10 bromine atoms attached to 2 aromatic rings, which results in 209 different congeners which are structurally similar to PCBs. Exposure to BFRs from indoor environments is of particular concern because of their widespread use within household interiors, building materials, electrical appliances, as well as rubber products. More specifically, house dust is thought to be a significant means of exposure to PBDEs for toddlers, children, teenagers, and adults, accounting for more than 50% of the total PBDE intake [45]. Widespread contamination of PBDEs in the environment and their detection in people and wildlife have raised concerns regarding adverse health effects [55]. Several reviews have suggested that BFRs, especially PBDEs, have potentially adverse effects on endocrine functions, the central nervous system, and reproductive systems in experimental studies [19, 54]. PBDEs and HBCDD have been listed as POPs in the Stockholm Convention because of their potentially negative influence on human health, their persistence in the environment, as well as bioaccumulation potential. In epidemiological studies, adverse effects on neurodevelopment [77], birth outcomes [17], changes in the levels of thyroid hormones [18, 77], and reproductive hormone levels [27] have been reported. As for immunological effects, however, experimental and epidemiological data is lacking. An in vitro study suggested that BFRs can induce or enhance immune or allergic responses by increasing antigen presentation-related molecule expression and IL-4 production [49]. A case-control study reported that, serum levels of BDE-209, which is the most widely used PBDE in China and was dominantly detected in the study population, was linked to an increased risk of asthma among children. However, levels of BDE-209 or other PBDEs in house dust were not associated with any allergic symptoms [14, 56].

3 Short Half-Lived Chemicals

3.1 Phthalates

Phthalates are plastic additives (plasticizers), which are added to plastics and perfumes and are widely contained in consumer products and personal care products (PCPs). Phthalates are nonpersistent, not bioaccumulative, and therefore short half-life compounds which are excreted in urine within hours to 2 days. Due to their endocrine-disrupting effects, some phthalates, such as di-2-ethylhexyl phthalate (DEHP) and di-n-butyl phthalate (DnBP), have been partly regulated for their use in food containers for fatty foods, as well as in children's toys and mouthing products. However, their use in other consumer products such as PCPs, furniture, and indoor materials is not regulated. We are exposed to phthalates from various consumer products on a daily basis. It is, therefore, important to investigate the possible associations between exposure to phthalates and allergic diseases. This is especially critical since the hand-to-mouth behavior of infants and toddlers is thought to be the main exposure route of phthalate exposure among young children. Moreover, phthalates are known to have adjuvant effects on allergies, which are consistent with experimental studies [48, 53]. In experimental studies, adjuvants induced production and differentiation of Th2 cells in mice, which in turn promoted

IgE and IgG1 production. In a human experimental study, healthy human participants showed no inflammatory responses to short-term inhalation of house dust which contains DEHP. Nevertheless, nasal exposure to dust mite in allergic participants showed elevated IL-5, IL-6, granulocyte-colony stimulating factor, and eosinophil cationic protein levels even after short-term exposure to low DEHP doses [23].

Epidemiological studies are mainly designed to use the levels of phthalate metabolites in urine or of phthalates in house dust as exposure assessments (Table 4). In human biological samples, both prenatal and postnatal exposure levels are considered; however, in dust samples, only postnatal time periods are investigated. Currently, evidence regarding the relations between prenatal exposure to phthalates in house dust and allergies in early childhood is lacking. Data generated using phthalates in house dust as a proxy for postnatal exposure assessment shows quite accordant results, in which higher house dust levels of butyl benzyl phthalate (BBzP), DEHP, and DnBP were linked to an increase in the risk for allergies among school-age children [1, 6, 8, 42, 51]. Some of these studies investigated the relations with urinary phthalate metabolite levels; however, no associations were found between urinary phthalate metabolites and allergies. In prenatal exposure, metabolites of diisononyl phthalate (DiNP) were associated with an increase in the risk for childhood asthma [7]. In this study, two spot urine samples were collected from pregnant women during the first and second trimester of pregnancy. Additionally, the prenatal exposure to diisodecyl phthalate (DiDP) was linked to wheeze at 5 years old [76]. Data seems to suggest that high molecular weight phthalates, such as DiNP and DIDP which are used as replacements for DEHP, are associated with asthma and respiratory symptoms. However, evidence for the effects of postnatal exposure to phthalates on childhood allergies is still very limited. Since phthalates are nonpersistent and short half-life compounds, the inconsistency of postnatal exposure to phthalates may be due to this and compounded by the fact that only one spot urine collection was used for assessing the effects of phthalate exposure. Intra- and interday variances of phthalate metabolites have been reported, and urine sampling in several time points is recommended. Therefore, only one spot urine collection is one of the limitations of exposure assessment of phthalates. On the other hand, levels of phthalates in house dust might not change dramatically on a daily basis, as well as intra-day basis. It is also quite challenging to collect urine samples from children at several time points. Nonetheless, further studies are needed to challenge this and to allow for robust analysis of postnatal phthalate exposure.

3.2 Phosphorus Flame Retardants and Plasticizers (PFRs)

Phosphorus flame retardants and plasticizers (PFRs) are mostly applied in polyurethane foam (PUF), thermoplastics, resins, polyvinyl chloride, synthetic rubbers, and textiles [75]. Tris(2-butoxyethyl) phosphate (TBOEP), which is used in waxes, floor polishes, and plasticizers in floor coverings, takes up the highest fraction of PFR concentrations in indoor dust [46]. PFR levels in house dust have been reported in

Table 4 Early-life exposure to phthalates and associations with allergies

Authors (year), country	No. of participants and age	Phthalates in house dust	Phthalates in urine	Results
Bornehag et al. (2004) Sweden	400 (3–8 years)	Dust: DMP, DEP, DiBP, DnBP, BBZP, DEHP, DiNP in children's bedrooms	–	Dust: BBzP was associated with rhinitis and eczema; DEHP was associated with asthma
Kolarik et al. (2008), Bulgaria	102 (2–7 years)	Dust: DMP, DEP, DnBP, BBZP, DEHP, DnOP in children's bedrooms	–	Dust: DEHP was higher in case houses than in control houses. DEHP was associated with wheezing in the 12 months
Beko et al. (2015) Denmark	500 (3–5 years)	Dust: DEP, DiBP, DnBP, BBZP, DEHP, DiNP in children's bedrooms	MEP, MnBP, MiBP, MBzP, MEHP, MEHHP, MEOHP, MECPP	Dust: DEHP and wheezing, DnBP, BBzP and asthma, rhino-conjunctivitis, atopic dermatitis were associated
			Daily intakes of DEP, DnBP, DiBP, BBzP, DEHP	Urine: MEP and atopic dermatitis were positively associated
Hsu et al. (2012) Taiwan	101 (3–9 years)	DMP, DEP, DBP, BBZP, DEHP, DiNP in children's activity rooms	MMP, MEP, MBP, MBzP, MEHP, MEHHP, MEOHP	Dust: BBzP increased risks of rhinitis and eczema.
				Urine: No association
Ait Bamai et al. (2014) Japan	526 inhabitants of new detached houses	DMP, DEP, DiBP, DnBP, BBZP, DEHP, DiNP in living room	–	Dust: DiBP and DnBP were associated with asthma, DEHP with allergic conjunctivitis, and DnBP, BBzP, and DEHP with atopic dermatitis. Associations were stronger in children than in adults
Ait Bamai et al. (2016) Japan	184 (6–12 years)		Daily intakes of DnBP, DiBP, BBzP, and DEHP	Dust: DEHP was associated with rhino-conjunctivitis
				Urine: No association
Bi et al. (2018) USA	54 children (mean age, 10.3 years) living in low-income homes	Dust: DMP, DEP, DnBP, BBZP, DEHP, DnOP in children's bedrooms	–	Dust: DEHP was associated with childhood asthma severity in summer
Bertelsen et al. (2013) Norway	623 (10 years)	–	MEP, MnBP, MiBP, MBzP, MEHP, MEHHP, MEOHP, MECPP, MCPP, MCOP, MCNP	Current asthma was associated with the highest quartiles of MCOP and MCNP

Table 5 Early-life exposure to phosphorous flame retardants and associations with allergies

Country	No. of participants and age	PFR	Outcome	Result
Japan, 2009–2010	128 (6–12 years)	TMP, TEP, TPP, TNBP, TCIPP, TCEP, TEHP, TBOEP, TDCIPP, TPHP, TMPP	Asthma, rhino-conjunctivitis, atopic dermatitis	TDCIPP in floor dust and eczema were strongly associated
				TDCIPP in house dust and urinary TDCIPP, TBOEP, and TCIPP metabolites were associated with allergies in children
USA, 2014–2015	54 children (mean age, 10.3 years) living in low-income homes	TNBP, TCIPP, TBOEP, TPHP, TDCIPP	Asthma, asthma symptoms	No association
Sweden	220 (110 children who developed asthma at 4 or at 8 years and 110 matched controls)	TCEP, TCIPP, TDCIPP, TBOEP, TPHP, EHDPHP, mmp-TMPP	Asthma at 4 or 8 years	Levels of TPHP and mmp-TMPP in dust were higher in control samples than in samples collected from homes of asthmatic children

several studies; however, human biomonitoring data is still rather limited. Studies investigating associations between PFRs and allergies are also very limited for both epidemiological and experimental studies (Table 5). Tris(1,3-dichloroisopropyl) phosphate (TDCIPP) found in dust was linked to noticeable rises in ORs of atopic dermatitis/eczema among elementary school children. Furthermore, in the same population, urinary TDCIPP, tris(2-chloroisopropyl) phosphate (TCIPP), and TBOEP metabolites were linked to eczema and/or rhinoconjunctivitis among elementary school children [4]. Metabolites of triphenyl phosphate (TPHP) and 2-ethylhexyl phenyl phosphate (EHPHP) and bis(2-butoxyethyl) phosphate (BBOEP) were linked to increased levels of oxidative stress biomarkers [2]. The allergy-inducing mechanisms of PFRs remain unclear. TBOEP, TCIPP, and TDCIPP cause mild to moderate skin irritation in rabbits [81, 82], while TCIPP and TDCIPP cause skin and eye irritation in rats [75, p. 1213]. A transcriptome study illustrated hepatic pro-inflammatory influence of TBOEP on the immune responses as well as on the lipid and steroid hormone metabolism [52]. Under in vitro conditions, TDCIPP and TPHP were found to be immunocytotoxic and induced oxidative stress [13]. Moreover, TDCIPP had antagonistic effects on androgen receptors, glucocorticoid receptors, and pregnane X receptors (PXRs). TBOEP and TCIPP also exhibited antagonistic activity against PXR [50]. These effects suggest that certain PFRs are likely to be endocrine disruptors. Nevertheless, the mechanisms underlying the immunological effects of PFRs in humans remain unknown. Further experimental and epidemiological researches are urgently required to elucidate these mechanisms.

3.3 Bisphenols (BPs)

Bisphenol A (BPA), a man-made chemical that is widely used for polycarbonate plastics and epoxy resins, can be found in certain food and beverage packaging, dental sealants, and receipts. With rising concerns regarding endocrine-disrupting effects on humans, the use of BPA in products has been phasing down, and other analogues, i.e., bisphenol F (BPF) and bisphenol S (BPS), are being used instead. Due to its widespread use, BPA is detected in more than 90% of human urine samples in Canadians [12], US children [59], and Asian populations (i.e., Chinese, Vietnamese, Malaysians, Indian, Japanese, and Korean people) [87]. Recent reviews have suggested that early-life exposure to BPA is linked to altered neurological developments leading to behavioral problems, low fetal growth, low birth weight, and thyroid dysfunction [9, 10, 66]. In regard to asthma, allergies, and immunological effects on humans, several epidemiological studies have been conducted. In a birth cohort of the Health Outcomes and Measures of the Environment (HOME) study, urine samples were collected from pregnant women twice during pregnancy (at 16 weeks and 26 weeks of gestation), and BPA levels were measured in each sample [69, 70]. Parent-reported child wheeze was assessed every 6 months until they were 5 years-old. Lung function was also assessed when the children were 4 and 5 years old. Maternal mean urinary BPA concentrations were not linked to wheeze under 3 years old; however, they were marginally linked to increased risk of wheezing at 5 years old. Moreover, maternal mean urinary BPA concentrations were linked to decreased lung function at 4 years old, but no relation was found at 5 years old. Urinary BPA concentrations in samples collected at 16 weeks, but not 26 weeks, were linked to increased risk of wheeze. Child urinary BPA concentrations were not linked to lung function or wheeze. Gascon et al. reported that prenatal exposure to BPA was linked to increased risk of wheeze as well as bronchitis under 7 years old [29]. Another birth cohort study in the USA reported that prenatal exposure to BPA was inversely linked to a risk of wheeze among 5-year-old children [26]. In the same study, postnatal exposure to BPA was also investigated. The data show that urinary BPA concentrations in 3-year-old children were linked with wheeze at 5 and 6 years of age. These epidemiological studies investigated both prenatal and postnatal exposure to BPA; however, the findings are inconsistent in each study. This may be due to BPA has a short half-life, resulting in variability in urinary BPA concentrations within and between days [10, 11, 74]. An additional confounding factor is that the timings of urine collections from pregnant women in these studies are different. Spanier et al. and Gascon et al. collected spot urine samples during the first and third trimester of pregnancy, and they used average concentrations of BPA as exposure assessments, while Donohue et al. collected samples during the third trimester.

Several experimental studies haves been suggested some direct mechanistic links between prenatal exposure to BPA and the influence on immune system. For example, pre- and postnatal developmental exposure to 50 μg/kgBW/day enhanced lung inflammation in the mucosal sensitization model [5]. Yang et al. demonstrated that prenatal exposure to BPA influences asthma risk through upregulation of Th2 pathways and possibly reduces regulatory T-cell counts [85]. Another possible mechanism suggests that BPA may bind to estrogen receptors to disrupt estrogen function and the response of immune cells [3]. However, regarding the other bisphenol analogues (e.g., BPF and BPS), no clear mechanism of action has been defined because of the limited research in this area. Although exposure levels of BPF and BPS are lower than BPA, it has been suggested that BPS and BPF could have equivalent or even greater toxicity than BPA [66]. In addition, the production and usage of BPA are reducing; however, BPF and BPS are increasing. Further epidemiological and experimental studies including other bisphenol analogues are needed to investigate both in detail.

4 Conclusions

In this section, the current epidemiological knowledge regarding the possible influence of environmental chemicals on childhood allergies were summarized. In spite of reported inconsistencies of the immunosuppressive effects of longer carbon-chain PFAS, PFOS, and PFOA, they showed consistent immunosuppressive effects on humans, which decreased risk of allergies and increased the risk of infectious diseases. Prenatal exposure to PCBs/PCDDs/PCDFs may modify the immune responses of children born to exposed mothers. Moreover, these children are at an increased risk of allergy and infection in their childhood and adolescence. Currently, there is insufficient evidence for the long-term effects of PCBs/PCDDs/PCDFs. Some BFRs have been banned due to widespread contaminations and concerns regarding the adverse health effects (e.g., neurodevelopment and reproductive) of BFRs in people. Despite a number of experimental and epidemiological studies, conclusive evidence on immune functions and allergies is very much lacking. Precise exposure assessment of short half-life compounds such as phthalate, PFRs, and bisphenols using human urine samples is difficult which may have led to inconsistent results within each epidemiological study. Nevertheless, even with the limited amount of available data, epidemiological and experimental studies have displayed that PFR exposure from house dust increases the risk of asthma and allergies in childhood. The influence of BPA on the developmental immune system is consistent within experimental studies; however, other bisphenols such as BPF and BPS have not yet been evaluated. Further investigation of the effects of these environmental chemicals, as well as alternative chemicals, on asthma and allergies are essential.

References

1. Ait Bamai Y, Araki A, Kawai T, Tsuboi T, Saito I, Yoshioka E, Cong S, Kishi R (2016) Exposure to phthalates in house dust and associated allergies in children aged 6–12years. Environ Int 96:16–23
2. Ait Bamai Y, Bastiaensen M, Araki A, Goudarzi H, Konno S, Ito S, Miyashita C, Yao Y, Covaci A, Kishi R (2019) Multiple exposures to organophosphate flame retardants alter urinary oxidative stress biomarkers among children: the Hokkaido Study. Environ Int 131:105003
3. Alonso-Magdalena P, Laribi O, Ropero AB, Fuentes E, Ripoll C, Soria B, Nadal A (2005) Low doses of bisphenol A and diethylstilbestrol impair Ca2+ signals in pancreatic alpha-cells through a nonclassical membrane estrogen receptor within intact islets of Langerhans. Environ Health Perspect 113:969–977
4. Araki A, Bastiaensen M, Ait Bamai Y, Van den Eede N, Kawai T, Tsuboi T, Ketema RM, Covaci A, Kishi R (2018) Associations between allergic symptoms and phosphate flame retardants in dust and their urinary metabolites among school children. Environ Int 119:438–446
5. Bauer SM, Roy A, Emo J, Chapman TJ, Georas SN, Lawrence BP (2012) The effects of maternal exposure to bisphenol A on allergic lung inflammation into adulthood. Toxicol Sci 130:82–93
6. Beko G, Callesen M, Weschler CJ, Toftum J, Langer S, Sigsgaard T, Host A, Kold Jensen T, Clausen G (2015) Phthalate exposure through different pathways and allergic sensitization in preschool children with asthma, allergic rhinoconjunctivitis and atopic dermatitis. Environ Res 137:432–439
7. Berger K, Eskenazi B, Balmes J, Kogut K, Holland N, Calafat AM, Harley KG (2019) Prenatal high molecular weight phthalates and bisphenol A, and childhood respiratory and allergic outcomes. Pediatr Allergy Immunol 30:36–46
8. Bornehag CG, Sundell J, Weschler CJ, Sigsgaard T, Lundgren B, Hasselgren M, Hagerhed-Engman L (2004) The association between asthma and allergic symptoms in children and phthalates in house dust: a nested case-control study. Environ Health Perspect 112:1393–1397
9. Braun JM (2017) Early-life exposure to EDCs: role in childhood obesity and neurodevelopment. Nat Rev Endocrinol 13:161–173
10. Braun JM, Hauser R (2011) Bisphenol A and children's health. Curr Opin Pediatr 23:233–239
11. Braun JM, Kalkbrenner AE, Calafat AM, Bernert JT, Ye X, Silva MJ, Barr DB, Sathyanarayana S, Lanphear BP (2011) Variability and predictors of urinary bisphenol A concentrations during pregnancy. Environ Health Perspect 119:131–137
12. Bushnik T, Haines D, Levallois P, Levesque J, Van Oostdam J, Viau C (2010) Lead and bisphenol A concentrations in the Canadian population. Health Rep 21:7–18
13. Canbaz D, Logiantara A, van Ree R, van Rijt LS (2017) Immunotoxicity of organophosphate flame retardants TPHP and TDCIPP on murine dendritic cells in vitro. Chemosphere 177:56–64
14. Canbaz D, van Velzen MJ, Hallner E, Zwinderman AH, Wickman M, Leonards PE, van Ree R, van Rijt LS (2016) Exposure to organophosphate and polybrominated diphenyl ether flame retardants via indoor dust and childhood asthma. Indoor Air 26:403–413
15. Candi E, Schmidt R, Melino G (2005) The cornified envelope: a model of cell death in the skin. Nat Rev Mol Cell Biol 6:328–340
16. Chao WY, Hsu CC, Guo YL (1997) Middle-ear disease in children exposed prenatally to polychlorinated biphenyls and polychlorinated dibenzofurans. Arch Environ Health 52:257–262
17. Chen L, Wang C, Cui C, Ding G, Zhou Y, Jin J, Gao Y, Tian Y (2015) Prenatal exposure to polybrominated diphenyl ethers and birth outcomes. Environ Pollut (Barking, Essex: 1987) 206:32–37
18. Chevrier J, Harley KG, Bradman A, Sjödin A, Eskenazi B (2011) Prenatal exposure to polybrominated diphenyl ether flame retardants and neonatal thyroid-stimulating hormone levels in the CHAMACOS study. Am J Epidemiol 174:1166–1174

19. Czerska M, Zieliński M, Kamińska J, Ligocka D (2013) Effects of polybrominated diphenyl ethers on thyroid hormone, neurodevelopment and fertility in rodents and humans. Int J Occup Med Environ Health 26:498–510
20. Dallaire F, Dewailly E, Muckle G, Vezina C, Jacobson SW, Jacobson JL, Ayotte P (2004) Acute infections and environmental exposure to organochlorines in Inuit infants from Nunavik. Environ Health Perspect 112:1359–1365
21. Dallaire F, Dewailly E, Vezina C, Muckle G, Weber JP, Bruneau S, Ayotte P (2006) Effect of prenatal exposure to polychlorinated biphenyls on incidence of acute respiratory infections in preschool Inuit children. Environ Health Perspect 114:1301–1305
22. Dalsager L, Christensen N, Husby S, Kyhl H, Nielsen F, Host A, Grandjean P, Jensen TK (2016) Association between prenatal exposure to perfluorinated compounds and symptoms of infections at age 1–4years among 359 children in the Odense Child Cohort. Environ Int 96:58–64
23. Deutschle T, Reiter R, Butte W, Heinzow B, Keck T, Riechelmann H (2008) A controlled challenge study on Di(2-ethylhexyl) phthalate (DEHP) in house dust and the immune response in human nasal mucosa of allergic subjects. Environ Health Perspect 116:1487–1493
24. Dong G-H, Zhang Y-H, Zheng L, Liu W, Jin Y-H, He Q-C (2009) Chronic effects of perfluorooctanesulfonate exposure on immunotoxicity in adult male C57BL/6 mice. Arch Toxicol 83:805–815
25. Dong GH, Tung KY, Tsai CH, Liu MM, Wang D, Liu W, Jin YH, Hsieh WS, Lee YL, Chen PC (2013) Serum polyfluoroalkyl concentrations, asthma outcomes, and immunological markers in a case-control study of Taiwanese children. Environ Health Perspect 121:507–513
26. Donohue KM, Miller RL, Perzanowski MS, Just AC, Hoepner LA, Arunajadai S, Canfield S, Resnick D, Calafat AM, Perera FP, Whyatt RM (2013) Prenatal and postnatal bisphenol A exposure and asthma development among inner-city children. J Allergy Clin Immunol 131:736–742
27. Eskenazi B, Rauch SA, Tenerelli R, Huen K, Holland NT, Lustig RH, Kogut K, Bradman A, Sjödin A, Harley KG (2017) In utero and childhood DDT, DDE, PBDE and PCBs exposure and sex hormones in adolescent boys: the CHAMACOS study. Int J Hyg Environ Health 220:364–372
28. Fromme H, Tittlemier SA, Volkel W, Wilhelm M, Twardella D (2009) Perfluorinated compounds – exposure assessment for the general population in Western countries. Int J Hyg Environ Health 212:239–270
29. Gascon M, Casas M, Morales E, Valvi D, Ballesteros-Gomez A, Luque N, Rubio S, Monfort N, Ventura R, Martinez D, Sunyer J, Vrijheid M (2015) Prenatal exposure to bisphenol A and phthalates and childhood respiratory tract infections and allergy. J Allergy Clin Immunol 135:370–378
30. Gascon M, Morales E, Sunyer J, Vrijheid M (2013) Effects of persistent organic pollutants on the developing respiratory and immune systems: a systematic review. Environ Int 52:51–65
31. Glynn A, Berger U, Bignert A, Ullah S, Aune M, Lignell S, Darnerud PO (2012) Perfluorinated alkyl acids in blood serum from primiparous women in Sweden: serial sampling during pregnancy and nursing, and temporal trends 1996-2010. Environ Sci Technol 46:9071–9079
32. Glynn A, Thuvander A, Aune M, Johannisson A, Darnerud PO, Ronquist G, Cnattingius S (2008) Immune cell counts and risks of respiratory infections among infants exposed pre- and postnatally to organochlorine compounds: a prospective study. Environ Health Glob 7
33. Goudarzi H, Miyashita C, Okada E, Kashino I, Chen CJ, Ito S, Araki A, Kobayashi S, Matsuura H, Kishi R (2017) Prenatal exposure to perfluoroalkyl acids and prevalence of infectious diseases up to 4 years of age. Environ Int 104:132
34. Goudarzi H, Miyashita C, Okada E, Kashino I, Kobayashi S, Chen CJ, Ito S, Araki A, Matsuura H, Ito YM, Kishi R (2016) Effects of prenatal exposure to perfluoroalkyl acids on prevalence of allergic diseases among 4-year-old children. Environ Int 94:124–132

35. Grandjean P, Andersen EW, Budtz-Jorgensen E, Nielsen F, Molbak K, Weihe P, Heilmann C (2012) Serum vaccine antibody concentrations in children exposed to perfluorinated compounds. JAMA 307:391–397
36. Granum B, Haug LS, Namork E, Stolevik SB, Thomsen C, Aaberge IS, van Loveren H, Lovik M, Nygaard UC (2013) Pre-natal exposure to perfluoroalkyl substances may be associated with altered vaccine antibody levels and immune-related health outcomes in early childhood. J Immunotoxicol 10:373–379
37. Guruge KS, Hikono H, Shimada N, Murakami K, Hasegawa J, Yeung LWY, Yamanaka N, Yamashita N (2009) Effect of perfluorooctane sulfonate (PFOS) on influenza A virus-induced mortality in female B6C3F1 mice. J Toxicol Sci 34:687–691
38. Hansen S, Strom M, Olsen SF, Dahl R, Hoffmann HJ, Granstrom C, Rytter D, Bech BH, Linneberg A, Maslova E, Kiviranta H, Rantakokko P, Halldorsson TI (2016) Prenatal exposure to persistent organic pollutants and offspring allergic sensitization and lung function at 20 years of age. Clin Exp Allergy: J Br Soc Allergy Clin Immunol 46:329–336
39. Hansen S, Strom M, Olsen SF, Maslova E, Rantakokko P, Kiviranta H, Rytter D, Bech BH, Hansen LV, Halldorsson TI (2014) Maternal concentrations of persistent organochlorine pollutants and the risk of asthma in offspring: results from a prospective cohort with 20 years of follow-up. Environ Health Perspect 122:93–99
40. Haug LS, Huber S, Schlabach M, Becher G, Thomsen C (2011) Investigation on per- and polyfluorinated compounds in paired samples of house dust and indoor air from Norwegian homes. Environ Sci Technol 45:7991–7998
41. Heilmann C, Grandjean P, Weihe P, Nielsen F, Budtz-Jorgensen E (2006) Reduced antibody responses to vaccinations in children exposed to polychlorinated biphenyls. PLoS Med 3:e311
42. Hsu NY, Lee CC, Wang JY, Li YC, Chang HW, Chen CY, Bornehag CG, Wu PC, Sundell J, Su HJ (2012) Predicted risk of childhood allergy, asthma, and reported symptoms using measured phthalate exposure in dust and urine. Indoor Air 22:186–199
43. Humblet O, Diaz-Ramirez LG, Balmes JR, Pinney SM, Hiatt RA (2014) Perfluoroalkyl chemicals and asthma among children 12-19 years of age: NHANES (1999–2008). Environ Health Perspect 122:1129–1133
44. Impinen A, Longnecker MP, Nygaard UC, London SJ, Ferguson KK, Haug LS, Granum B (2019) Maternal levels of perfluoroalkyl substances (PFASs) during pregnancy and childhood allergy and asthma related outcomes and infections in the Norwegian Mother and Child (MoBa) cohort. Environ Int 124:462–472
45. Johnson-Restrepo B, Kannan K (2009) An assessment of sources and pathways of human exposure to polybrominated diphenyl ethers in the United States. Chemosphere 76:542–548
46. Kanazawa A, Saito I, Araki A, Takeda M, Ma M, Saijo Y, Kishi R (2010) Association between indoor exposure to semi-volatile organic compounds and building-related symptoms among the occupants of residential dwellings. Indoor Air 20:72–84
47. Kaneko H, Matsui E, Shinoda S, Kawamoto N, Nakamura Y, Uehara R, Matsuura N, Morita M, Tada H, Kondo N (2006) Effects of dioxins on the quantitative levels of immune components in infants. Toxicol Ind Health 22:131–136
48. Koike E, Yanagisawa R, Sadakane K, Inoue K, Ichinose T, Takano H (2010) Effects of diisononyl phthalate on atopic dermatitis in vivo and immunologic responses in vitro. Environ Health Perspect 118:472–478
49. Koike E, Yanagisawa R, Takigami H, Takano H (2013) Brominated flame retardants stimulate mouse immune cells in vitro. J Appl Toxicol 33:1451–1459
50. Kojima H, Takeuchi S, Itoh T, Iida M, Kobayashi S, Yoshida T (2013) In vitro endocrine disruption potential of organophosphate flame retardants via human nuclear receptors. Toxicology 314:76–83
51. Kolarik B, Naydenov K, Larsson M, Bornehag CG, Sundell J (2008) The association between phthalates in dust and allergic diseases among Bulgarian children. Environ Health Perspect 116:98–103

52. Krivoshiev BV, Beemster GTS, Sprangers K, Cuypers B, Laukens K, Blust R, Husson SJ (2018) Toxicogenomics of the flame retardant tris (2-butoxyethyl) phosphate in HepG2 cells using RNA-seq. Toxicol in Vitro 46:178–188
53. Larsen ST, Lund RM, Nielsen GD, Thygesen P, Poulsen OM (2002) Adjuvant effect of di-n-butyl-, di-n-octyl-, di-iso-nonyl- and di-iso-decyl phthalate in a subcutaneous injection model using BALB/c mice. Pharmacol Toxicol 91:264–272
54. Linares V, Bellés M, Domingo JL (2015) Human exposure to PBDE and critical evaluation of health hazards. Arch Toxicol 89:335–356
55. Lyche JL, Rosseland C, Berge G, Polder A (2015) Human health risk associated with brominated flame-retardants (BFRs). Environ Int 74:170–180
56. Meng G, Nie Z, Feng Y, Wu X, Yin Y, Wang Y (2016) Typical halogenated persistent organic pollutants in indoor dust and the associations with childhood asthma in Shanghai, China. Environ Pollut 211:389–398
57. Miyashita C, Bamai YA, Araki A, Itoh S, Minatoya M, Kobayashi A, Kajiwara J, Hori T, Kishi R (2018) Prenatal exposure to dioxin-like compounds is associated with decreased cord blood IgE and increased risk of wheezing in children aged up to 7 years: The Hokkaido study. Sci Total Environ 610:191–199
58. Miyashita C, Sasaki S, Saijo Y, Washino N, Okada E, Kobayashi S, Konishi K, Kajiwara J, Todaka T, Kishi R (2011) Effects of prenatal exposure to dioxin-like compounds on allergies and infections during infancy. Environ Res 111:551–558
59. Morgan MK, Jones PA, Calafat AM, Ye X, Croghan CW, Chuang JC, Wilson NK, Clifton MS, Figueroa Z, Sheldon LS (2011) Assessing the quantitative relationships between preschool children's exposures to bisphenol A by route and urinary biomonitoring. Environ Sci Technol 45:5309–5316
60. Nagayama J, Tsuji H, Iida T, Nakagawa R, Matsueda T, Hirakawa H, Yanagawa T, Fukushige J, Watanabe T (2007) Immunologic effects of perinatal exposure to dioxins, PCBs and organochlorine pesticides in Japanese infants. Chemosphere 67:S393–S398
61. Okada E, Kashino I, Matsuura H, Sasaki S, Miyashita C, Yamamoto J, Ikeno T, Ito YM, Matsumura T, Tamakoshi A, Kishi R (2013) Temporal trends of perfluoroalkyl acids in plasma samples of pregnant women in Hokkaido, Japan, 2003–2011. Environ Int 60:89–96
62. Okada E, Sasaki S, Kashino I, Matsuura H, Miyashita C, Kobayashi S, Itoh K, Ikeno T, Tamakoshi A, Kishi R (2014) Prenatal exposure to perfluoroalkyl acids and allergic diseases in early childhood. Environ Int 65:127–134
63. Okada E, Sasaki S, Saijo Y, Washino N, Miyashita C, Kobayashi S, Konishi K, Ito YM, Ito R, Nakata A, Iwasaki Y, Saito K, Nakazawa H, Kishi R (2012) Prenatal exposure to perfluorinated chemicals and relationship with allergies and infectious diseases in infants. Environ Res 112:118–125
64. Park HY, Hertz-Picciotto I, Petrik J, Palkovicova L, Kocan A, Trnovec T (2008) Prenatal PCB exposure and thymus size at birth in neonates in Eastern Slovakia. Environ Health Perspect 116:104–109
65. Potaczek DP, Harb H, Michel S, Alhamwe BA, Renz H, Tost J (2017) Epigenetics and allergy: from basic mechanisms to clinical applications. Epigenomics 9:539–571
66. Rochester JR (2013) Bisphenol A and human health: A review of the literature. Reprod Toxicol 42:132–155
67. Sandilands A, Terron-Kwiatkowski A, Hull PR, O'Regan GM, Clayton TH, Watson RM, Carrick T, Evans AT, Liao H, Zhao Y, Campbell LE, Schmuth M, Gruber R, Janecke AR, Elias PM, van Steensel MA, Nagtzaam I, van Geel M, Steijlen PM, Munro CS, Bradley DG, Palmer CN, Smith FJ, McLean WH, Irvine AD (2007) Comprehensive analysis of the gene encoding filaggrin uncovers prevalent and rare mutations in ichthyosis vulgaris and atopic eczema. Nat Genet 39:650–654
68. Smit LA, Lenters V, Hoyer BB, Lindh CH, Pedersen HS, Liermontova I, Jonsson BA, Piersma AH, Bonde JP, Toft G, Vermeulen R, Heederik D (2015) Prenatal exposure to environmental chemical contaminants and asthma and eczema in school-age children. Allergy 70:653–660

69. Spanier AJ, Kahn RS, Kunselman AR, Hornung R, Xu Y, Calafat AM, Lanphear BP (2012) Prenatal exposure to bisphenol A and child wheeze from birth to 3 years of age. Environ Health Perspect 120:916–920
70. Spanier AJ, Kahn RS, Kunselman AR, Schaefer EW, Hornung R, Xu Y, Calafat AM, Lanphear BP (2014) Bisphenol a exposure and the development of wheeze and lung function in children through age 5 years. JAMA Pediatr 168:1131–1137
71. Stein CR, McGovern KJ, Pajak AM, Maglione PJ, Wolff MS (2016) Perfluoroalkyl and polyfluoroalkyl substances and indicators of immune function in children aged 12–19 y: National Health and Nutrition Examination Survey. Pediatr Res 79:348–357
72. Sunyer J, Torrent M, Munoz-Ortiz L, Ribas-Fito N, Carrizo D, Grimalt J, Anto JM, Cullinan P (2005) Prenatal dichlorodiphenyldichloroethylene (DDE) and asthma in children. Environ Health Perspect 113:1787–1790
73. ten Tusscher GW, Steerenberg PA, van Loveren H, Vos JG, von dem Borne AE, Westra M, van der Slikke JW, Olie K, Pluim HJ, Koppe JG (2003) Persistent hematologic and immunologic disturbances in 8-year-old Dutch children associated with perinatal dioxin exposure. Environ Health Perspect 111:1519–1523
74. Townsend MK, Franke AA, Li X, Hu FB, Eliassen AH (2013) Within-person reproducibility of urinary bisphenol A and phthalate metabolites over a 1 to 3 year period among women in the Nurses' Health Studies: a prospective cohort study. Environ Health 12:80
75. van der Veen I, de Boer J (2012) Phosphorus flame retardants: properties, production, environmental occurrence, toxicity and analysis. Chemosphere 88:1119–1153
76. Vernet C, Pin I, Giorgis-Allemand L, Philippat C, Benmerad M, Quentin J, Calafat AM, Ye X, Annesi-Maesano I, Siroux V, Slama R, Group, E.M.C.C.S (2017) In utero exposure to select phenols and phthalates and respiratory health in five-year-old boys: a prospective study. Environ Health Perspect 125:097006
77. Vuong AM, Braun JM, Webster GM, Thomas Zoeller R, Hoofnagle AN, Sjödin A, Yolton K, Lanphear BP, Chen A (2018a) Polybrominated diphenyl ether (PBDE) exposures and thyroid hormones in children at age 3 years. Environ Int 117:339–347
78. Wang M, Park JS, Petreas M (2011) Temporal changes in the levels of perfluorinated compounds in California women's serum over the past 50 years. Environ Sci Technol 45:7510–7516
79. Weisglas-Kuperus N, Patandin S, Berbers GA, Sas TC, Mulder PG, Sauer PJ, Hooijkaas H (2000) Immunologic effects of background exposure to polychlorinated biphenyls and dioxins in Dutch preschool children. Environ Health Perspect 108:1203–1207
80. Weisglas-Kuperus N, Vreugdenhil HJ, Mulder PG (2004) Immunological effects of environmental exposure to polychlorinated biphenyls and dioxins in Dutch school children. Toxicol Lett 149:281–285
81. WHO (1998) Frame Retardants: Tris(chloropropyl)phosphate and Tris(2-chloroethyl) Phosphate. World Health Organization, Geneva
82. WHO (2000) Flame Retardants: Tris (2-butoxyethyl) phosphate, Tris (2-ethylhexyl)phosphate and Tetrakis (hydroxymethyl)phosphonium salt. World Health Organization, Geneva
83. WHO (2012) Endocrine disruptoers and child health: possible developmental early effects of endocrine disrupters on child health. World Health Organization, Geneva
84. WHO/UNEP. State of the science of endocrine disrupting chemicals – 2012. 2013
85. Yan H, Takamoto M, Sugane K (2008) Exposure to Bisphenol A prenatally or in adulthood promotes T(H)2 cytokine production associated with reduction of CD4CD25 regulatory T cells. Environ Health Perspect 116:514–519
86. Zeng XW, Bloom MS, Dharmage SC, Lodge CJ, Chen D, Li S, Guo Y, Roponen M, Jalava P, Hirvonen MR, Ma H, Hao YT, Chen W, Yang M, Chu C, Li QQ, Hu LW, Liu KK, Yang BY, Liu S, Fu C, Dong GH (2019) Prenatal exposure to perfluoroalkyl substances is associated with lower hand, foot and mouth disease viruses antibody response in infancy: findings from the Guangzhou Birth Cohort Study. Sci Total Environ 663:60–67
87. Zhang Z, Alomirah H, Cho HS, Li YF, Liao C, Minh TB, Mohd MA, Nakata H, Ren N, Kannan K (2011) Urinary bisphenol A concentrations and their implications for human exposure in several Asian countries. Environ Sci Technol 45:7044–7050

Early-Life Social and Economic Adversities on Health

Omar Ben Forge Risk, Hein Tun, Logan Manikam, and Monica Lakhanpaul

1 Introduction

With more than 9 out of 10 pollution-related deaths occurring in low- and middle-income countries, the Lancet Commission on pollution and health states it bluntly: pollution disproportionately kills the poor and the vulnerable [1] with children at higher risk due to the cumulative effects of antenatal and early life exposure. This chapter aims to delineate the mechanisms through which these exposures, in particular during the first 1000 days of life, influence children's health throughout the life course. Key concepts such as the life course approach, social determinants of health, and health inequity are explained alongside their relevance to environmental health and disease using a case study of informal settlements in Freetown, Sierra Leone.

O. B. F. Risk (✉) · M. Lakhanpaul
Population, Policy and Practice Research and Teaching Department, UCL Great Ormond Street Institute of Child Health, University College London, London, UK
e-mail: o.risk@ucl.ac.uk

H. Tun
HKU-Pasteur Research Pole, School of Public Health, Li Ka Shing Faculty of Medicine, The University of Hong Kong, Pok Fu Lam, Hong Kong

L. Manikam
Research Department of Epidemiology & Public Health, UCL Institute of Epidemiology & Health Care, University College London Institute of Child Health, London, UK

Aceso Global Health Consultants Ltd, Delhi, India

Y. Xia (ed.), *Early-life Environmental Exposure and Disease*,
https://doi.org/10.1007/978-981-15-3797-4_10

Box 1 Types of Environmental Pollutants Associated with Health Risks [1]

- Air
  - Household air
  - Ambient particulate
  - Ambient ozone
- Water
  - Unsafe sanitation
  - Unsafe source
- Occupational
  - Carcinogens
  - Particulates
- Lead
- Soil, heavy metals, and chemicals

2 Sustainable Development, Child Health, and Pollution

Pollution, child health, and early life adversity are closely linked. This is recognised explicitly in the Sustainable Development Goals (SDGs), the United Nation's accountable targets to equitably and sustainably improve the lives of the world's population [2]. The SDGs are a set of 17 goals that make global and interconnected commitments to improve human health and well-being, through specific targets that act on inequality, climate change, pollution, and peace (Box 2). Within goal 3 (good health and well-being), target 3.9 is a specific call to environmental action in the context of health to "substantially reduce the number of deaths and illnesses from hazardous chemicals and air, water, and soil pollution and contamination". In the UNICEF 2019 report "Progress for Every Child", these targets are organised into five child-relevant domains. Within one of these domains, *every child lives in a clean and safe environment* (with indicators on reliance on clean fuels; deaths from air pollution and disasters; and access to safe drinking water, sanitation, and hygiene), it finds that progress worldwide towards every child living in a clean and safe environment by 2030 is mixed, with many indicators requiring acceleration to be achieved (Fig. 1).

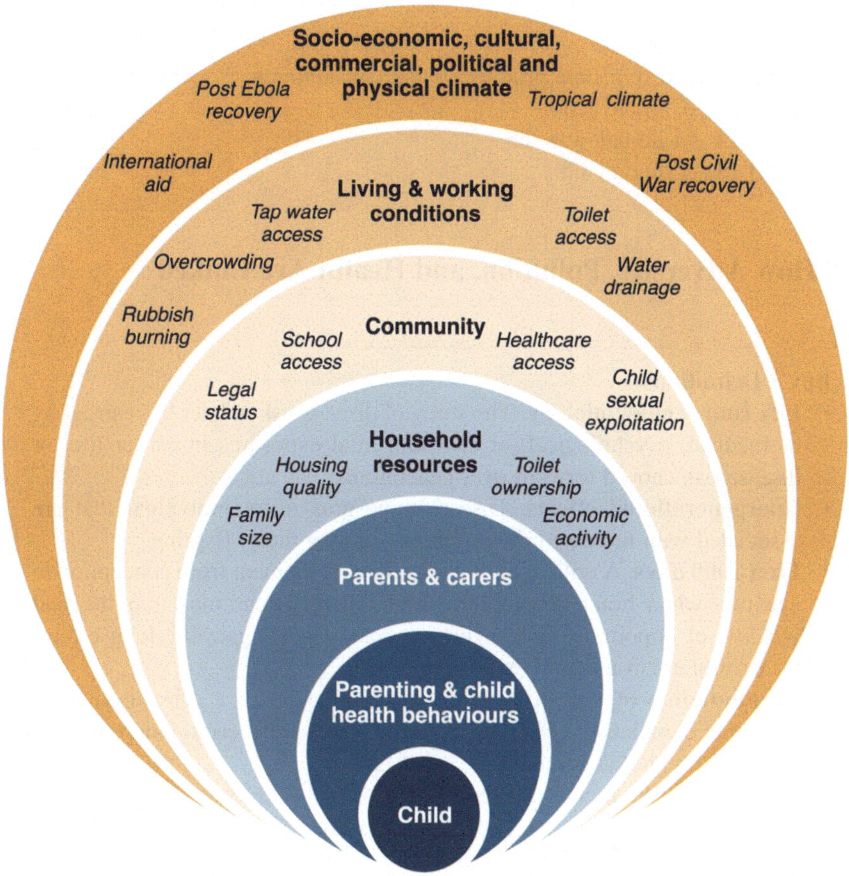

Fig. 1 This is a socioecological model of determinants of child health [3] using examples from the case study on informal settlements in Sierra Leone. The child is represented at the centre, and concentric circles represent a hierarchy of increasingly structural factors

Box 2 Pollution-related Sustainable Development Goals

- **Target 2.4** – "…progressively improve land and soil quality"
- **Target 3.9** – "substantially reduce the number of deaths and illnesses from hazardous chemicals and air, water, and soil pollution and contamination"
- **Goal 6** – Clean water and sanitation
- **Goal 7** – Affordable and clean energy
- **Target 9.4** – "…adoption of clean and environmentally sound technologies and industrial processes…"
- **Goal 11** – Sustainable cities and communities

(continued)

Box 2 (continued)

- **Goal 12** – Responsible production and consumption
- **Goal 13** – Climate action
- **Goal 14** – Life below water
- **Goal 15** – Life on land

3 How Adversity, Pollution, and Health Are Linked

Box 3 Definitions

- **Life course epidemiology**: The study of disease risk in later life carried by biomedical, psychological, or environmental exposures in earlier life; or disease risk carried forward over generations
- **Intergenerational effects**: Disease exposures in an individual that are associated with increased risk of disease among their offspring
- **First 1000 days**: A critical period in child development from conception to age two when brain development and growth occur most rapidly, and window of opportunity when interventions can mitigate life-long effects of harmful environmental exposures
- **Accumulation of risk**: The increasing probability of a disease outcome with the cumulative effect of multiple exposures, each independently associated with that outcome
- **Chains of risk**: Increasing probability of a disease outcome as certain exposures increase the risk of further exposures

Individual health is influenced by societal factors. These are known as the social determinants of health: the material, psychosocial, structural, and behavioural "conditions in which we are born, grow up, work and live" [3] that exert protective or harmful downstream effects on individual health. Put simply, they are the potentially modifiable "causes of the causes" of ill-health [4], interacting to mitigate or exacerbate one another (Fig. 2).

Identifying how societal factors influence health can be complex, especially if exposures are separated from outcomes by long periods of time. Life course epidemiology originated from the *foetal origins* hypothesis that antenatal exposures during critical periods of in utero life "programmed" organs and systems to be more vulnerable to chronic disease in adulthood, as opposed to a focus on adult health behaviours alone predicting adult health outcomes. The emphasis is on the timing and links between different exposures and disease at different stages of the life course. [5] A key concept is the *accumulation of risk* or *chains of risk* from repeated or multiple different exposures over time. This is visualised in Fig. 3 [5].

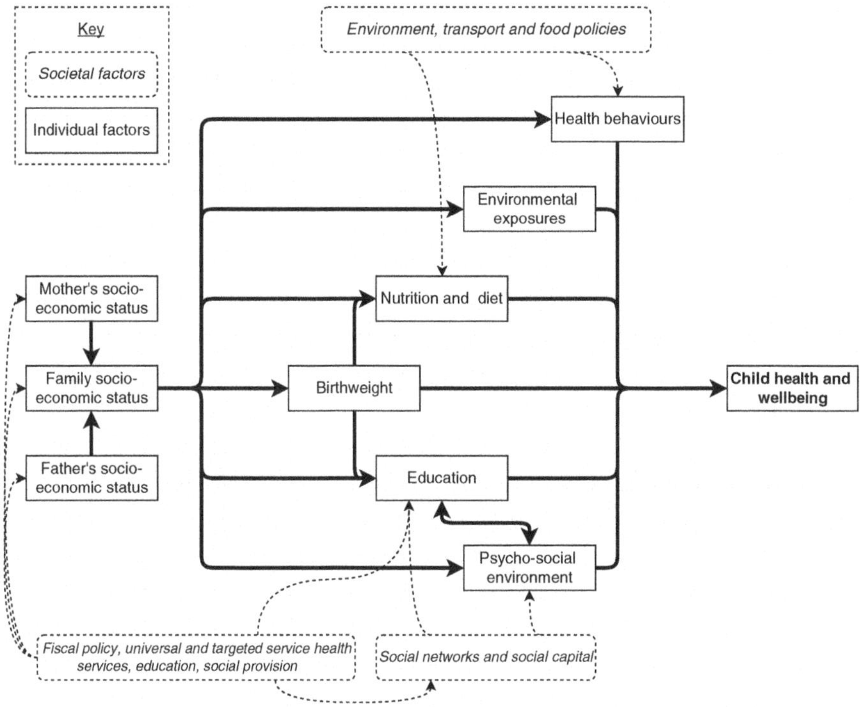

Fig. 2 This flow diagram is replicated from a review of the social determinants of child health [7]. The researchers used observational data to propose an explanatory pathway for how social risk factors exert influence on health outcomes throughout the life course, including the temporal relationship between these factors, such as intergenerational effects. In the diagram, "environmental exposures" refers to pollution, which we define here in Box 1. Infections such as diarrhoeal diseases, respiratory disease, and malaria play a crucial role in child health and well-being but are not directly referenced

The case study below highlights how children growing up in poverty face the double jeopardy of increased exposure to toxic pollutants. During the first 1000 days from a child's conception to their second birthday, children are particularly vulnerable to toxic environmental exposures. Examples include the disease risk carried by teratogens in utero and neurotoxins during infancy. This critical period is a time when the brain is developing most rapidly and is becoming more complex, interconnected, and organised. During this period, it is thought to be more malleable under environmental influence, either for better or for worse. Exposures are embodied and carry long-term disease risks. If not corrected during this period, stunting tends to be irreversible, with effects throughout the life course and across generations. Stunted growth in girls is carried forward in adulthood and in their offspring [6]. Conversely, the first 1000 days can also be thought of a *window of opportunity* to intervene to mitigate socially patterned disease exposures. Positive interventions in

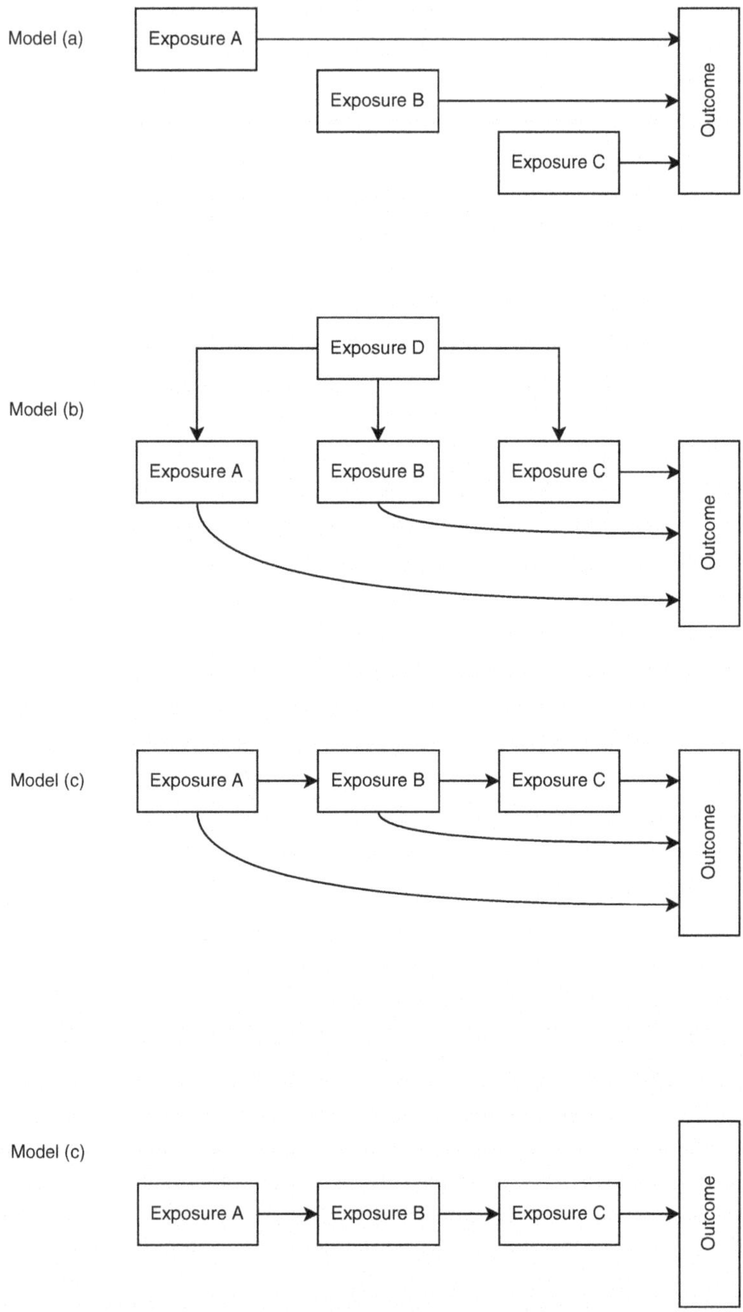

Fig. 3 Accumulation of risk [5]
Model (a) shows that multiple different exposures may occur sequentially but be independently associated with the outcome of interest.
Alternatively, as per Model (b), exposures may group together because they are each associated with some other risk factor as well as with the long-term outcome.

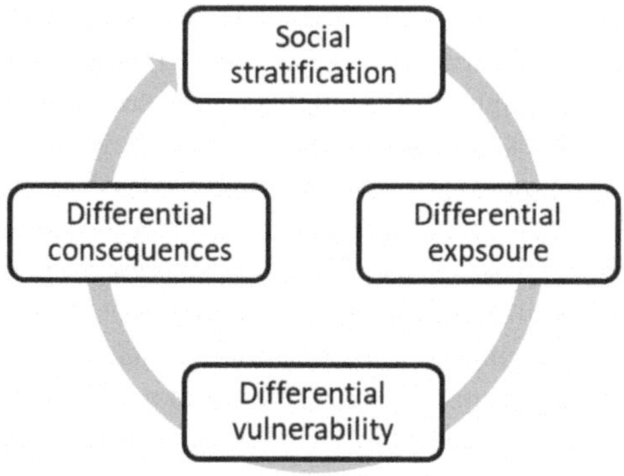

Fig. 4 Mechanisms of health inequity
Social stratification: Individual children's socioeconomic circumstances are made unequal by prevailing political, cultural, and economic structures
Differential exposure: Disadvantaged children take a greater share of health risks
Differential vulnerability: Early life adversity exposes children to worse outcomes from the same risk factors compared with their counterparts
Differential consequences: Impacts of ill-health have greater effects on the well-being and life chances of disadvantaged children

this period can have long-lasting effects to improve health throughout life and across generations.

4 Case Study: Informal Settlements in Freetown, Sierra Leone

This case study considers informal settlements in Freetown, Sierra Leone, as an example of how environmental injustice interacts with health inequity and mediates health risks. Informal settlements in the Sierra Leonean capital Freetown proliferated during the horrific 1992–2002 civil war when people living in rural areas were displaced to the relative safety of the Freetown peninsular. Since the war, economic forces have meant that internal migration and urbanisation have continued for Sierra Leone's population of 7,396,000 people. Densely populated informal settlements such as Dwarzak and Moyiba in the hills around Freetown and on reclaimed

Fig. 3 (continued) Another key concept is chains of risk whereby certain exposures give rise to a given probability of further exposures, as in Models (c) and (d). Model (c) implies each exposure independently carries a risk of disease, as well as accumulating risk by increasing the probability of further exposures;
Model (d) implies a causative chain leading to a trigger event which leads to disease whereby earlier exposures have minimal influence on risk without the final link.

mangroves in its coastal areas such as Cockle Bay, Kroobay, and Portee-Rokupa are home to large proportion of Freetown's urban poor (Picture 1).

Sierra Leone has very high child mortality rates, despite drastic improvements versus one and two decades ago (see Table 1). In Freetown's informal settlements, rates are likely to be even more dire. Child mortality in Sierra Leone is largely driven by infection in the first 1000 days and beyond, particularly malaria, lower respiratory infections, and diarrhoeal diseases (see Table 2). Epidemiological and demographic data at the local level is difficult to collect in these areas, but one study of verbal autopsies sought from community members in Freetown informal settlements suggested that the leading reported cause of death in neonates was pneumonia, and in children up to 5 years was malaria followed by pneumonia [10]. The Sierra Leone Urban Research Centre [11] recently reported the findings of their mixed methods study on the health impacts of living in Freetown's informal settlements, which informs the following discussion of the multitude of socially mediated pollution exposures that harm child health.

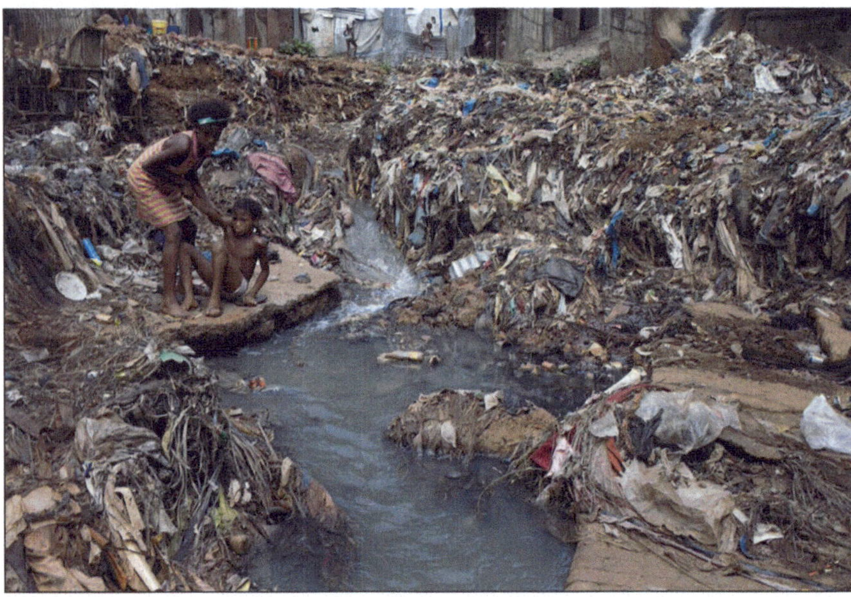

Picture 1 Crocodile River, Kroobay, Freetown, Sierra Leone. Photographer: Dominic Chavez

Table 1 Mortality estimates for Sierra Leone [8]

Deaths/1000 live births (90% CI)	1998	2008	2018
Neonatal: First 28 days of life	52 (45 to 59)	44 (38 to 50)	33 (24 to 43)
Infant: Birth to age 1	147 (139 to 155)	117 (110 to 124)	78 (66 to 91)
Under 5: Birth to age 5	244 (227 to 262)	180 (167 to 195)	105 (85 to 128)

Table 2 Top five causes of death by age in Sierra Leone, 2008 to 2017 [9]

1 to 7 days	8 to 28 days	29 days to 1 year	1 to 4 years
Neonatal disorders	Neonatal disorders	Malaria	Malaria
Congenital birth defects	Lower respiratory infections	Lower respiratory infections	Lower respiratory infections
Lower respiratory infections	Malaria	Diarrhoeal diseases	Diarrhoeal diseases
Syphilis	Congenital birth defects	Congenital birth defects	Protein-energy malnutrition
Diarrhoeal diseases	Diarrhoeal diseases	Protein-energy malnutrition	Congenital birth defects

Local geography makes the Freetown peninsular one of the rainiest parts of West Africa, and flooding is a constant risk for residents: however, the inhabitants of informal settlements are extremely vulnerable in particular. Deforestation and dense settlement in the hills around Freetown undermine the soil structure, increasing the risk of flooding and landslides. This is compounded by a lack of effective drainage. Landslides and flash flooding in 2017 killed at least 500 people and displaced over 5900. The most significant event was a six-kilometre mudslide that destroyed 300 homes. Although not directly related to pollution as defined here (see Box 1), environmental factors like deforestation and housing quality that have a direct deleterious effect on the health of children and their families are interacting with social factors like population density, urban migration, and poverty.

Informal settlements located on reclaimed mangroves in coastal areas of Freetown are less than a metre above sea level leaving children and their families at constant risk of flooding. Pools of standing water provide ideal conditions for Anopheles mosquitoes, with malaria being one of the leading causes of childhood mortality in Sierra Leone (see Table 2). Water distribution through PVC piping, which is vulnerable to damage, runs through areas where open defecation takes place, leaving children and their families with limited access to clean water sources and vulnerable to diarrhoeal disease. Water pumped from boreholes is highly saline and residents face long waits for tap water with variable availability. The burden of collecting water often falls to boys and girls: adolescent girls are coerced into what one author describes as "transactional sex" in return for quicker access to water [12]. This exposes them to the possibility of adolescent pregnancy and the health risks associated with it for both the mother and her child, as well as psychological trauma, injury, and sexually transmitted infections.

Diarrhoeal diseases are a leading driver of child mortality in Sierra Leone (see Table 2). Cholera, typhoid, and coliforms are spread rapidly in part because of a lack of good quality sewerage infrastructure. In general, toilet ownership for residents in these communities is uncommon with shared toilets being the norm. Most human waste is destined for pits, streams, or the sea. This leads to significant coliform contamination of water sources, which is compounded by flooding during rainy season. The same streams which are contaminated with human waste are regularly used as water sources for laundry and bathing.

In the absence of effective infrastructure for household waste disposal, these communities face a build-up of refuse. Children often play in piles of waste, which include not only domestic waste but especially hazardous materials like clinical waste from health facilities. This potentially exposes them to the risk of injury, heavy metal poisoning, chemical burns, and infections. If waste has not been discarded into the streams, it is discarded into the sea as a form of land reclamation.

Commonly, this household waste is piled up and burnt in the open. Regularly seen rising from certain areas of the city, smog is a visual reminder of the poisonous cocktail of particulates and invisible noxious gases accumulating from several different combustion sources. As seen in Table 2, pneumonia is a leading cause of childhood death in Sierra Leone. From 2018 to 2019, a diesel burning power station on a converted cargo ship was moored close to the shore of Kroobay to meet Freetown's energy deficit. There is strong evidence that ambient air pollution, diesel in particular, harms the respiratory health of children especially; for example through pneumonia and exacerbations of asthma, and through life course effects via maternal exposure during pregnancy and via laying the foundation for cardiovascular disease in adulthood [13–16]. At the same time, solid fuels are the primary energy and cooking source for many households. Solid fuel use is strongly associated with childhood pneumonia and bronchiolitis, with children and women particularly vulnerable to exposure [17–19].

5 Child Health Inequity and Its Mechanisms

Box 4 Definitions

- **Horizontal equity**: a group of people with equal need are treated in an equal way
- **Vertical equity**: different groups with different needs are treated in proportionately different ways
- **Inequity**: "differences among groups that are unnecessary, avoidable, unfair and unjust" [20].
- **Health inequity**: unjust and avoidable differences in how the burden of health outcomes such as low birth weight, under five mortality, infectious disease, or asthma are shared in society
- **Child health equity**: a goal that sees all children having an equal opportunity to be healthy, regardless of the circumstances in which they are born; related to a domain of Sustainable Development Goals, that *every child thrives and survives* [21].

The increased exposure to toxic pollutants described in the case study is driven by poverty and other social factors. It leads to increased burden of disease among children growing up in these informal settlements. Not only is this increased burden unfair, it is also avoidable. It is estimated that under five mortality among Freetown's urban poor could be reduced by 80% through improvements in children's living environment [22]. These socially determined health inequities are thought to be mediated by four overarching mechanisms [23].

The principal mechanism is *social stratification*, whereby inhabitants of Freetown's informal settlements lack the social, financial, and political capital to escape hazardous and perilous living conditions. This leads to *differential exposure*, with wealthier communities in Freetown able to afford to have clean water delivered, or live in accommodation with a safe functioning toilet, reducing children's exposure to harmful environmental hazards. This is compounded by *differential vulnerability*, for example their increased exposure to ambient and household air pollution and associated risk of respiratory infection is made worse by their stunted physiological reserve due to poor nutrition or low birth weight. Early life adversity leads to *differential consequences*. When they get sick, their access to medical care is not adequate. Because they have not received planning permission, these settlements are seen by local and central government as illegal, which disempowers poor families even further and inhibits communities' access to the limited amount of public services that do exist. These factors in turn have effects on school attendance, work-readiness, and future employment, embedding social inequalities yet deeper to lead to *further social stratification* and perpetuate the *chain of risk* across generations.

6 Conclusion

Box 5 Key Points of This Chapter

- Health risks and health outcomes are not distributed equally in society
- Children living in poverty are disproportionately affected by the health risks of pollution
- Health and disease are in part socially determined, as opposed to being influenced only by individual factors
- The social determinants of health are the multifactorial "causes of the causes" of disease and interact with each other to have downstream effects on health
- Early life exposures have effects throughout the life course as well across generations, and there are epidemiological tools to establish these associations

This chapter has hopefully highlighted how environmental exposures in childhood, especially in the first 1000 days, interact with poverty and other social factors to impact on children's health throughout the life course. The early years are a critical period. Growing up in poverty and challenging environments leads to exposure to pollutants. These have a direct adverse effect on health through infection, growth, and brain development, as well as interacting with the indirect effects of social factors such as poor quality housing and dense population. These factors have a feedback effect, for example a child who has poor light and who can't concentrate due to malnutrition will be less work ready and less able to have the means to mitigate these factors to improve the health of their own children. Improvements in child health require improvements in the social milieu in which they grow up. There are opportunities to intervene during this period to reduce burden of disease both in childhood and in later life.

References

1. Landrigan PJ, Fuller R, Acosta NJR et al (2018) The lancet commission on pollution and health. Lancet 391(10119):462–512
2. United Nations. Transforming our world: the 2030 agenda for sustainable development. In: Assembly G, ed. Vol 12015
3. Pearce A, Dundas R, Whitehead M, Taylor-Robinson D (2019) Pathways to inequalities in child health. Arch Dis Child 104(10):998–1003
4. Marmot M (2015) The health gap: the challenge of an unequal world. Lancet 386 (10011):2442–2444
5. Kuh D, Ben-Shlomo Y, Lynch J, Hallqvist J, Power C (2003) Life course epidemiology. J Epidemiol Community Health 57(10):778–783
6. Georgiadis A, Penny ME (2017) Child undernutrition: opportunities beyond the first 1000 days. Lancet Public Health 2(9):e399
7. Spencer N (2018) The social determinants of child health. Paediatr Child Health 28(3):138–143
8. UN Inter-agency Group for Child Mortality Estimation. https://childmortality.org/. Published 2019. Accessed
9. The Global Burden of Disease Collaborative (2018) Global, regional, and national age-sex-specific mortality for 282 causes of death in 195 countries and territories, 1980–2017: a systematic analysis for the Global Burden of Disease Study 2017. The Lancet 392 (10159):1736–178
10. Hutain J, Perry HB, Koffi AK et al (2019) Engaging communities in collecting and using results from verbal autopsies for child deaths: an example from urban slums in Freetown, Sierra Leone. J Glob Health 9(1):010419
11. Macarthy JC A, Sellu S, Heinrich L. (2018) Health impacts of the living conditions of people residing in informal settlements in Freetown
12. November L, Sandall J (2018) 'Just because she's young, it doesn't mean she has to die': exploring the contributing factors to high maternal mortality in adolescents in Eastern Freetown; a qualitative study. Reprod Health 15(1):31
13. Cohen AJ, Brauer M, Burnett R et al (2017) Estimates and 25-year trends of the global burden of disease attributable to ambient air pollution: an analysis of data from the global burden of diseases study 2015. Lancet 389(10082):1907–1918

14. Nhung NTT, Amini H, Schindler C et al (2017) Short-term association between ambient air pollution and pneumonia in children: a systematic review and meta-analysis of time-series and case-crossover studies. Environ Pollut 230:1000–1008
15. Lelieveld J, Haines A, Pozzer A (2018) Age-dependent health risk from ambient air pollution: a modelling and data analysis of childhood mortality in middle-income and low-income countries. Lancet Planet Health 2(7):e292–e300
16. Liu NM, Grigg J (2018) Diesel, children and respiratory disease. BMJ Paediatrics Open 2(1): e000210
17. Bates MN, Chandyo RK, Valentiner-Branth P et al (2013) Acute lower respiratory infection in childhood and household fuel use in Bhaktapur, Nepal. Environ Health Perspect 121 (5):637–642
18. Gordon SB, Bruce NG, Grigg J et al (2014) Respiratory risks from household air pollution in low and middle income countries. Lancet Respir Med 2(10):823–860
19. Simkovich SM, Goodman D, Roa C et al (2019) The health and social implications of household air pollution and respiratory diseases. NPJ Prim Care Respir Med 29(1):12–12
20. Whitehead M (1992) The concepts and principles of equity and health. Int J Health Serv 22 (3):429–445
21. UNICEF (2019) Progress for every child in the SDG Era: are we on track to achieve the SDGs for children? The situation in 2019
22. UN-HABITAT (2006) The Improvement of Slums and Informal Settlements in Freetown
23. Diderichsen F, Evans T, Whitehead M (2001) The social basis of disparities in health. In: Evans T (ed) Challenging inequities in health from ethics to action. Oxford University Press, Oxford

Endocrine-Disrupting Chemical Exposure and Later-Onset Diseases

Di Wu and Guizhen Du

1 Introduction

The 'developmental origins of health and disease' (DOHaD) concept posits that adverse environmental factors in early life can affect one's health status and increase disease risks in childhood and adult life. Originally based on association studies between in utero nutrition and childhood health, the concept has now given rise to a field that brings together a wide range of factors, including lifestyle, nutrition, chemical exposure, and genetic heredity [1].

In the past half century, chemicals were used widely in plastics, flame retardants, pesticides, industrial solvents, and pharmaceuticals to improve life quality, which caused widespread exposure to these chemicals among children across the world. Most of these chemicals can cross the placenta and interact with genetic and epigenetic mechanisms to alter the course of normal development [2, 3]. The term endocrine-disrupting chemicals (EDCs) has risen from total obscurity to becoming nearly a household term now. EDCs, as exogenous chemicals, can affect the endocrine system through multiple pathways that target different levels of the hypothalamic-pituitary-gonad, thyroid and adrenal axes, ranging from altering hormone synthesis to affecting hormone metabolism. Therefore, they can increase or inhibit normal endocrine function and have far-reaching health implications throughout the entire lifetime [2].

Early-life exposures are especially of concern because children undergo rapid development that is susceptible to even small doses of environmental stressors. Compared to adults, they have frequent hand-to-mouth or object-to-mouth activities, thus increasing their chances of exposure to contaminated soil and dust. There is evidence that prenatal and/or early postnatal EDC exposure during development

D. Wu · G. Du (✉)
School of Public Health, Nanjing Medical University, Nanjing, China
e-mail: guizhendu@njmu.edu.cn

Y. Xia (ed.), *Early-life Environmental Exposure and Disease*,
https://doi.org/10.1007/978-981-15-3797-4_11

may have lifelong ramifications, increasing the risk of developing chronic diseases including diabetes, obesity, cardiovascular disease, cancer, and infertility later in life. Thus, this review provides a brief introduction to several common EDCs and an overview of their adverse effects on later-onset health problems. Given the important role of epigenetics in the relationship between EDC exposure and later-onset diseases, our review will first give an overview about the EDC exposure and later-onset diseases and then highlight several represented EDCs and their potential epigenetic mechanisms in diseases.

2 BPA Exposure and Later Health

BPA is one of the well-studied EDCs that had been shown to have an impact on epigenetic regulation of gene expression. BPA is a high-production chemical with estrogenic activity used in food cans, bottle tops, and drink packaging, such as plastic water containers and baby bottles. BPA is also detected in medical equipment, as infants in the neonatal intensive care unit have been shown to have elevated exposure levels [4]. It has been known to be weakly estrogenic for 75 years, and recent animal studies have reported a diverse variety of developmental problems following early-life exposure such as altered reproductive organ development and neurobehavioral effects. There is increasing evidence from animal studies that in utero and/or neonatal exposure to BPA produces a broad range of adverse adult outcomes, including impaired sexual behavior and reproductive function, immune system dysregulation, and cancer [5–8].

In utero BPA exposure may induce alterations in the gene expression in multiple tissues, including brain and spleen, that may persist into adulthood. Data from recent studies indicate that early-life exposure to BPA can affect postnatal developmental landmarks such as weight of the pups at birth and reduced anogenital distance [9]. The developmental exposure of rats to low-dose BPA has been also found to increase prostate gland susceptibility to adult-onset precancerous lesions and hormonal carcinogenesis [8]. Environmentally relevant doses of BPA exposure in the critical window of prostate development resulted in increasing susceptibility to carcinogenesis [10].

3 Perfluorinated Compound (PFC) Exposure and Later Health

PFCs are man-made fluorinated chemicals used in numerous industrial and consumer products. PFCs are persistent, and some of the substances bioaccumulate in the environment. Perfluorooctanesulfonic acid (PFOS) and perfluorooctanoic acid (PFOA), often referred to as reference or key substances for the PFCs, have been most intensively studied from a toxicological standpoint. Perfluorinated alkyl substances (PFAs, such as PFOA and PFOS) are almost universally detected in the serum of pregnant women, neonates, and children worldwide, which indicates that exposure is ubiquitous and these chemicals can cross the placenta [11, 12]. Unlike BPA, PFAs have long biological half-life in humans, which range from 3.8 to 7.3 years [13]. The sources and relative contributions of different PFAs to human exposure vary according to age-related behavioral factors and dietary patterns. PFA exposures during infancy can be equal or exceed prenatal exposures derived from the mother [14]. For instance, breast milk and formula might contribute almost exclusively to an infant's exposure, as PFAs are found in breast milk and water, and infants consume up to sixfold more fluid than adults (150 versus 26 mL/kg/day) [15].

Numerous evidences exist, suggesting that prenatal exposure to PFAs could affect fetal growth and subsequent risk of childhood obesity. In a recent meta-analysis, increasing prenatal PFOA exposure was associated with a 19 g decrease in birth weight [16]. These results in humans are similar to those observed in animal studies where each 1 mg/kg/day increase in PFOA exposure was associated with a 0.023 g decrease in pup birth weight [17]. Altered fetal growth patterns related to PFA exposure might increase the risk of subsequent obesity and cardio-metabolic disorders, as earlier studies have shown that fetal growth deceleration and infant growth acceleration are associated with increased adiposity and levels of cardiometabolic risk markers in later childhood [18, 19]. Consistent with this statement, prospective cohort data showed that prenatal PFA exposure was associated with alterations in infant or child growth and increased adiposity during childhood and adulthood [20, 21], while other studies reported contradictory findings [22].

Although the association study identified a relationship between PFA exposure and later weight gain, the potential mechanisms are still not fully determined. PFA exposure was reported to be associated with hypomethylation in sperm cells, suggesting that PFAs are potential germline epimutagens and could be tied to preconception exposure [23, 24]. PFA exposures were also associated with changes in the expression of genes involved in cholesterol metabolism, including peroxisome proliferator-activated receptors (PPARs) [25–27]. PPARs (PPARα, PPARβ, and PPARγ) belong to the class of nuclear receptors that are regulated by different lipophilic molecules ranging from xenobiotics to drugs to nutrients. PFOA and PFOS can bind to and activate PPARα or PPARγ to increase adipocyte differentiation and increase body fat [28–30].

4 Triclosan (TCS) Exposure and Later Health

TCS, as an antimicrobial chemical, is widely used in household and personal care products (PCPs) such as hand soaps, toothpastes, and deodorants. It is one of the most frequently detected and highly concentrated chemicals in the environment and in humans [31]. Compared with other EDCs, TCS does not persist, has a biological half-life of <24 h, and is primarily excreted in the urine as a glucuronide or sulfate conjugate [32]. TCS has been found in human samples including urine, serum, plasma, and human breast milk [33, 34]. TCS was detected in more than 70% of the US population, with urine concentrations ranging from 7.9 nM to 13.1 μM [35]. In China, a study showed that 80% of a sample of 209 participants tested displayed detectable levels of TCS in their urine [36]. In Australia, TCS was detected in all 2400 urine samples, with concentrations ranging from 0.08 to 0.71 μM between 2012 and 2013 [37]. In addition, females tended to exhibit higher TCS concentrations than males, and the age group with the highest TCS concentrations were people in their 20s [36, 37]. All these results indicate that TCS is widely exposed and readily absorbed into the body.

TCS was reported to be embryotoxic in cardiogenesis and osteogenesis at environmental concentrations [38, 39]. Chronic TCS exposure leads to severe toxic effects on the growth and development of blood vessels in zebrafish through dysregulation of miRNAs, which also suggested the potential molecular mechanisms of TCS-induced cardiovascular diseases [40]. A recent longitudinal study showed that prenatal exposure to TCS caused girls to experience puberty at younger ages [41]. Urinary concentrations of TCS were also associated with allergic sensitization, in particular to inhalant allergens, as well as with current rhinitis among the children [42]. There are still contradictory findings about TCS exposure and childhood obesity or excess adiposity [43–45]. Xue et al. measured the TCS urinary levels in obese and non-obese children and found no correlation between TCS exposure and obesity [43]. Li et al. used data from National Health and Nutrition Examination Survey (NHANES) 2003–2010, which included 2898 children (6–19 years old), and found that TCS exposure was inversely associated with BMI and waist circumference [44]. Another cross-sectional study from the NHANES (2007–2010) found no association between urinary TCS concentrations and BMI z-score, waist circumference, or prevalence of overweight or obesity [45]. Currently, few epidemiological studies have directly examined the neurotoxicity of early-life TCS exposure. TCS exposure might reduce serum thyroxine concentrations during pregnancy, causing adverse neurodevelopment, given the important role that thyroxine has in fetal brain development [46]. Additionally, given TCS's antimicrobial activity, it might be capable of altering the gut microbiota, which is now also considered a cause of neural diseases.

5 Particular Matter Exposure and Later Health

PM (particular matter) refers to a heterogeneous mixture of substances of air pollutants, which includes EDCs and metals, and PM2.5 is a group of PM $\leq$2.5 μm in aerodynamic diameter. PM2.5 pollution is now a global health problem, which has been reported that PM2.5 exposure affected the fetal development and caused dysfunctions of circulation system through reprogramming the heart development [47]. In rodents, exposure to PM2.5 caused cardiomyopathy, increased cardiomyocyte membrane permeability, heart failure, and myocardial fibrosis. Theses indicated that EDCs in the air pollution-induced adverse cardiorenal health later in life may begin from the fetal stage. During early development, the fetal is exposed to the maternal environment, and any stress from the EDCs will disturb the niche of the embryo and change the susceptibility to the later-onset disease. Recent epidemiological study found that exposure to PM2.5 during the earth gestation stage was significantly correlated with blood pressure in the later life, while this observation was also sex dependent and only in boys [48]. This suggested that early PM2.5 exposure can predict the adult cardiorenal health in later life.

Besides the blood pressure, PM2.5 exposure was associated with gestational diabetes mellitus [49]. Using the cohort of 3612 pregnant women in Australia during 2012–2015, Melody et al. found that nearly 20% of the cohort was exposed to the smoke event caused by the Hazelwood coal mine fire. The researcher quantified the PM2.5 exposure and found that increasing PM2.5 exposure was significantly associated with increased gestational diabetes mellitus (GDM) risk, especially in the second trimester [49]. Proposed mechanisms are that the components of PM2.5 contain numerous EDCs and evidences support the effects of EDC exposure on pancreatic β cell and GDM [50]. GDM will change the metabolic status of embryo permanently and caused the obesity and metabolic syndrome in the later life. Intrauterine exposure to GDM had significantly increased BMI, waist circumference, and blood pressure in the offspring. Unexposed offspring have a lower risk of cardiovascular disease with decreased levels of circulating cellular adhesion molecules, which are biomarkers of early stages of atherosclerosis [51].

6 EDCs and Epigenetics

The DOHaD concept has been confirmed by both animal and human epidemiological studies over the last 20 years [52, 53], while the mechanisms underlying developmental programming of adult disease remain poorly understood. Increasing evidence has suggested that epigenetic regulation might be involved in developmental programming of late-onset pathologies such as asthma, obesity, and cancers. Epigenetics is defined as changes in gene expression that occur without changes in DNA sequence and can be transmitted to offspring [53]. Two common epigenetic mechanisms are DNA methylation and post-translational modifications of histone proteins (histone modifications), and they collectively make up the major components of the epigenome.

DNA methylation is a crucial epigenetic control mechanism in mammals that can influence gene expression by regulating accessibility of transcription factors, histone modifiers, and transcriptional machinery to chromatin [54, 55]. This modification is itself highly regulated by multiple components adding and removing methyl groups. DNA methyltransferases (DNMTs) can add a methyl group from the donor S-adenosyl methionine (SAM) to the carbon-5 position of the cytosine (5 mC), while the ten-eleven translocation enzyme (TET) dioxygenase family can actively reverse this process through oxidation of 5 mC to 5-hydroxymethylcytosine (5 hmC) [54]. Besides DNA methylation, the other main epigenetic mechanism contributing to transcriptional regulation is post-translational histone modification [55]. Multiple modifications can be made to these histones including acetylation, methylation, phosphorylation, and ubiquitination, primarily on N-terminal histone tails. Epigenetic writers, readers, and erasers can recognize specific combinations of histone modification to provide a dynamic system for modulating gene expression.

EDCs affect the epigenome through the enzymes regulating epigenetic modifications and the levels of their cofactors. Neonatal exposure to diethylstilbestrol (DES) decreased both Tet1 mRNA expression and 5 hmC across the genome in the uterus of adult mice [56]. In another study, bisphenol A (BPA) treatment reduced the nuclear localization of TET2 protein in murine gonadotropin-releasing hormone (GnRH) neurons in vitro, which correlated with decreased H3K4 trimethylation at the GnRH promoter and decreased GnRH protein expression [57]. SAM is the methyl donor for virtually all methylation reactions in the cell, including methylation of DNA and histone tails. Processes that deplete intracellular SAM thus lead to a global reduction of methylation capacity. Dietary methyl donors such as folic acid mitigated DNA hypomethylation induced by BPA in the agouti mouse model [58], suggesting that SAM production is involved in the epigenetic effects of BPA. Changes to histone-modifying enzymes, particularly histone deacetylases (HDACs) and histone methyltransferases (HMTs), following exposure to EDCs have also been reported. BPA-induced histone demethylation via phosphorylation and inhibition of the repressing histone methyltransferase EZH2 has been reported [59]. Conversely, BPA-induced histone methylation via phosphorylation and activation of the histone-activating methyltransferase MLL1 has also been shown [60].

7 EDCs Affect Later Health Through Epigenetic Mechanisms

During early ontogenesis, different sets of genes are activated or deactivated in a sequential manner, providing numerous targets for environmental exposures. Therefore, the developmental period is a critically sensitive window of vulnerability because the epigenome is more labile than during adulthood. In mammalian development, gametogenesis and early embryogenesis are two main periods of enhanced sensitivity of the epigenome to environmental stimuli. In human beings, the window of epigenetic developmental plasticity extends from preconception to early childhood and involves epigenetic responses to environmental changes, which exert their effects during life-history phase transitions. The developmentally established epigenetic marks are stably maintained through somatic cell divisions and create unique, lineage-specific patterns of gene expression. Prenatal and early postnatal exposure to environmental toxicants was repeatedly found to be associated with aberrant DNA methylation of regulatory sequences in susceptible genes, leading to inappropriate gene expression and disease pathogenesis in later life.

In utero BPA exposure may induce alterations in the gene expression through epigenetic modifications. MiRNA-224 was found upregulated in BPA's effect on long-term ovarian dysfunction [9]. Besides, in utero BPA exposure increased all-trans-retinoic acid concentration and expression levels of Adh1, Aox1 and Cyp1a2 (biosynthesis of retinoic acid) in the offspring liver, which showed altered pancreatic function and impaired glucose metabolism during adulthood [61]. BPA exposure resulted in permeant promoter demethylation of PDE4D4, which is an enzyme responsible for intracellular signal induction, and upregulation of this gene increased the later-onset susceptibilities to prostate gland carcinogenesis [10]. Further complicating the study of DNA methylation and BPA exposure, fetal liver methylation alterations associated with prenatal exposure to BPA displayed a nonmonotonic association with BPA level [62, 63]. Researchers also observed significant alterations in BPA-exposed female but not male fetal livers, which indicated that prenatal exposure to BPA disrupts the mouse fetal liver maturation in a sex-specific manner [63]. In gene-specific analyses of CpG methylation as it relates to prenatal BPA exposure, differentially methylated loci associated with BPA were the small nucleolar RNA (SNORD) complex of genes, sulfotransferase family 2A member 1 (SULT2A1), and catechol-O-methyltransferase (COMT) [64].

Taking together, evidence supports sexual dimorphism and a nonmonotonic dose response of DNA methylation associated with BPA, resulting in a need for more research to understand the complicated functional consequences of BPA-associated DNA methylation alterations. Experimental evidence also showed that early-life exposure to BPA led to hypermethylation of the estrogen receptor promoter region in the adult testis, indicating that epigenetic changes may be one of the mechanisms contributing to BPA-induced adverse effects on spermatogenesis and fertility [65].

8 Conclusion

The DOHaD concept suggests that potential chemical exposures during critical windows of human development induce epigenetic changes that may lead to later-life adverse health outcomes. Not surprisingly, recent works also highlight the relationships between early EDC exposure and later-onset diseases, which demonstrate an important role for the epigenome in regulating human health against environmental signals (Fig. 1). It is a challenge to detect effects that are induced by early-life exposures but manifest as health issues later in life, or even in subsequent generations. Although the adverse effects of early exposure have been better understood as our knowledge of the epigenetics has improved, many of the details of the potential mechanisms remain unclear. Epigenetic modifications induced by EDCs can precede adverse phenotypic outcomes with/without additional stressors to act on the same pathway. Thus, epigenetic changes could also serve both as early markers of subsequent disease development and as predictive markers of increased

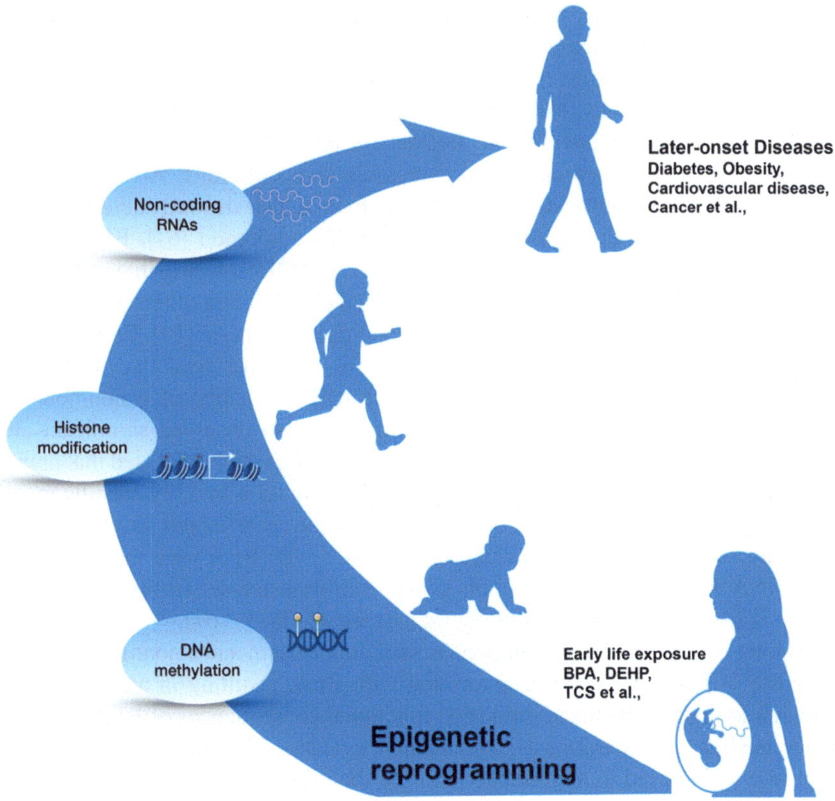

Fig. 1 EDCs exposure and later-onset diseases

susceptibility to further exposures to chemicals and other agents. Further complicating this biological picture, lifestyle, health status, and combinations of exposures also regulate the epigenome and alter later-onset diseases. Therefore, further studies deciphering effects from specific EDCs that affect the host epigenome will provide new insights in understanding the causal relationship between exposure and diseases and lead to new mechanistic insights into EDCs' risk assessment for health protection.

Acknowledgments This study was supported by the National Natural Science Foundation of China (81402706), the Natural Science Foundation of Jiangsu Province (BK20181366).

References

1. Goyal D, Limesand SW, Goyal R (2019) Epigenetic responses and the developmental origins of health and disease. J Endocrinol 242(1):T105–T119

2. Vaiserman A (2014) Early-life exposure to endocrine disrupting chemicals and later-life health outcomes: an epigenetic bridge? Aging Dis 5(6):419–429
3. Bollati V, Baccarelli A (2010) Environmental epigenetics. Heredity (Edinb) 105(1):105–112
4. Calafat AM, Weuve J, Ye X, Jia LT, Hu H, Ringer S et al (2009) Exposure to bisphenol A and other phenols in neonatal intensive care unit premature infants. Environ Health Perspect 117 (4):639–644
5. Doherty LF, Bromer JG, Zhou Y, Aldad TS, Taylor HS (2010) In utero exposure to diethylstilbestrol (DES) or bisphenol-A (BPA) increases EZH2 expression in the mammary gland: an epigenetic mechanism linking endocrine disruptors to breast cancer. Horm Cancer 1 (3):146–155
6. Veiga-Lopez A, Luense LJ, Christenson LK, Padmanabhan V (2013) Developmental programming: gestational bisphenol-A treatment alters trajectory of fetal ovarian gene expression. Endocrinology 154(5):1873–1884
7. Abi Salloum B, Steckler TL, Herkimer C, Lee JS, Padmanabhan V (2013) Developmental programming: impact of prenatal exposure to bisphenol-A and methoxychlor on steroid feedbacks in sheep. Toxicol Appl Pharmacol 268(3):300–308
8. Ho SM, Tang WY, Belmonte de Frausto J, Prins GS (2006) Developmental exposure to estradiol and bisphenol A increases susceptibility to prostate carcinogenesis and epigenetically regulates phosphodiesterase type 4 variant 4. Cancer Res 66(11):5624–5632
9. Lite C, Ahmed S, Santosh W, Seetharaman B (2019) Prenatal exposure to bisphenol-A altered miRNA-224 and protein expression of aromatase in ovarian granulosa cells concomitant with elevated serum estradiol levels in F1 adult offspring. J Biochem Mol Toxicol 33(6):e22317
10. Prins GS, Tang WY, Belmonte J, Ho SM (2008) Perinatal exposure to oestradiol and bisphenol A alters the prostate epigenome and increases susceptibility to carcinogenesis. Basic Clin Pharmacol Toxicol 102(2):134–138
11. Woodruff TJ, Zota AR, Schwartz JM (2011) Environmental chemicals in pregnant women in the United States: NHANES 2003–2004. Environ Health Perspect 119(6):878–885
12. Braun JM, Kalkbrenner AE, Just AC, Yolton K, Calafat AM, Sjodin A et al (2014) Gestational exposure to endocrine-disrupting chemicals and reciprocal social, repetitive, and stereotypic behaviors in 4- and 5-year-old children: the HOME study. Environ Health Perspect 122 (5):513–520
13. Olsen GW, Burris JM, Ehresman DJ, Froehlich JW, Seacat AM, Butenhoff JL et al (2007) Half-life of serum elimination of perfluorooctanesulfonate, perfluorohexanesulfonate, and perfluorooctanoate in retired fluorochemical production workers. Environ Health Perspect 115(9):1298–1305
14. Sunderland EM, Hu XC, Dassuncao C, Tokranov AK, Wagner CC, Allen JG (2019) A review of the pathways of human exposure to poly- and perfluoroalkyl substances (PFASs) and present understanding of health effects. J Expo Sci Environ Epidemiol 29(2):131–147
15. Post GB, Cohn PD, Cooper KR (2012) Perfluorooctanoic acid (PFOA), an emerging drinking water contaminant: a critical review of recent literature. Environ Res 116:93–117
16. Johnson PI, Sutton P, Atchley DS, Koustas E, Lam J, Sen S et al (2014) The navigation guide – evidence-based medicine meets environmental health: systematic review of human evidence for PFOA effects on fetal growth. Environ Health Perspect 122(10):1028–1039
17. Koustas E, Lam J, Sutton P, Johnson PI, Atchley DS, Sen S et al (2014) The navigation guide – evidence-based medicine meets environmental health: systematic review of nonhuman evidence for PFOA effects on fetal growth. Environ Health Perspect 122(10):1015–1027
18. Jaddoe VW, de Jonge LL, Hofman A, Franco OH, Steegers EA, Gaillard R (2014) First trimester fetal growth restriction and cardiovascular risk factors in school age children: population based cohort study. BMJ 348:g14
19. Perng W, Hajj H, Belfort MB, Rifas-Shiman SL, Kramer MS, Gillman MW et al (2016) Birth size, early life weight gain, and midchildhood cardiometabolic health. J Pediatr 173:122–130. e121

20. Braun JM, Chen A, Romano ME, Calafat AM, Webster GM, Yolton K et al (2016) Prenatal perfluoroalkyl substance exposure and child adiposity at 8 years of age: the HOME study. Obesity (Silver Spring) 24(1):231–237
21. Hoyer BB, Ramlau-Hansen CH, Vrijheid M, Valvi D, Pedersen HS, Zviezdai V et al (2015) Anthropometry in 5- to 9-year-old Greenlandic and Ukrainian children in relation to prenatal exposure to perfluorinated alkyl substances. Environ Health Perspect 123(8):841–846
22. Barry V, Darrow LA, Klein M, Winquist A, Steenland K (2014) Early life perfluorooctanoic acid (PFOA) exposure and overweight and obesity risk in adulthood in a community with elevated exposure. Environ Res 132:62–69
23. Consales C, Toft G, Leter G, Bonde JP, Uccelli R, Pacchierotti F et al (2016) Exposure to persistent organic pollutants and sperm DNA methylation changes in Arctic and European populations. Environ Mol Mutagen 57(3):200–209
24. Leter G, Consales C, Eleuteri P, Uccelli R, Specht IO, Toft G et al (2014) Exposure to perfluoroalkyl substances and sperm DNA global methylation in Arctic and European populations. Environ Mol Mutagen 55(7):591–600
25. Guerrero-Preston R, Goldman LR, Brebi-Mieville P, Ili-Gangas C, Lebron C, Witter FR et al (2010) Global DNA hypomethylation is associated with in utero exposure to cotinine and perfluorinated alkyl compounds. Epigenetics 5(6):539–546
26. Watkins DJ, Wellenius GA, Butler RA, Bartell SM, Fletcher T, Kelsey KT (2014) Associations between serum perfluoroalkyl acids and LINE-1 DNA methylation. Environ Int 63:71–76
27. Fletcher T, Galloway TS, Melzer D, Holcroft P, Cipelli R, Pilling LC et al (2013) Associations between PFOA, PFOS and changes in the expression of genes involved in cholesterol metabolism in humans. Environ Int 57–58:2–10
28. Vanden Heuvel JP, Thompson JT, Frame SR, Gillies PJ (2006) Differential activation of nuclear receptors by perfluorinated fatty acid analogs and natural fatty acids: a comparison of human, mouse, and rat peroxisome proliferator-activated receptor-alpha, -beta, and -gamma, liver X receptor-beta, and retinoid X receptor-alpha. Toxicol Sci 92(2):476–489
29. Taxvig C, Dreisig K, Boberg J, Nellemann C, Schelde AB, Pedersen D et al (2012) Differential effects of environmental chemicals and food contaminants on adipogenesis, biomarker release and PPARgamma activation. Mol Cell Endocrinol 361(1–2):106–115
30. Bastos Sales L, Kamstra JH, Cenijn PH, van Rijt LS, Hamers T, Legler J (2013) Effects of endocrine disrupting chemicals on in vitro global DNA methylation and adipocyte differentiation. Toxicol in Vitro 27(6):1634–1643
31. Wang CF, Tian Y (2015) Reproductive endocrine-disrupting effects of triclosan: population exposure, present evidence and potential mechanisms. Environ Pollut 206:195–201
32. Sandborgh-Englund G, Adolfsson-Erici M, Odham G, Ekstrand J (2006) Pharmacokinetics of triclosan following oral ingestion in humans. J Toxicol Environ Health A 69(20):1861–1873
33. Allmyr M, Adolfsson-Erici M, McLachlan MS, Sandborgh-Englund G (2006) Triclosan in plasma and milk from Swedish nursing mothers and their exposure via personal care products. Sci Total Environ 372(1):87–93
34. Wang X, Chen X, Feng X, Chang F, Chen M, Xia Y et al (2015) Triclosan causes spontaneous abortion accompanied by decline of estrogen sulfotransferase activity in humans and mice. Sci Rep 5:18252
35. Calafat AM, Ye X, Wong LY, Reidy JA, Needham LL (2008) Urinary concentrations of triclosan in the U.S. population: 2003–2004. Environ Health Perspect 116(3):303–307
36. Yin J, Wei L, Shi Y, Zhang J, Wu Q, Shao B (2016) Chinese population exposure to triclosan and triclocarban as measured via human urine and nails. Environ Geochem Health 38 (5):1125–1135
37. Heffernan AL, Baduel C, Toms LM, Calafat AM, Ye X, Hobson P et al (2015) Use of pooled samples to assess human exposure to parabens, benzophenone-3 and triclosan in Queensland, Australia. Environ Int 85:77–83

38. Cheng W, Yang S, Liang F, Wang W, Zhou R, Li Y et al (2019) Low-dose exposure to triclosan disrupted osteogenic differentiation of mouse embryonic stem cells via BMP/ERK/Smad/Runx-2 signalling pathway. Food Chem Toxicol 127:1–10
39. Du G, Yu M, Wang L, Hu W, Song L, Lu C et al (2018) Transcriptome and DNA Methylome dynamics during Triclosan-induced cardiomyocyte differentiation toxicity. Stem Cells Int 2018:8608327
40. Ma Y, Zang L, Wang D, Jiang J, Wang C, Wang X et al (2019) Effects of miR-181a-5p abnormal expression on zebrafish (Danio rerio) vascular development following triclosan exposure. Chemosphere 223:523–535
41. Harley KG, Berger KP, Kogut K, Parra K, Lustig RH, Greenspan LC et al (2019) Association of phthalates, parabens and phenols found in personal care products with pubertal timing in girls and boys. Hum Reprod 34(1):109–117
42. Bertelsen RJ, Longnecker MP, Lovik M, Calafat AM, Carlsen KH, London SJ et al (2013) Triclosan exposure and allergic sensitization in Norwegian children. Allergy 68(1):84–91
43. Xue J, Wu Q, Sakthivel S, Pavithran PV, Vasukutty JR, Kannan K (2015) Urinary levels of endocrine-disrupting chemicals, including bisphenols, bisphenol a diglycidyl ethers, benzophenones, parabens, and triclosan in obese and non-obese Indian children. Environ Res 137:120–128
44. Li S, Zhao J, Wang G, Zhu Y, Rabito F, Krousel-Wood M et al (2015) Urinary triclosan concentrations are inversely associated with body mass index and waist circumference in the US general population: experience in NHANES 2003–2010. Int J Hyg Environ Health 218 (4):401–406
45. Buser MC, Murray HE, Scinicariello F (2014) Association of urinary phenols with increased body weight measures and obesity in children and adolescents. J Pediatr 165(4):744–749
46. Gyllenberg D, Sourander A, Surcel HM, Hinkka-Yli-Salomaki S, McKeague IW, Brown AS (2016) Hypothyroxinemia during gestation and offspring schizophrenia in a national birth cohort. Biol Psychiatry 79(12):962–970
47. Gorr MW, Velten M, Nelin TD, Youtz DJ, Sun Q, Wold LE (2014) Early life exposure to air pollution induces adult cardiac dysfunction. Am J Physiol Heart Circ Physiol 307(9):H1353–H1360
48. Rosa MJ, Hair GM, Just AC, Kloog I, Svensson K, Pizano-Zarate ML et al (2019) Identifying critical windows of prenatal particulate matter (PM2.5) exposure and early childhood blood pressure. Environ Res 182:109073
49. Melody SM, Ford JB, Wills K, Venn A, Johnston FH (2019) Maternal exposure to fine particulate matter from a large coal mine fire is associated with gestational diabetes mellitus: a prospective cohort study. Environ Res:108956
50. Hectors TL, Vanparys C, van der Ven K, Martens GA, Jorens PG, Van Gaal LF et al (2011) Environmental pollutants and type 2 diabetes: a review of mechanisms that can disrupt beta cell function. Diabetologia 54(6):1273–1290
51. West NA, Crume TL, Maligie MA, Dabelea D (2011) Cardiovascular risk factors in children exposed to maternal diabetes in utero. Diabetologia 54(3):504–507
52. Barker DJ (2007) The origins of the developmental origins theory. J Intern Med 261 (5):412–417
53. Grandjean P, Barouki R, Bellinger DC, Casteleyn L, Chadwick LH, Cordier S et al (2015) Life-long implications of developmental exposure to environmental stressors: new perspectives. Endocrinology 156(10):3408–3415
54. Wu X, Zhang Y (2017) TET-mediated active DNA demethylation: mechanism, function and beyond. Nat Rev Genet 18(9):517–534
55. Bernstein BE, Meissner A, Lander ES (2007) The mammalian epigenome. Cell 128(4):669–681
56. Jefferson WN, Chevalier DM, Phelps JY, Cantor AM, Padilla-Banks E, Newbold RR et al (2013) Persistently altered epigenetic marks in the mouse uterus after neonatal estrogen exposure. Mol Endocrinol 27(10):1666–1677

57. Kurian JR, Louis S, Keen KL, Wolfe A, Terasawa E, Levine JE (2016) The Methylcytosine dioxygenase ten-eleven Translocase-2 (tet2) enables elevated GnRH gene expression and maintenance of male reproductive function. Endocrinology 157(9):3588–3603
58. Dolinoy DC, Huang D, Jirtle RL (2007) Maternal nutrient supplementation counteracts bisphenol A-induced DNA hypomethylation in early development. Proc Natl Acad Sci U S A 104(32):13056–13061
59. Greathouse KL, Bredfeldt T, Everitt JI, Lin K, Berry T, Kannan K et al (2012) Environmental estrogens differentially engage the histone methyltransferase EZH2 to increase risk of uterine tumorigenesis. Mol Cancer Res 10(4):546–557
60. Wang Q, Trevino LS, Wong RL, Medvedovic M, Chen J, Ho SM et al (2016) Reprogramming of the epigenome by MLL1 links early-life environmental exposures to prostate cancer risk. Mol Endocrinol 30(8):856–871
61. Esteban J, Serrano-Macia M, Sanchez-Perez I, Alonso-Magdalena P, Pellin MC, Garcia-Arevalo M et al (2019) In utero exposure to bisphenol-A disrupts key elements of retinoid system in male mice offspring. Food Chem Toxicol 126:142–151
62. Faulk C, Kim JH, Jones TR, McEachin RC, Nahar MS, Dolinoy DC et al (2015) Bisphenol A-associated alterations in genome-wide DNA methylation and gene expression patterns reveal sequence-dependent and non-monotonic effects in human fetal liver. Environ Epigenet 1(1): dvv006
63. DeBenedictis B, Guan H, Yang K (2016) Prenatal exposure to bisphenol A disrupts mouse fetal liver maturation in a sex-specific manner. J Cell Biochem 117(2):344–350
64. Nahar MS, Kim JH, Sartor MA, Dolinoy DC (2014) Bisphenol A-associated alterations in the expression and epigenetic regulation of genes encoding xenobiotic metabolizing enzymes in human fetal liver. Environ Mol Mutagen 55(3):184–195
65. Doshi T, Mehta SS, Dighe V, Balasinor N, Vanage G (2011) Hypermethylation of estrogen receptor promoter region in adult testis of rats exposed neonatally to bisphenol A. Toxicology 289(2–3):74–82

Paternal-Specific Exposure and Child Health

Hong Qian, Wei Wu, Francis Manyori Bigambo, and Chuncheng Lu

1 Introduction

5.9 million children (16,000 per day) died in 2015 of diseases which can be prevented and treated [1, 2]. We are still facing the challenges on how to reduce the child mortality rate [3]. This has led to increased demand for child health promotion. Many diseases are threatening the healthy growth of children. Some of them are preventable if effective measures can be taken early. In children, infectious diseases such as diarrhea and pneumonia account for the majority of childhood morbidity and mortality [4]. In addition to diarrhea and pneumonia, childhood illnesses also include respiratory symptom, respiratory infections, and asthma [5]. These diseases impose a heavy health and economic burden on society. According to the WHO European Region, although the child mortality rate is gradually declining, the rate of children dying from cancer is disappointingly increasing [6]. No matter which age group, leukemia is firmly the first cause of death of childhood cancer followed by brain cancer and non-Hodgkin's lymphoma.

It has been known to the public that the parents' healthy status and the environment which they contact most frequently can substantially impact children's health [7]. For example, more than 600,000 people die each year from secondhand smoke, 28% of whom are children. The source of secondhand smoke in the home is mostly from their parents [8]. In addition to smoke, several studies have reported that maternal and paternal exposures to POPs and radiation have an association with birth outcomes and childhood diseases [9–12]. The public is comparatively aware that maternal exposures to unhealthy lifestyle and toxic chemicals may have effects on childhood health. However, paternal exposure, which is anything the father of the baby is exposed to before or during his partner's pregnancy, has been omitted for a

H. Qian · W. Wu · F. M. Bigambo · C. Lu (✉)
School of Public Health, Nanjing Medical University, Nanjing, China
e-mail: chunchenglu@njmu.edu.cn

Y. Xia (ed.), *Early-life Environmental Exposure and Disease*,
https://doi.org/10.1007/978-981-15-3797-4_12

long time. Recently, researchers are beginning to recognize the significance of paternal exposure.

In this chapter, we summarize the paternal exposure effects of some common chemicals and physical agents on child health, especially POPs, radiation, and tobacco smoke. We have investigated the association and possible pathophysiological mechanisms of the exposed factors on adverse health outcomes in children.

2 Paternal Exposure to Persistent Organic Pollutants (POPs)

According to the U.S. Environmental Protection Agency (EPA), POPs are chemicals which exhibit toxic characteristics that can adversely affect human health and the environment around the world. They include intentionally produced chemicals currently or once used in agriculture, disease control, manufacturing, or industrial processes and unintentionally produced chemicals, such as dioxins [13, 14]. They have ability to biomagnify in the ecosystems and to bioaccumulate in humans and animals [14–16]. Because of the stable durability and potential for long-range transport of persistent organic pollutants, they are widely distributed in the world today, and they can be found even in places where they have not been used [15, 17, 18]. As a result, human exposure to POPs may occur via numerous ways. For example, exposure to POPs can occur through the environments such as food, drinking water, the outdoor and indoor air and at the work place (Fig. 1) [19]. They deserve global concern for their possibility of long-term existence in the environment, as well as their significant hazardous effects on human or animal health and the environment [19, 20].

Previous studies have suggested that potential exposure to POPs may have effects on child health, even at low-dose exposure level, such as metabolic health among children [16, 21]. Furthermore, several epidemiological studies have shown that maternal exposures to POPs have a contact with factors related to child development, such as birth weight and birth size [9, 22]. However, the health of an offspring is also linked to paternal exposure (Table 1). Few studies have shown that paternal occupational exposure to POP, such as 2,3,7,8-tetrachlorodibenzo-p-dioxin (TCDD), may increase the body weight of the offspring [25]. More evidence has shown that paternal exposure to dioxin-contaminated chlorophenols was related to the development of certain birth defect in the offspring [26]. Limited results indicate that POP is likely to increase the risk of low birth weight or infant death due to paternal exposure [25, 28]. This does not mean that paternal exposure to POPs may not result in serious consequences for child health. Many previous researches which focused on paternal exposure to POPs and the outcomes of child health suffer from inaccurate exposure methods or no access to the needed information. More studies are necessary to be designed to explore the relationship between POP exposure and birth weight, birth size, congenital anomalies, or infant death. All of them play an important role on the

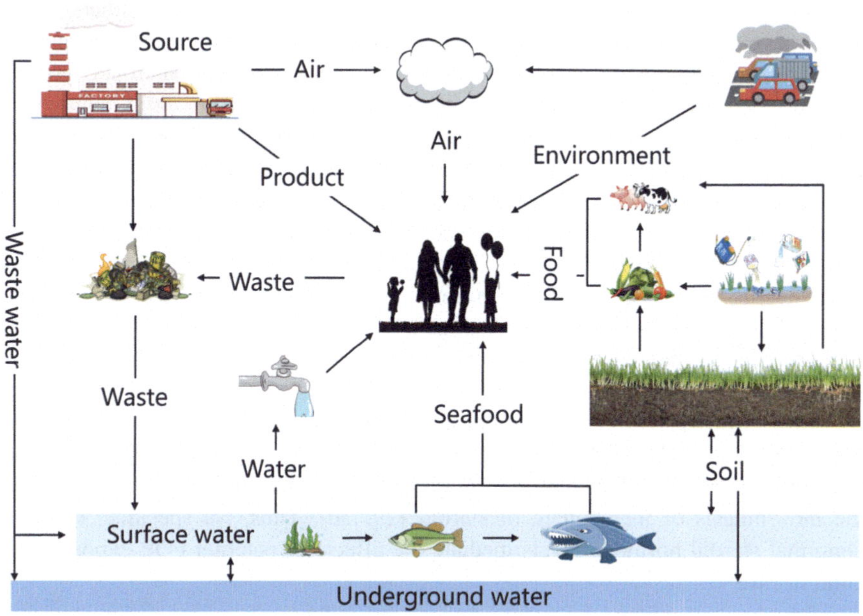

Fig. 1 The exposure pathways of POPs

Table 1 Paternal exposure of POPs and associations with child health

No. of participants	Exposure	Results	References
234 couples (from 2005 to 2009)	PBDEs(183,66,99)	PCB 195 and infant size: −6.94 (−102.96, 89.07)∗(girls); −148.39 (281.69, −15.08)∗ (boys)	[23]
	PCBs (167, 172,195)	*p,p´*-DDE and infant size: 0.12 (0.02, 0.22)∗(girls); 0.01 (−0.06, 0.07)∗(boys)	
	p,p´-DDE	Significant associations between parental concentrations of PCBs and birth size were more frequent among boys	
300 couples (from 1973 to 1974)	PCB	Combined parents' enrollment PBB exposure increased the odds of a male birth but did not reach statistical significance	[24]
1117 babies (from 1987 to 1988)	TCDD	Paternal exposure to TCDD yielded a nonstatistically significant increase in infant birth weight	[25]
9512 fathers and 19,675 births	Dioxincontaminated chlorophenols	Increased the risk of developing congenital anomalies of the eye and birth defects such as congenital anomalies of genital organs	[26]
398 fathers-infant	Organic solvents	Increased the risk of low birth weight children	[27]

*P value <0.05 was considered the threshold for significance

development of child health. Researchers used a statistical model to estimate quantitative exposure measures on the data from Dutch Trade Union for Construction Workers, the Netherlands, 2001. They draw a conclusion that the paternal exposure to POP has been exposed to a positive corollary link with child congenital malformations [27]. A prospective pregnancy study with preconception enrollment of couples takes maternal and paternal serum concentrations into account and found that paternal serum concentrations of POPs, such as polychlorinated biphenyls (PCBs) and polybrominated diphenyl ethers (PBDEs), were significantly associated with birth size [23]. However, there is limited evidence of whether the associations were specific to paternal serum concentrations in other populations. Therefore, there is a need for more comprehensive investigations of the associations between paternal exposures and child development and growth when considering the correlation between parental exposures and child health.

Some experimental studies suggested that POPs, the potential endocrine-disrupting chemicals (EDCs), interact with steroid hormone levels which resulted in disturbing the hormone balance through binding to steroid receptor or disrupting the biosynthesis or metabolism of steroid [29, 30]. Thus, we speculate that the abnormal steroid hormone levels mediate the effects of paternal POP exposure on child health.

3 Paternal Exposure to Radiation

Radiation is energy that comes from a source and travels through space and may be able to penetrate various materials. There are many types of radiation. For example, shortwave radiation is widely used in wireless communications, radar observations, industrial manufacturing, and medical and other fields, which are closely related to our life [31]. Several studies suggested that short-term, low-level exposure of shortwave radiation has few adverse effects on human health [32]. More investigations are needed to focus on long-term, low- or high-level exposure of radiation. Attention should be focused on the people who are in radiation-related occupations, such as the workers in nuclear power plants or who live near a source of radiation.

Exposure to a high level of radiation to children is one of the known risk factors of childhood cancers [33], which has caught a great deal of attention in the public (Table 2). Gardner et al. have designed a case-control study to explore the relationship between paternal exposure to radiation and childhood tumors [10]. In the study, the children who were born near Sellafield nuclear plant and the children whose fathers were employed at the plant, particularly those exposed to high radiation dose before their child's conception, have a higher risk of developing tumors compared to the control. A study published in 2003 conducted analysis by using the data of 34,538 childhood cancer cases diagnosed in the UK between 1952 and 1986 [34]. The results of analysis supported the conclusion from Gardner et al. that there is a large connection between the risk of childhood cancer and paternal employment as a radiation worker. A follow-up study suggested an increased

Table 2 Paternal exposure to radiation and childhood cancer

The research methods	Country	Study population	Cancer	References
A case-control study	UK	People who live near Sellafield nuclear plant	Leukemia and non-Hodgkin's lymphoma	[10]
A case-control study	UK	Parents from National Registry for radiation workers	Malignant neoplasm or brain tumor	[34]
A case-control study	UK	Parents and children from the National Registry of Childhood Tumors	Leukemia and non-Hodgkin's lymphoma	[35]

morbidity of childhood leukemia and non-Hodgkin's lymphoma among the children of male parents who were exposed to radiation. However, the study did not reveal the correlation with radiation doses [35]. These observations in human populations suggested that different levels of exposure will lead to inconsistent incidence of childhood cancers. The possible mechanisms of the associations between paternal exposure to radiation and child cancers have been presented. The radiation can result in a germline mutation in the father or mother before conception or affect the developing fetus in utero directly [36]. More rigorous experimental designs are needed to provide more convincing evidence to persuade the public.

4 Paternal Exposure to Tobacco Smoking

In 1964, the U.S. General Surgeon released the first report to demonstrate the negative effects of tobacco use on health [37]. Thereafter, numerous investigations were conducted to identify the possible association between child health and maternal and paternal exposure to tobacco smoking. For example, a review published in 2017 aims to explore the role of tobacco smoke exposure in causing harm to children [38], including negative impact on fetal growth and birth outcomes [39], sudden infant death syndrome (SIDS) [40, 41], childhood obesity and related effects [42], and brain development and neurobehavioral disorders [11]. However, in those reviews, the child health outcomes were studied from maternal exposure to tobacco smoke and not from secondhand smoke. Secondhand smoke has been one of the established reasons for a variety of adverse health effects, such as children's cough, sputum [43], asthma [44], breathing difficulties, and lung function decline [45]. The source of secondhand smoke is not only from mothers but also from fathers. More studies focused on the association between paternal exposure to tobacco smoke and childhood diseases.

A birth cohort study was conducted between May 2009 and May 2010 in Nha Trang, Vietnam, by using the neonates' data of 1999 to explore the association between paternal tobacco smoking as a risk factor and infectious and non-infectious diseases among infants [46]. The epidemiological evidence indicated that paternal exposure to tobacco smoking independently increased the risk of lower respiratory tract infection. According to different studies, if we take actions to prohibit paternal tobacco smoking in the place where children are present, the lower respiratory tract infection-related hospitalizations will be reduced in this epidemiological setting.

Birth length, head circumference, and low birth weight are major parameters of fetal growth measurement [12]. A study published in 2013 using the nationwide Longitudinal Survey of Babies in the twenty-first Century in Japan, indicating the importance of birth length as a screening index of child health, reported that birth length had a relationship with the incidence of hospitalization due to all causes between 6 and 18 months of age, and the association was stronger than that with birth weight [47]. Maternal exposure to tobacco smoking has adverse effects on a series of birth outcomes, which has been widely accepted by the public [12]. Formerly, the child health effects of paternal exposure to smoking were examined as a passive risk factor during the period of fetus development in some studies [48–50]. These studies were unable to conclude the relationship between paternal smoking exposure and adverse birth outcomes in children. Inoue et al. conducted a follow-up hospital-based study from pregnancy to delivery of 1997–2010 with parents and newborn infants who delivered at a large hospital in Hamamatsu, Japan [12]. They suggested that the individual effects of paternal exposure to smoking are associated with short birth length and small head circumference. In addition to evaluating the independent effects, the study examined the interaction effect of parental smoking. This is an important detail in assessing the impact of parental exposure to tobacco smoking on children.

The animal models have also supported the association between paternal exposure to smoking and adverse child health outcomes including infertility, birth defects, and childhood cancers. The model of cigarette smoke condensate (CSC) exposure to paternal mice demonstrates testicular toxicity and developmental defects in the offspring. This study showed that CSC induced testicular DNA damage and cytotoxicity due to the accumulation of benzo(a)pyrene and cotinine [51]. More researches are needed to focus on exploring the mechanism of the genetic effects of parental exposure to tobacco smoking to provide convincing evidence. Then, we can develop more targeted prevention measures and methods.

5 Conclusion and Future Prospects

Exposures to unhealthy lifestyles and environmental risk factors during the period of fetal development can lead to adverse consequences for child health. The source of exposure is not only from the mother, but also from the father, or a combination of both parents. Many previous studies have reported the adverse effect of maternal exposure to these risk factors on birth weight, fetal toxicity, fetal growth, etc. [25, 52]. In this chapter, we briefly describe the possible adverse effects of paternal exposure on the health of children. Epidemiological studies showed that the fathers with potentially high exposure to toxic and harmful chemicals, such as PCBs, TCDD, etc., physical agents, and high-risk behavior in the environment may have an increased risk of the congenital malformations, child cancer, or other adverse outcomes to their offspring compared to low or no exposure ones.

Limited results from functional studies imply the critical roles of paternal exposure effects on child health [53]. Paternal exposure, such as POPs, participate in the epigenetic biological process of the paternal germ line, involving DNA methylation, histone modifications or retention, etc. For example, pesticide dichlorodiphenyltrichloroethane (DDT) can induce intergenerational perturbation of sperm miRNAs [54, 55]. In the future, epidemiological and functional studies need to be performed to uncover the trans-generational mechanism of the paternal exposures and supply new insight into the pertinent intervention that can mitigate the effect of such exposures.

Acknowledgments This work was supported by National Natural Science Foundation of China (No. 81671461) and the Priority Academic Program for the Development of Jiangsu Higher Education Institutions (Public Health and Preventive Medicine).

References

1. UNICEF (2015) Monitoring the situation for women and children. http://data.unicef.org/resources/committing-to-child-survival-a-promise-renewed-2015.html
2. Victora CG, Requejo JH, Barros AJ, Berman P, Bhutta Z, Boerma T, Chopra M, de Francisco A, Daelmans B, Hazel E et al (2016) Countdown to 2015: a decade of tracking progress for maternal, newborn, and child survival. Lancet (London, England) 387 (10032):2049–2059
3. Steenhoff AP, Crouse HL, Lukolyo H, Larson CP, Howard C, Mazhani L, Pak-Gorstein S, Niescierenko ML, Musoke P, Marshall R et al (2017) Partnerships for global child health. Pediatrics 140(4):e20163823
4. Walker CLF, Rudan I, Liu L, Nair H, Theodoratou E, Bhutta ZA, O'Brien KL, Campbell H, Black RE (2013) Global burden of childhood pneumonia and diarrhoea. Lancet (London, England) 381(9875):1405–1416
5. Kotecha SJ, Watkins WJ, Lowe J, Henderson AJ, Kotecha S (2016) Effect of early-term birth on respiratory symptoms and lung function in childhood and adolescence. Pediatr Pulmonol 51 (11):1212–1221
6. Kyu HH, Stein CE, Boschi Pinto C, Rakovac I, Weber MW, Dannemann Purnat T, Amuah JE, Glenn SD, Cercy K, Biryukov S et al (2018) Causes of death among children aged 5–14 years in the WHO European region: a systematic analysis for the global burden of disease study 2016. Lancet Child Adolesc Health 2(5):321–337
7. Goodman DM (2017) Family health is child health. J Pediatr 181:1–2
8. Kleier JA, Mites-Campbell M, Henson-Evertz K (2017) Children's exposure to secondhand smoke, parental nicotine dependence, and motivation to quit smoking. Pediatr Nurs 43 (1):35–39

9. Karmaus W, Zhu X (2004) Maternal concentration of polychlorinated biphenyls and dichlorodiphenyl dichlorethylene and birth weight in Michigan fish eaters: a cohort study. Environ Health 3(1):1
10. Gardner MJ, Snee MP, Hall AJ, Powell CA, Downes S, Terrell JD (1990) Results of case-control study of leukaemia and lymphoma among young people near Sellafield nuclear plant in West Cumbria. BMJ 300(6722):423–429
11. Zhu JL, Olsen J, Liew Z, Li J, Niclasen J, Obel C (2014) Parental smoking during pregnancy and ADHD in children: the Danish national birth cohort. Pediatrics 134(2):e382–e388
12. Inoue S, Naruse H, Yorifuji T, Kato T, Murakoshi T, Doi H, Subramanian SV (2017) Impact of maternal and paternal smoking on birth outcomes. J Public Health (Oxf) 39(3):1–10
13. EPA (Environmental Protection Agency) (2009) Persistent organic pollutants: a global issue, a global response. https://www.epa.gov/international-cooperation/persistent-organic-pollutants-global-issue-global-response#pops
14. Ashraf MA (2017) Persistent organic pollutants (POPs): a global issue, a global challenge. Environ Sci Pollut R 24(5):4223–4227
15. Wu BZ, Chen GY, Yak HK, Liao WS, Chiu KH, Peng SM (2016) Degradation of lindane and hexachlorobenzene in supercritical carbon dioxide using palladium nanoparticles stabilized in microcellular high-density polyethylene. Chemosphere 152:345–352
16. Lee HA, Park SH, Hong YS, Ha EH, Park H (2016) The effect of exposure to persistent organic pollutants on metabolic health among Korean children during a 1-year follow-up. Int J Env Res Pub He 13(3):270
17. Grgic M, Maletic S, Beljin J, Isakovski MK, Roncevic S, Tubic A, Agbaba J (2019) Lindane and hexachlorobenzene sequestration and detoxification in contaminated sediment amended with carbon-rich sorbents. Chemosphere 220:1033–1040
18. Munoz-Morales M, Braojos M, Saez C, Canizares P, Rodrigo MA (2017) Remediation of soils polluted with lindane using surfactant-aided soil washing and electrochemical oxidation. J Hazard Mater 339:232–238
19. WHO (World Health Organization) (2011) Persistent organic pollutants (POPs). https://www.who.int/foodsafety/areas_work/chemical-risks/pops/en/
20. Tombesi N, Pozo K, Harner T (2014) Persistent organic pollutants (POPs) in the atmosphere of agricultural and urban areas in the province of Buenos Aires in Argentina using PUF disk passive air samplers. Atmos Pollut Res 5(2):170–178
21. Sanders AP, Saland JM, Wright RO, Satlin L (2018) Perinatal and childhood exposure to environmental chemicals and blood pressure in children: a review of literature 2007–2017. Pediatr Res 84(2):165–180
22. Farhang L, Weintraub JM, Petreas M, Eskenazi B, Bhatia R (2005) Association of DDT and DDE with birth weight and length of gestation in the child health and development studies, 1959–1967. Am J Epidemiol 162(8):717–725
23. Robledo CA, Yeung E, Mendola P, Sundaram R, Maisog J, Sweeney AM, Barr DB, Louis GM (2015) Preconception maternal and paternal exposure to persistent organic pollutants and birth size: the LIFE study. Environ Health Perspect 123(1):88–94
24. Terrell ML, Berzen AK, Small CM, Cameron LL, Wirth JJ, Marcus M (2009) A cohort study of the association between secondary sex ratio and parental exposure to polybrominated biphenyl (PBB) and polychlorinated biphenyl (PCB). Environ Health 8:35
25. Lawson CC, Schnorr TM, Whelan EA, Deddens JA, Dankovic DA, Piacitelli LA, Sweeney MH, Connally LB (2004) Paternal occupational exposure to 2,3,7,8-tetrachlorodibenzo-p-dioxin and birth outcomes of offspring: birth weight, preterm delivery, and birth defects. Environ Health Perspect 112(14):1403–1408
26. Dimich-Ward H, Hertzman C, Teschke K, Hershler R, Marion SA, Ostry A, Kelly S (1996) Reproductive effects of paternal exposure to chlorophenate wood preservatives in the sawmill industry. Scand J Work Environ Health 22(4):267–273

27. Hooiveld M, Haveman W, Roskes K, Bretveld R, Burstyn I, Roeleveld N (2006) Adverse reproductive outcomes among male painters with occupational exposure to organic solvents. Occup Environ Med 63(8):538–544
28. Michalek JE, Rahe AJ, Boyle CA (1998) Paternal dioxin, preterm birth, intrauterine growth retardation, and infant death. Epidemiology 9(2):161–167
29. Sharpe RM, Irvine DS (2004) How strong is the evidence of a link between environmental chemicals and adverse effects on human reproductive health? BMJ 328(7437):447–451
30. Vested A, Giwercman A, Bonde JP, Toft G (2014) Persistent organic pollutants and male reproductive health. Asian J Androl 16(1):71–80
31. Yu C, Peng RY (2017) Biological effects and mechanisms of shortwave radiation: a review. Mil Med Res 4:24
32. Larsen AI, Olsen J, Svane O (1991) Gender-specific reproductive outcome and exposure to high-frequency electromagnetic radiation among physiotherapists. Scand J Work Environ Health 17(5):324–329
33. Kendall GM, Bithell JF, Bunch KJ, Draper GJ, Kroll ME, Murphy MFG, Stiller CA, Vincent TJ (2018) Childhood cancer research in oxford III: the work of CCRG on ionising radiation. Br J Cancer 119(6):771–778
34. Sorahan T, Haylock RG, Muirhead CR, Bunch KJ, Kinlen LJ, Little MP, Draper GJ, Kendall GM, Lancashire RJ, English MA (2003) Cancer in the offspring of radiation workers: an investigation of employment timing and a reanalysis using updated dose information. Br J Cancer 89(7):1215–1220
35. Draper GJ, Little MP, Sorahan T, Kinlen LJ, Bunch KJ, Conquest AJ, Kendall GM, Kneale GW, Lancashire RJ, Muirhead CR et al (1997) Cancer in the offspring of radiation workers: a record linkage study. BMJ 315(7117):1181–1188
36. De Roos AJ, Teschke K, Savitz DA, Poole C, Grufferman S, Pollock BH, AFJE O (2001) Parental occupational exposures to electromagnetic fields and radiation and the incidence of neuroblastoma in offspring. Epidemiology 12(5):508–517
37. United States. Surgeon General's Advisory Committee on Smoking and Health (1964) Smoking and health; report of the advisory committee to the Surgeon General of the Public Health Service. Washington, DC: U.S. Department of Health, Education, and Welfare, Public Health Service; for sale by the Superintendent of Documents, U.S. Government Printing Office
38. Peterson LA, Hecht SS (2017) Tobacco, e-cigarettes, and child health. Curr Opin Pediatr 29 (2):225–230
39. Aagaard-Tillery K, Spong CY, Thom E, Sibai B, Wendel G Jr, Wenstrom K, Samuels P, Simhan H, Sorokin Y, Miodovnik M et al (2010) Pharmacogenomics of maternal tobacco use: metabolic gene polymorphisms and risk of adverse pregnancy outcomes. Obstet Gynecol 115 (3):568–577
40. Dietz PM, England LJ, Shapiro-Mendoza CK, Tong VT, Farr SL, Callaghan WM (2010) Infant morbidity and mortality attributable to prenatal smoking in the U.S. Am J Prev Med 39 (1):45–52
41. Lahr MB, Rosenberg KD, Lapidus JA (2005) Bedsharing and maternal smoking in a population-based survey of new mothers. Pediatrics 116(4):e530–e542
42. Behl M, Rao D, Aagaard K, Davidson TL, Levin ED, Slotkin TA, Srinivasan S, Wallinga D, White MF, Walker VR et al (2013) Evaluation of the association between maternal smoking, childhood obesity, and metabolic disorders: a national toxicology program workshop review. Environ Health Perspect 121(2):170–180
43. Haberg SE, Stigum H, Nystad W, Nafstad P (2007) Effects of pre- and postnatal exposure to parental smoking on early childhood respiratory health. Am J Epidemiol 166(6):679–686
44. Hugg TT, Jaakkola MS, Ruotsalainen RO, Pushkarev VJ, Jaakkola JJ (2008) Parental smoking behaviour and effects of tobacco smoke on children's health in Finland and Russia. Eur J Pub Health 18(1):55–62
45. United States. Public Health Service. Office of the Surgeon General (2014) The health consequences of smoking–50 years of progress: a report of the Surgeon General: Executive summary.

Rockville: U.S. Department of Health and Human Services, Public Health Service, Office of the Surgeon General
46. Miyahara R, Takahashi K, Anh NT, Thiem VD, Suzuki M, Yoshino H, Tho LH, Moriuchi H, Cox SE, Yoshida LM et al (2017) Exposure to paternal tobacco smoking increased child hospitalization for lower respiratory infections but not for other diseases in Vietnam. Sci Rep 7:45481
47. Kato T, Yorifuji T, Inoue S, Doi H, Kawachi I (2013) Association of birth length and risk of hospitalisation among full-term babies in Japan. Paediatr Perinat Epidemiol 27(4):361–370
48. Thacher JD, Gruzieva O, Pershagen G, Neuman A, Wickman M, Kull I, Melen E, Bergstrom A (2014) Pre- and postnatal exposure to parental smoking and allergic disease through adolescence. Pediatrics 134(3):428–434
49. Ahluwalia IB, Grummer-Strawn L, Scanlon KS (1997) Exposure to environmental tobacco smoke and birth outcome: increased effects on pregnant women aged 30 years or older. Am J Epidemiol 146(1):42–47
50. Newman RB, Momirova V, Dombrowski MP, Schatz M, Wise R, Landon M, Rouse DJ, Lindheimer M, Caritis SN, Sheffield J et al (2010) The effect of active and passive household cigarette smoke exposure on pregnant women with asthma. Chest 137(3):601–608
51. Esakky P, Hansen DA, Drury AM, Felder P, Cusumano A, Moley KH (2016) Paternal exposure to cigarette smoke condensate leads to reproductive sequelae and developmental abnormalities in the offspring of mice. Reprod Toxicol 65:283–294
52. Govarts E, Nieuwenhuijsen M, Schoeters G, Ballester F, Bloemen K, de Boer M, Chevrier C, Eggesbo M, Guxens M, Kramer U et al (2012) Birth weight and prenatal exposure to polychlorinated biphenyls (PCBs) and Dichlorodiphenyldichloroethylene (DDE): a meta-analysis within 12 European birth cohorts. Environ Health Perspect 120(2):162–170
53. Nomura T (1982) Parental exposure to x rays and chemicals induces heritable tumours and anomalies in mice. Nature 296(5857):575–577
54. Herst PM, Dalvai M, Lessard M, Charest PL, Navarro P, Joly-Beauparlant C, Droit A, Trasler JM, Kimmins S, MacFarlane AJ et al (2019) Folic acid supplementation reduces multigenerational sperm miRNA perturbation induced by in utero environmental contaminant exposure. Environ Epigenet 5(4):dvz024
55. Maamar MB, King SE, Nilsson E, Beck D, Skinner MK (2020) Epigenetic transgenerational inheritance of parent-of-origin allelic transmission of outcross pathology and sperm epimutations. Dev Biol 458(1):106–119

Molecular Mechanism of Early-Life Chemical Exposure-Induced Harmful Effects

Hua Wang and De-Xiang Xu

1 Introduction

Early developmental stages are more sensitive to environmental chemicals, such as nicotine, ethanol, heavy metals, endocrine disruptors, pesticides, and so on [1]. Accumulating data have demonstrated that exposure to environmental chemicals in early life produces short-term and long-term harmful effects, such as metabolic diseases, neurodevelopmental defects, male infertility, etc. [2–4]. Other works further identified intergenerational and transgenerational effects of environmental chemicals [2, 5]. On one hand, some chemicals enter fetuses and neonates across either placental or blood milk barriers and directly impair fetal and neonatal development. On the other hand, early-life chemical exposure causes indirectly toxic effects via impairing placenta or germlines. In the past decade, great progress has been made in molecular mechanisms by which early-life chemical exposure induces adverse health outcomes later in life. This chapter will summarize the role of genetic mutation, epigenetic alterations, oxidative stress, inflammation, and glucocorticoid on the latent effects of early-life exposure.

2 Genetic Mutation

Genetic mutation refers to the processes that chemical agents alter genetic information. There is more and more evidence indicating that early-life exposure to chemicals can induce genetic mutation. An epidemiological study showed that higher arsenic exposure elevated micronucleus content in peripheral blood

H. Wang · D.-X. Xu (✉)
Key Laboratory of Environmental Toxicology of Anhui Higher Education Institutes and Department of Toxicology, School of Public Health, Anhui Medical University, Hefei, China

Y. Xia (ed.), *Early-life Environmental Exposure and Disease*,
https://doi.org/10.1007/978-981-15-3797-4_13

lymphocytes from children [6]. Another study found that maternal smoking during pregnancy was positively associated with DNA damage in lymphocytes of their newborns [7]. Later animal experiment demonstrated that early-life exposure to cadmium induced DNA damage in embryos of terrestrial snails [8]. A recent experiment found that early-life exposure to dichlorobenzoquinone elevated the level of 8-hydroxydeoxyguanosine in zebrafish [9].

Genetic mutation plays a key role in chemical-induced developmental toxicity. According to a recent study, gestational exposure to ethanol caused deficits of bone development mainly through osteoblast DNA injury and micronucleus formation in neonatal rats [10]. Moreover, prenatal co-exposure to copper and cadmium induced embryo spinal and cardiovascular deformities in *Oryzias latipes*, which was correlated with the increased DNA damage [11]. Another recent study found that developmental exposure to diethylstilbestrol elevated the incidence of uterine fibroids through altering DNA repair in myometrial stem cells [12]. An earlier research reported that ascorbic acid protected against cyclophosphamide-induced embryonic resorptions via inhibiting structural chromosomal aberrations in mice [13]. In addition, *N*-acetylcysteine alleviated cadmium-induced embryonic lethality through rescuing DNA mismatch repair in zebrafish embryos [14].

3 Epigenetic Alterations

Epigenetics was defined as heritable alterations in gene expression without underlying changes in DNA sequence. Increasing evidence has demonstrated that epigenetic modifications, such as DNA methylation, histone modification and noncoding RNA, play key roles in controlling gene expression through time- and space-dependent manner. Indeed, embryonic stem cells and their differentiated cells owned different biological functions due to selective gene expression affected by epigenetic modifications. During the embryonic development, cell differentiation and lineage commitment are determined by epigenetic reprogramming. Early-life exposure to toxic chemicals may disrupt epigenetic reprograming and cause persistent changes and even transgenerational impacts [15]. The Norwegian Mother and Child Cohort Study (n = 1062) showed that maternal smoking during pregnancy was associated with the differential methylation in AHRR, CYP1A1, and GFI1 in neonatal cord blood [16]. The Genome-wide Consortium Meta-analysis including 13 cohorts (n = 6685) found that over 6000 CpGs were differentially methylated in blood from newborns or older children whose mothers smoked during pregnancy [17]. An earlier animal experiment showed that perinatal nicotine exposure enhanced the susceptibility of HI-induced brain injury via DNA methylation of the AT2R gene in neonatal male rats [18]. Indeed, Pb-induced neurodevelopmental toxicity and subsequent epigenetic alterations was also a good example. This study found that early postnatal exposure to Pb markedly reduced the levels of DNMT1 and MECP2 in mouse cerebral cortex across life span [19]. In line with above data, an in vitro experiment showed that Pb altered the global DNA methylation profile in human embryonic stem cells and subsequently impaired neuronal differentiation [20]. According to an observational study, gestational Pb exposure altered the DNA methylation profiles in fetal germ cells and persistently modified DNA methylation status in grandchildren's neonatal blood [21]. This group also found that Pb exposure in infancy upregulated H3K9Ac and H3K4me2 proteins (marks for gene activation) but downregulated H3K27me3 (marks for gene repression) in older primate and mouse brains [19, 22]. Additional study reported that miR-106b, which targeted the APP mRNA, was significantly reduced in the brain of mice whose mothers were exposed to Pb during lactation [23].

Epigenetic alterations in the germline, including sperm and egg, were essential for transmitting transgenerational effects. Numerous studies found that exposure to environmental chemicals in early life caused intergenerational and transgenerational effects, which was associated with epigenetic alterations in germlines [2, 24]. The earliest study reported that prenatal exposure to vinclozolin and methoxychlor, two environment endocrine disruptors, induced transgenerational actions of male fertility through altering sperm DNA methylation [5]. Consistent with alteration of sperm DNA methylation, Dnmt3a and Dnmt3l were altered in the testes of fetal rats (F1–F3) whose mothers were exposed to vinclozolin during pregnancy [25]. Further work found that alteration of sperm noncoding RNA, such as piRNAs, miRNAs and lncRNAs, and histone H3K27me3 methylation were observed in vinclozolin-induced epigenetic transgenerational inheritance of phenotypes [26, 27]. Recently, several studies demonstrated that sperm transfer RNA-derived small RNAs (tsRNAs) were involved in environment chemical-induced intergenerational inheritance of acquired metabolic disorders [4, 28].

4 Oxidative Stress

Oxidative stress results from imbalance between reactive oxygen species (ROS) overproduction and endogenous antioxidants. Excessive ROS causes oxidative injury to intracellular macromolecules, such as DNA, lipids and proteins. Accumulating evidence has demonstrated that early-life exposure to toxic chemicals triggers oxidative stress and even oxidative damage of intracellular macromolecules. An early report showed that urinary 8-hydroxydeoxyguanosine (8-OHdG) in infants was positively linked with cadmium level in both urine and breast milk [29]. Several animal experiments found that early-life exposure to dichlorobenzoquinone and cyhalofop-butyl triggered excess ROS production, upregulated activity of superoxide dismutase (SOD), and elevated the levels of 8-OHdG and malondialdehyde (MDA) in zebrafish [9, 30]. A recent study indicated that paternal arsenic exposure elevated MDA/GSH ratio in hypothalamic-pituitary-gonadal (HPG) axis of adolescent male mouse offspring [31].

Numerous studies have demonstrated that exposure to toxic chemicals induces oxidative stress in adult offspring. An early report showed that prenatal ethanol exposure caused hypothalamic oxidative stress and neuroendocrine alterations in adult rat offspring [32]. Another early study indicated that prenatal co-exposure to ethanol and smoking impaired learning and memory abilities, which was associated with oxidative stress in cerebral cortex of adult offspring [33]. Moreover, antenatal nicotine exposure caused vascular dysfunction and enhanced oxidative stress in adult offspring [34]. Pretreatment with apocynin, an NAPDH oxidase inhibitor, and tempol, an SOD mimetic, improved vascular contractions in adult offspring whose mothers were exposed to nicotine in pregnancy [34]. Additionally, supplementation with MitoQ, a mitochondria-targeted antioxidant, protected against chronic kidney disease in adult mouse offspring whose mothers were exposed to smoking [35]. The modulatory subunit of glutamate cysteine ligase (GCLM) is the key enzyme of GSH synthesis. A recent study showed that Gclm KO mice were more sensitive to pharmacological stimuli as compared with WT mice [36]. Oxidative stress triggered by pharmacological stimuli in preweaning or pubertal Gclm KO mice reduced the number of parvalbumin-immunoreactive interneurons, but not in adult Gclm KO mice [36]. Further observation found that pretreatment with *N*-acetylcysteine reversed early-life stimuli-impaired parvalbumin interneurons via inhibiting oxidative stress in Gclm KO mice [36].

5 Inflammation

Inflammation is a biological response of immune system upon pathogens, damaged cells, or chemicals. The inflammatory process mainly includes vascular permeability changes, leukocyte recruitment, the release of inflammatory cytokines, the resolution of inflammation, and organ-specific inflammatory response [37, 38]. In response to inflammatory stimuli, acute or chronic inflammation occurs in target organs, potentially resulting in tissue injury and diseases [39]. Increasing data demonstrate that early-life exposure to chemicals triggers inflammation. A recent population study found that systemic inflammatory response of schoolchildren was associated with chronic exposure to air pollution [40]. Another population study reported that early gestational co-exposure to the mixture of phenols, phthalates, and metals was linked with altered inflammatory cytokines in maternal and neonatal blood [41]. Several earlier studies indicated that early-life exposure to endocrine-disrupting chemicals, including bisphenol A, caused inflammatory response in different target tissues [42, 43]. Later animal experiments demonstrated that early-life exposure to acetaminophen or 1-nitropyrene increased airway inflammation and susceptibility of allergic asthma in adult offspring [44, 45]. The NF-κB and MAPK are the key signaling pathways for modulating inflammatory mediators and cytokines in inflammatory cells [39]. A recent study indicated that prenatal LPS exposure caused activation of NF-κB signaling, resulting in prenatally programmed hypertension in adult offspring [46]. Moreover, maternal inflammation-mediated p38 MAPK activation predisposes offspring to heart injury caused by isoproterenol via augmenting ROS generation [47].

Various experimental studies have demonstrated that inflammation mediates the harmful effects induced by early-life exposure to chemicals. Maternal dioctyl sodium sulfosuccinate (DOSS) exposure during pregnancy elevated the circulating level of IL-6 and increased susceptibility of adiposity, metabolic disorders, and dyslipidemia in adult male offspring [48]. In utero exposure to lipopolysaccharide (LPS) increased the level of pro-inflammatory cytokines in the postnatal brain and caused the alteration of the glial cells in the developing amygdala [49]. Melatonin, an anti-inflammatory agent, protected mice from placental insufficiency and fetal cardiovascular compromise via downregulating IL-1β and TNF-α [50]. Supplementation with vitamin D3 inhibited IFN-γ production, thereby improving alveolar development in LPS-induced bronchopulmonary dysplasia (BPD) in rats [51].

6 Glucocorticoid Overexposure

Glucocorticoid (GC) is an adrenal steroid hormone that controls a variety of physiological processes such as development, metabolism, immune response, cardiovascular activity and brain function [52–54]. However, excessive GC exposure during pregnancy impairs fetal development. Indeed, increasing evidence has demonstrated that early-life chemical exposure may cause active GC overexposure. According to a birth cohort study in Chile, maternal urinary arsenic concentration during gestation was positively associated with the level of salivary cortisol in infants [55]. Several animal experiments demonstrated that prenatal exposure to caffeine or cadmium (Cd) caused fetal overexposure to active GC [56, 57]. An in vitro study confirmed that Cd downregulated expression of 11β-HSD2 and inhibited 11β-HSD2 promoter activity in human placental trophoblasts [58].

Numerous studies reported that early-life exposure to chemical caused abnormality in adult period maybe through excess exposure to active GC. Several studies showed that prenatal caffeine exposure increased circulatory GC level, changed peripheral glucose and lipid metabolic pathways, and caused hypercholesterolemia and osteoporosis in adult offspring [56, 59, 60]. Gestational ethanol exposure enhanced the susceptibility of offspring rats to glomerulosclerosis and hypercholesterolemia via programming glucocorticoid-insulin-like growth factor 1 (GC-IGF1) axis [61–63]. The Comparative Genomic Enrichment Method (CGEM) found that prenatal co-exposure to arsenic and cadmium altered the expression of glucocorticoid receptor (GR)-regulated target genes related to infectious disease [64]. Additional study found that cortexolone, a GR inhibitor, protected against arsenic-induced neural tube defects [65]. However, postnatal or perinatal exposure to toxic chemicals inhibits GC/GR signaling. According to a recent report, cigarette smoke during lactation lowered glucocorticoid level in male adult offspring [66]. Moreover, both perinatal exposure to arsenic and lactational exposure to benzpyrene reduced the level of serum GR in offspring [67, 68]. Indeed, GC reduction impairs the function of hypothalamic-pituitary-thyroid (HPT) and hypothalamic-pituitary-adrenal (HPA) function, whereas the latter is the cause of

Fig. 1 Molecular mechanism of early-life chemical exposure-induced harmful effects

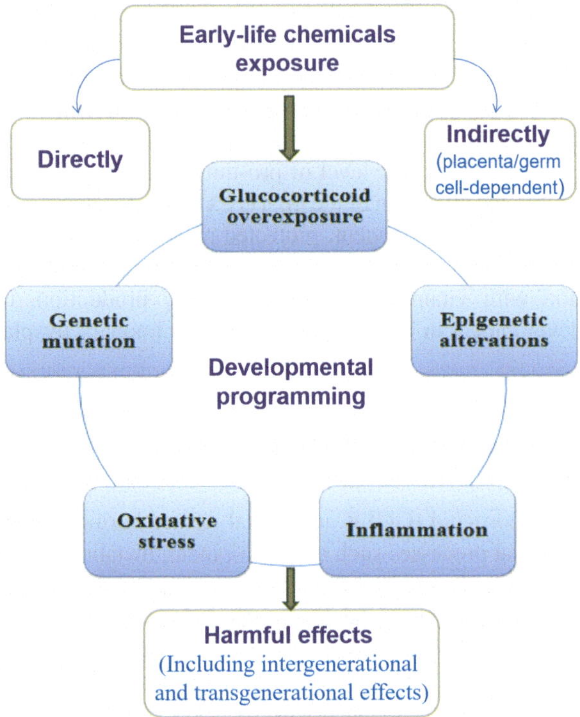

behavior alteration in rat offspring [69, 70]. Interestingly, gestational supplementation with betaine attenuates GC-induced hepatic lipid accumulation and activation of lipolytic genes in adipose tissue through epigenetic modification in adult offspring rats. In addition, postnatal supplementation with omega-3 fatty acid reversed GC-programmed adiposity, hypertension, and hyperlipidemia in high-fat diet-fed male offspring [71–73].

7 Conclusions and Future Prospect

The molecular mechanisms, such as genetic mutation, epigenetic alterations, oxidative stress, inflammation, and glucocorticoid overexposure, are involved in the harmful effects of early-life chemical exposure (Fig. 1). Although great progress has been made in the molecular mechanisms of early-life chemical exposure-induced harmful effects in adult period, further work is needed to elucidate following issues:

(1) The interaction among genetic mutation, epimutation, and other molecular mechanisms remains elusive, (2) the exact mechanism by which early-life chemical exposure induces intergenerational and transgenerational effects needs to be determined, (3) the mechanisms underlying enhanced disease susceptibility of offspring

to the second hit remain unclear, and (4) how to transform the molecular mechanisms into the predictive biomarkers remains uncertain. As above, additional work is required to explore the novel molecular mechanisms by which exposure to toxic chemicals in early life induces harmful effects in later life.

Acknowledgments This work was supported by National Natural Science Foundation of China (81930093, 81973079 and 81473016).

References

1. Martin EM, Fry RC (2018) Environmental influences on the epigenome: exposure-associated DNA methylation in human populations. Annu Rev Public Health 39:309–333
2. Barouki R, Melen E, Herceg Z, Beckers J, Chen J et al (2018) Epigenetics as a mechanism linking developmental exposures to long-term toxicity. Environ Int 114:77–86
3. Hogg K, Price EM, Hanna CW, Robinson WP (2012) Prenatal and perinatal environmental influences on the human Fetal and placental Epigenome. Clin Pharmacol Ther 92:716–726
4. Chen Q, Yan W, Duan E (2016) Epigenetic inheritance of acquired traits through sperm RNAs and sperm RNA modifications. Nat Rev Genet 17:733–743
5. Anway MD, Cupp AS, Uzumcu M, Skinner MK (2005) Epigenetic transgenerational actions of endocrine disruptors and mate fertility. Science 308:1466–1469
6. Bandyopadhyay AK, Paul S, Adak S, Giri AK (2016) Reduced LINE-1 methylation is associated with arsenic-induced genotoxic stress in children. Biometals 29:731–741
7. de Assis KR, Ladeira MS, Bueno RC, Dos Santos BF, Dalben I et al (2009) Genotoxicity of cigarette smoking in maternal and newborn lymphocytes. Mutat Res 679:72–78
8. Baurand PE, de Vaufleury A, Scheifler R, Capelli N (2013) Coupling of random amplified polymorphic DNA profiles analysis and high resolution capillary electrophoresis system for the assessment of chemical genotoxicity. Environ Sci Technol 47:9505–9513
9. Sun HJ, Zhang Y, Zhang JY, Lin H, Chen J et al (2019) The toxicity of 2, 6-dichlorobenzoquinone on the early life stage of zebrafish: A survey on the endpoints at developmental toxicity, oxidative stress, genotoxicity and cytotoxicity. Environ Pollut 245:719–724
10. Carvalho IC, Dutra TP, Andrade DP, Balducci I, Pacheco-Soares C et al (2016) High doses of alcohol during pregnancy cause DNA damages in osteoblasts of newborns rats. Birth Defects Res A Clin Mol Teratol 106:122–132
11. Barjhoux I, Baudrimont M, Morin B, Landi L, Gonzalez P et al (2012) Effects of copper and cadmium spiked-sediments on embryonic development of Japanese medaka (Oryzias latipes). Ecotoxicol Environ Saf 79:272–282
12. Prusinski Fernung LE, Yang Q, Sakamuro D, Kumari A, Mas A et al (2018) Endocrine disruptor exposure during development increases incidence of uterine fibroids by altering DNA repair in myometrial stem cells. Biol Reprod 99:735–748
13. Kola I, Vogel R, Spielmann H (1989) Co-administration of ascorbic acid with cyclophosphamide (CPA) to pregnant mice inhibits the clastogenic activity of CPA in preimplantation murine blastocysts. Mutagenesis 4:297–301
14. Hsu T, Huang KM, Tsai HT, Sung ST, Ho TN (2013) Cadmium(Cd)-induced oxidative stress down-regulates the gene expression of DNA mismatch recognition proteins MutS homolog 2 (MSH2) and MSH6 in zebrafish (Danio rerio) embryos. Aquat Toxicol 126:9–16
15. Faulk C, Dolinoy DC (2011) Timing is everything the when and how of environmentally induced changes in the epigenome of animals. Epigenetics 6:791–797

16. Joubert BR, Haberg SE, Nilsen RM, Wang XT, Vollset SE et al (2012) 450K Epigenome-wide scan identifies differential DNA methylation in newborns related to maternal smoking during pregnancy. Environ Health Perspect 120:1425–1431
17. Joubert BR, Felix JF, Yousefi P, Bakulski KM, Just AC et al (2016) DNA methylation in Newborns and maternal smoking in pregnancy: genome-wide consortium meta-analysis. Am J Hum Genet 98:680–696
18. Li Y, Xiao DL, Dasgupta C, Xiong FX, Tong WN et al (2012) Perinatal nicotine exposure increases vulnerability of hypoxic-ischemic brain injury in neonatal rats role of Angiotensin II receptors. Stroke 43:2483–2490
19. Eid A, Bihaqi SW, Renehan WE, Zawia NH (2016) Developmental lead exposure and lifespan alterations in epigenetic regulators and their correspondence to biomarkers of Alzheimer's disease. Alzheimers Dement (Amst) 2:123–131
20. Senut MC, Sen A, Cingolani P, Shaik A, Land SJ et al (2014) Lead exposure disrupts global DNA methylation in human embryonic stem cells and alters their neuronal differentiation. Toxicol Sci 139:142–161
21. Sen A, Heredia N, Senut MC, Land S, Hollocher K et al (2015) Multigenerational epigenetic inheritance in humans: DNA methylation changes associated with maternal exposure to lead can be transmitted to the grandchildren. Sci Rep 5:14466
22. Bihaqi SW, Huang H, Wu JF, Zawia NH (2011) Infant exposure to Lead (Pb) and epigenetic modifications in the aging primate brain: implications for Alzheimer's disease. J Alzheimers Dis 27:819–833
23. Masoud AM, Bihaqi SW, Machan JT, Zawia NH, Renehan WE (2016) Early-life exposure to Lead (Pb) alters the expression of microRNA that target proteins associated with Alzheimer's disease. J Alzheimers Dis 51:1257–1264
24. Cavalli G, Heard E (2019) Advances in epigenetics link genetics to the environment and disease. Nature 571:489–499
25. Anway MD, Rekow SS, Skinner MK (2008) Transgenerational epigenetic programming of the embryonic testis transcriptome. Genomics 91:30–40
26. Ben Maamar M, Sadler-Riggleman I, Beck D, Skinner MK (2018) Epigenetic transgenerational inheritance of altered sperm histone retention sites. Sci Rep 8(1):1–10
27. Ben Maamar M, Sadler-Riggleman I, Beck D, McBirney M, Nilsson E et al (2018) Alterations in sperm DNA methylation, non-coding RNA expression, and histone retention mediate vinclozolin-induced epigenetic transgenerational inheritance of disease. Environ Epigenet 4: dvy010
28. Chen Q, Yan MH, Cao ZH, Li X, Zhang YF et al (2016) Sperm tsRNAs contribute to intergenerational inheritance of an acquired metabolic disorder. Science 351:397–400
29. Kippler M, Hossain MB, Lindh C, Moore SE, Kabir I et al (2012) Early life low-level cadmium exposure is positively associated with increased oxidative stress. Environ Res 112:164–170
30. Zhu L, Mu X, Wang K, Chai T, Yang Y et al (2015) Cyhalofop-butyl has the potential to induce developmental toxicity, oxidative stress and apoptosis in early life stage of zebrafish (Danio rerio). Environ Pollut 203:40–49
31. Ommati MM, Heidari R, Manthari RK, Tikka Chiranjeevi S, Niu R et al (2019) Paternal exposure to arsenic resulted in oxidative stress, autophagy, and mitochondrial impairments in the HPG axis of pubertal male offspring. Chemosphere 236:124325
32. Dembele K, Yao XH, Chen L, Nyomba BL (2006) Intrauterine ethanol exposure results in hypothalamic oxidative stress and neuroendocrine alterations in adult rat offspring. Am J Phys Regul Integr Comp Phys 291:R796–R802
33. Li Y, Wang H (2004) In utero exposure to tobacco and alcohol modifies neurobehavioral development in mice offspring: consideration a role of oxidative stress. Pharmacol Res 49:467–473
34. Xiao D, Huang X, Yang S, Zhang L (2011) Antenatal nicotine induces heightened oxidative stress and vascular dysfunction in rat offspring. Br J Pharmacol 164:1400–1409

35. Sukjamnong S, Chan YL, Zakarya R, Nguyen LT, Anwer AG et al (2018) MitoQ supplementation prevent long-term impact of maternal smoking on renal development, oxidative stress and mitochondrial density in male mice offspring. Sci Rep 8:6631
36. Cabungcal JH, Steullet P, Kraftsik R, Cuenod M, Do KQ (2013) Early-life insults impair parvalbumin interneurons via oxidative stress: reversal by N-acetylcysteine. Biol Psychiatry 73:574–582
37. Nathan C, Ding A (2010) Nonresolving inflammation. Cell 140:871–882
38. Chertov O, Yang D, Howard OM, Oppenheim JJ (2000) Leukocyte granule proteins mobilize innate host defenses and adaptive immune responses. Immunol Rev 177:68–78
39. Chen L, Deng H, Cui H, Fang J, Zuo Z et al (2018) Inflammatory responses and inflammation-associated diseases in organs. Oncotarget 9:7204–7218
40. Li X, Zhang X, Zhang Z, Han L, Gong D et al (2019) Air pollution exposure and immunological and systemic inflammatory alterations among schoolchildren in China. Sci Total Environ 657:1304–1310
41. Kelley AS, Banker M, Goodrich JM, Dolinoy DC, Burant C et al (2019) Early pregnancy exposure to endocrine disrupting chemical mixtures are associated with inflammatory changes in maternal and neonatal circulation. Sci Rep 9:5422
42. Dietert RR (2012) Misregulated inflammation as an outcome of early-life exposure to endocrine-disrupting chemicals. Rev Environ Health 27:117–131
43. Roy A, Bauer SM, Lawrence BP (2012) Developmental exposure to bisphenol A modulates innate but not adaptive immune responses to influenza A virus infection. PLoS One 7:e38448
44. Lu X, Tan ZX, Wang B, Li J, Hu B et al (2019) Maternal 1-nitropyrene exposure during pregnancy increases susceptibility of allergic asthma in adolescent offspring. Chemosphere 243:125356
45. Karimi K, Kessler T, Thiele K, Ramisch K, Erhardt A et al (2015) Prenatal acetaminophen induces liver toxicity in dams, reduces fetal liver stem cells, and increases airway inflammation in adult offspring. J Hepatol 62:1085–1091
46. Deng Y, Deng Y, He X, Chu J, Zhou J et al (2016) Prenatal inflammation-induced NF-kappaB dyshomeostasis contributes to renin-angiotensin system over-activity resulting in prenatally programmed hypertension in offspring. Sci Rep 6:21692
47. Zhang Q, Deng Y, Lai W, Guan X, Sun X et al (2016) Maternal inflammation activated ROS-p38 MAPK predisposes offspring to heart damages caused by isoproterenol via augmenting ROS generation. Sci Rep 6:30146
48. Temkin AM, Bowers RR, Ulmer CZ, Penta K, Bowden JA et al (2019) Increased adiposity, inflammation, metabolic disruption and dyslipidemia in adult male offspring of DOSS treated C57BL/6 dams. Sci Rep 9:1530
49. O'Loughlin E, Pakan JMP, Yilmazer-Hanke D, McDermott KW (2017) Acute in utero exposure to lipopolysaccharide induces inflammation in the pre- and postnatal brain and alters the glial cytoarchitecture in the developing amygdala. J Neuroinflammation 14:212
50. Lee JY, Li S, Shin NE, Na Q, Dong J et al (2019) Melatonin for prevention of placental malperfusion and fetal compromise associated with intrauterine inflammation-induced oxidative stress in a mouse model. J Pineal Res 67:e12591
51. Liu C, Chen Z, Li W, Huang L, Zhang Y (2017) Vitamin D enhances alveolar development in antenatal lipopolysaccharide-treated rats through the suppression of interferon-gamma production. Front Immunol 8:1923
52. Jellyman JK, AJW F, Fowden AL, Giussani DA (2019) Glucocorticoid maturation of fetal cardiovascular function. Trends Mol Med 26:170–184
53. Bivol S, Owen SJ, Rose Meyer RB (2016) Glucocorticoid-induced changes in glucocorticoid receptor mRNA and protein expression in the human placenta as a potential factor for altering fetal growth and development. Reprod Fertil Dev 29:845–854
54. Quinn MA, McCalla A, He B, Xu X, Cidlowski JA (2019) Silencing of maternal hepatic glucocorticoid receptor is essential for normal fetal development in mice. Commun Biol 2:104

55. Valdes Salgado MA, Schisterman E, Pino P, Bangdiwala S, Munoz MP et al (2019) Is prenatal arsenic exposure associated with salivary cortisol in infants in Arica, Chile? An exploratory cohort study. Ann Agric Environ Med 26:266–272
56. Liu YS, Xu D, Feng JH, Kou H, Liang G et al (2013) Fetal rat metabonome alteration by prenatal caffeine ingestion probably due to the increased circulatory glucocorticoid level and altered peripheral glucose and lipid metabolic pathways (vol 262, pg 205, 2012). Toxicol Appl Pharmacol 273:691
57. Ronco AM, Urrutia M, Montenegro M, Llanos MN (2009) Cadmium exposure during pregnancy reduces birth weight and increases maternal and foetal glucocorticoids. Toxicol Lett 188:186–191
58. Yang K, Julan L, Rubio F, Sharma A, Guan H (2006) Cadmium reduces 11 beta-hydroxysteroid dehydrogenase type 2 activity and expression in human placental trophoblast cells. Am J Physiol Endocrinol Metab 290:E135–EE42
59. Xu D, Luo HWW, Hu W, Hu SWW, Yuan C et al (2018) Intrauterine programming mechanism for hypercholesterolemia in prenatal caffeine-exposed female adult rat offspring. FASEB J 32:5563–5576
60. Shangguan Y, Wen Y, Tan Y, Qin J, Jiang H et al (2018) Intrauterine programming of glucocorticoid-insulin-like growth Factor-1 Axis-mediated developmental origin of osteoporosis susceptibility in female offspring rats with prenatal caffeine exposure. Am J Pathol 188:2863–2876
61. Chen H, Zhu Y, Zhao X, He H, Luo J et al (2019) Prenatal ethanol exposure increased the susceptibility of adult offspring rats to glomerulosclerosis. Toxicol Lett 321:44–53
62. Hu S, Qin J, Zhou J, Magdalou J, Chen L et al (2019) Glucocorticoid programming mechanism for hypercholesterolemia in prenatal ethanol-exposed adult offspring rats. Toxicol Appl Pharmacol 375:46–56
63. He H, Xiong Y, Li B, Zhu Y, Chen H et al (2019) Intrauterine programming of the glucocorticoid-insulin-like growth factor 1 (GC-IGF1) axis mediates glomerulosclerosis in female adult offspring rats induced by prenatal ethanol exposure. Toxicol Lett 311:17–26
64. Rager JE, Yosim A, Fry RC (2014) Prenatal exposure to arsenic and cadmium impacts infectious disease-related genes within the glucocorticoid receptor signal transduction pathway. Int J Mol Sci 15:22374–22391
65. Ahir BK, Sanders AP, Rager JE, Fry RC (2013) Systems biology and birth defects prevention: blockade of the glucocorticoid receptor prevents arsenic-induced birth defects. Environ Health Perspect 121:332–338
66. Novaes Soares P, Silva Tavares Rodrigues V, Cherem Peixoto T, Calvino C, Aparecida Miranda R et al (2018) Cigarette smoke during breastfeeding in rats changes glucocorticoid and vitamin D status in obese adult offspring. Int J Mol Sci 19:3084
67. Csaba G, Inczefi-Gonda A (1994) Breastmilk can mediate chemical imprinting. Benzpyrene exposure during lactation reduces the thymic glucocorticoid receptor density of the offspring. Gen Pharmacol 25:603–606
68. Martinez-Finley EJ, Goggin SL, Labrecque MT, Allan AM (2011) Reduced expression of MAPK/ERK genes in perinatal arsenic-exposed offspring induced by glucocorticoid receptor deficits. Neurotoxicol Teratol 33:530–537
69. Wilcoxon JS, Redei EE (2007) Maternal glucocorticoid deficit affects hypothalamic-pituitary-adrenal function and behavior of rat offspring. Horm Behav 51:321–327
70. Slone-Wilcoxon J, Redei EE (2004) Maternal-fetal glucocorticoid milieu programs hypothalamic-pituitary-thyroid function of adult offspring. Endocrinology 145:4068–4072
71. Zhao NN, Yang S, Jia YM, Sun B, He B et al (2018) Maternal betaine supplementation attenuates glucocorticoid-induced hepatic lipid accumulation through epigenetic modification in adult offspring rats. J Nutr Biochem 54:105–112

72. Zhao N, Yang S, Sun B, Feng Y, Zhao R (2019) Maternal betaine protects rat offspring from glucocorticoid-induced activation of lipolytic genes in adipose tissue through modification of DNA methylation. Eur J Nutr. https://doi.org/10.1007/s00394-019-02025-1
73. Zulkafli IS, Waddell BJ, Mark PJ (2013) Postnatal dietary omega-3 fatty acid supplementation rescues glucocorticoid-programmed adiposity, hypertension, and hyperlipidemia in male rat offspring raised on a high-fat diet. Endocrinology 154:3110–3117

Transgenerational Epigenetic Inheritance of Developmental Origins of Health and Disease

Wei Wu, Peihao Wu, Qiuqin Tang, and Chuncheng Lu

1 Introduction

For the past few years, the national economy has been booming on people's living conditions, especially on the way of development. The incidence of some metabolic diseases like obesity has increased. At the same time, diseases like neurodegeneration and mental diseases are seriously threatening human health. The emergence of the developmental origins of health and disease theory provides a feasible means for disease prevention and treatment, and the relationship between the theory and transgenerational inheritance has attracted the attention and discussion of researchers.

2 Development History of DOHaD

In the 1970s, Forsdahl was the first to report that the risk of death which resulted from coronary heart disease has something to do with poverty and prosperity and indicated that a close relationship has been seen between permanent damage to the body caused by nutritional deficiency during pregnancy and such a phenomenon. Subsequently, studies launched by Barker and his colleagues showed that nutritional deficiency during pregnancy was closely related to the occurrence of cardiovascular risks, high blood pressure, abnormal blood fat, and central obesity along with

W. Wu (✉) · P. Wu · C. Lu
School of Public Health, Nanjing Medical University, Nanjing, China
e-mail: wwu@njmu.edu.cn

Q. Tang
Department of Obstetrics, The Affiliated Obstetrics and Gynecology Hospital of Nanjing Medical University, Nanjing Maternity and Child Health Care Hospital, Nanjing, China

Y. Xia (ed.), *Early-life Environmental Exposure and Disease*,
https://doi.org/10.1007/978-981-15-3797-4_14

disordered glucose metabolism in later generations [1]. Based on this research, the hypothesis of FOAD was used to portray the possible relationship between adult disease and fetal period. Further studies found that fetal growth restriction and postnatal growth patterns caused by an adverse intrauterine environment has significant effects on adult onset. Thus, the study of the origin of health and disease was formally introduced in 2003.

Currently, with modern medicine and some related disciplines growing rapidly beneath our eyes, DOHaD theory has been constantly improved, and harmful factors are unfolded before people's eyes gradually. Definitely, maternal pregnancy has a greater influence on the health and disease of one's offspring than paternal factors [2]. According to animal models and epigenetic theory, fathers also contribute to disease and health of the offspring [3]. However, people still have a shallow understanding of the impact of fathers on the health of their offspring. At the Latsis Symposium 2017 seminar, this issue was in depth discussed and much attention should be taken by the field of public health. Early-life exposure is mainly transmitted through maternal exposures or traits [4, 5].

3 Intergeneration Effect and Transgenerational Inheritance

3.1 Intergenerational Effect

Genetic information independent of DNA sequence, acknowledged as epigenetic data, tends to be inherited between adjacent generations [6, 7]. Through animal models, researchers call the complex information layer outside the DNA sequence epigenetic markers. This marker can be passed from parent to child through gametes for intergenerational inheritance [8]. Moreover, nutritional conditions during uterine development have a permanent impact on the subsequent development of the fetus, such as metabolic diseases mentioned above [9] (Table 1).

Although epidemiological studies and related animal model studies support the hypothesis of "thrifty phenotype," to date, most studies have focused on epigenetic effects between generations rather than on epigenetic effects represented by segregation. Studies have shown that exposure to pollutants, alcohol, tobacco, and other environments can affect the normal development of the fetus, and even the improper experiences of young children during their development may have a great impact on their mental health in adulthood [2, 9, 17].

Table 1 Examples of epigenetic intergenerational inheritance

Environmentally induced intergenerational inheritance	References
Paternally indeed transgenerational inheritance of susceptibility to diabetes in mammals (rats; prediabetes increases the susceptibility to diabetes in offspring)	[7]
Thee Gpr1/Zdbf2 locus provides new paradigms for transient and dynamic genomic imprinting in mammals (locus; paternal sDMR provides lifelong, paternal specificity)	[8]
Maternal exposures to persistent organic pollutants are associated with DNA methylation of thyroid hormone-related genes in placenta differently by infant sex (Korea mothers; placental epigenetic changes of key thyroid regulating genes)	[28]
A low DNA methylation epigenotype in lung squamous cell carcinoma and its association with idiopathic pulmonary fibrosis and poorer prognosis (patients with IPF; low-methylation lung SCC that significantly correlates with IPF shows unfavorable outcome)	[32]
DNA methylation links prenatal smoking exposure to later life health outcomes in offspring (the offspring of smokers during pregnancy; an increased risk of inflammatory bowel disease or schizophrenia)	[41]
Maternal and post-weaning high-fat diets produce distinct metabolic pathways within specific genomic contexts (male Sprague-Dawley rats; maternal and post-weaning HF exposure differentially affect the epigenome within specific genomic contexts)	[48]

3.2 *Transgenerational Inheritance*

It has been found that some of the epigenetic markers are essentially removable [10]; however, epigenetic modifications are not invariably eliminated thoroughly within generations [11, 12]. Reproductive cell reprogramming is an important stage of biological development for intergenerational inheritance. Sperms carries its genetic modification into the egg, and few times after fertilization, the epigenetic modification except for the imprinted region is removed [13, 14]. The ICM cells begin to differentiate, and the epigenetic modification is implanted. When primordial germ cells and somatic cells diverge, almost all of the epigenetic modifications, including imprinted regions, are removed together. Finally, epigenetic modifications are implanted during sperm development.

There are two threads for the strict transgenerational inheritance effects. First, in males, the F0 generation is exposed to specific toxins and nutrients that can induce epigenetic effects, and the second generation (F2 generation) may acquire epigenetic effects; second, while in females, the third generation (F3 generation) may acquire epigenetic effects ultimately. The reason is that the above exposure environment will affect the male and reproductive lines of F0 generation, and also affect the female and reproductive lines of F0 generation and F1 generation. Therefore, the epigenetic characteristics acquired by these generations are not truly segregated to represent epigenetic inheritance. This review screens and distinguishes intergenerational and transgenerational inheritance (Fig. 1).

Does the DOHaD theory have something to do with transgenerational inheritance? The answer is yes. Substantial experiments of animal models indicate that

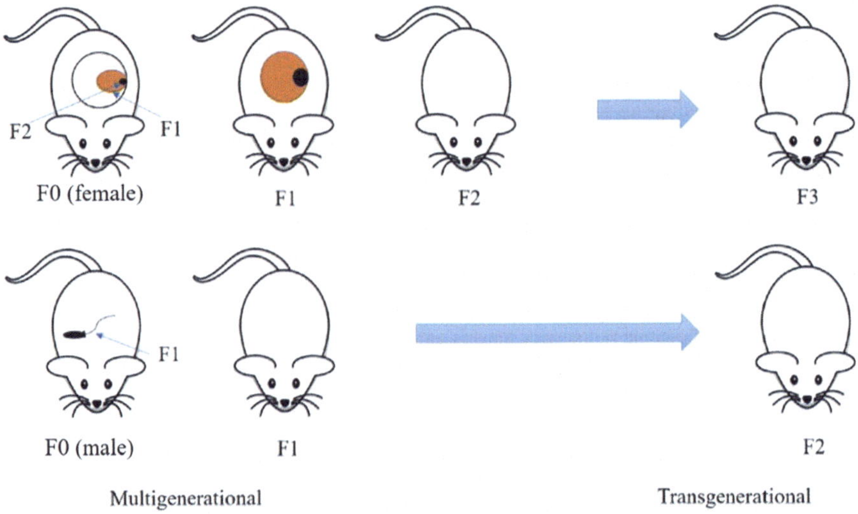

Fig. 1 Schematic of how the environmental exposure affects transgenerational inheritance. Strict transgenerational epigenetic inheritance, as shown in the figure, requires epigenetic characteristics acquired by F3 generations of female lines and F2 generations of male lines after exposure

DOHaD has transgenerational and multigenerational effects [15]. Morrison et al. [16] conducted a guinea pig model experiment and it is noteworthy that the F0 generation did not show the corresponding epigenetic characteristics, while the F2 and F3 generations showed the epigenetic characteristics. DDT has been shown to give impetus to transgenerational inheritance in adult diseased rats. Stephanie et al. exposed pregnant F0 female rats to DDT for a short time and then measured the incidence of some diseases in the subsequent F1, F2, and F3 generations. The finding was that in F2 generations, testicular diseases were more common in males than in adolescents, and in F3 generations, ovarian and kidney diseases increased [17]. Similarly, Anway and Skinner et al. [18, 19] used EDCs like vinclozolin to induce sperm epigenetic mutation to elucidate that epigenetic effects exist in the genesis and development of reproductive lines which may be related to transgenerational diseases.

But in the final analysis, the transgenerational genetic mechanism cannot be separated from the support of epigenetics, especially DNA methylation, histone modification, and the role of ncRNA [20] (Table 2).

Table 2 Examples of epigenetic transgenerational inheritance

Environmentally induced transgenerational inheritance	References
Correlation between altered DNA methylation of intergenic regions of ITPR3 and development of delayed cerebral ischemia in patients with subarachnoid hemorrhage (patients with SAH and DCI; higher levels of methylation intensity)	[10]
Stable inheritance of an acquired behavior in *Caenorhabditis elegans* (*C. elegans*: produce life-long olfactory imprints)	[13]
Primordial germ cell development and epigenetic reprogramming in mammals (rats; reveal the critical steps during PGC development)	[14]
Sperm epimutation biomarkers of obesity and pathologies following DDT-induced epigenetic transgenerational inheritance of disease (rats; inherited disease)	[17]
Transgenerational sperm DNA methylation epimutation developmental origins follow ancestral vinclozolin exposure (rats; developmental programming of the transgenerational epigenetic inheritance phenomenon occurs throughout the development of the germline)	[19]

4 Epigenetic Mechanism

4.1 What Is Epigenetic

In 1957, Conrad Waddington put forward the theory of "Waddington's epigenetic landscape" to clarify the concept of developmental biology. This theory has been processed and perfected by later generations, thus becoming epigenetics that we are now familiar with [21]. This theory implies that genetic changes occur when the nucleotide sequence of a gene does not change [22–24]. The term "epigenetics" does not refer to an additional layer above a gene; rather it is a process of gene development in which genes are expressed by different choices to gradually construct individuals [25]. Epigenetics has been used for a proper explanation of the difficult and incomprehensible problems of biology. Also it can be used to explain a long-standing mystery. By revealing how gene expression is regulated, we can better understand how genetic and non-genetic factors coordinate to determine our characteristics [26, 27]. The non-genetic factors are mainly regulated by a series of epigenetic markers. Currently, many researchers associate epigenetics with many complex diseases, such as methylation in DNA as well as RNA analysis in peripheral blood cells of patients with some diseases [28] and have made some breakthroughs, which provide a new perspective for looking at aging and various diseases [29]. Of course, the explanation of the DOHaD theory is inseparable from the study of epigenetics. At present, epigenetic studies have been carried out in areas such as neurodegeneration, cancer, metabolic diseases, and allergic diseases, which have renewed understanding and insights into the occurrence and treatment of diseases [30–35].

Epigenetic mechanisms mainly include DNA methylation, regulation of ncRNA, and histone modification. These mechanisms make a great difference in DOHaD [36–39].

4.2 DNA Methylation

Enzymes that produce, distinguish, or clear DNA methylation are classified into three categories: writers, erasers, and readers. The writer catalyzes methyl addition to cytosine residues, eraser modifies and removes methyl, and the reader recognizes and binds to methyl to affect gene output. It is through these mechanisms that DNA methylation affects DOHaD [40–42].

DNMT1, DNMT3A, and DNMT3B can directly add methyl to DNA in the DNMT (methyltransferase) family that compiles DNA methylation [43]. DNMT1 has its particularity that tends to methylate semi-methylated DNA in the process of DNA replication. DNMT1 methylate, according to the pre-replication methylation mode, can repair methylation, thus maintaining the stability of methylation of a gene [44, 45]. However, it is still unclear how methyltransferases target specific gene loci.

DNA methylation reduces the expression of some gene fragments by blocking the combination of transcriptional activators. It is worth investigating thoroughly that DNA methylation can be recognized by three family proteins: MBD protein, UHRF protein, and zinc finger protein. When methylation is recognized by these proteins, gene transcription is suppressed [46, 47].

4.3 Histone Modification

Modification of histone can be multifarious, especially when propionylation, methylation, and acetylation are included. Abnormal histone modification can lead to various pathological changes [48].

The interaction of DNA methylation and histone modification on mitochondria results in genomic imprinting. It is due to the epigenetic modification of the allele derived from a parent or its chromosome that the two alleles from different parents express differently in progeny cells [49–51] (Fig. 2).

4.4 Noncoding RNA

Through improved methodologies, researchers have found that parts of the genome that do not encode proteins do transcribe a lot, but are initially misunderstood as "transcriptional that has a firm foothold beside proteins." However, their different roles cannot be ignored [52–54]. Studies have confirmed that ncRNAs can silence multiple genes by binding to chromatin and recruiting modification elements. This counts a lot in the process of random inactivation of the X chromosome and can also be seen in DNA damage repair. An increasing number of studies have found that ncRNAs function by forming nucleic acid-protein interactions [55, 56].

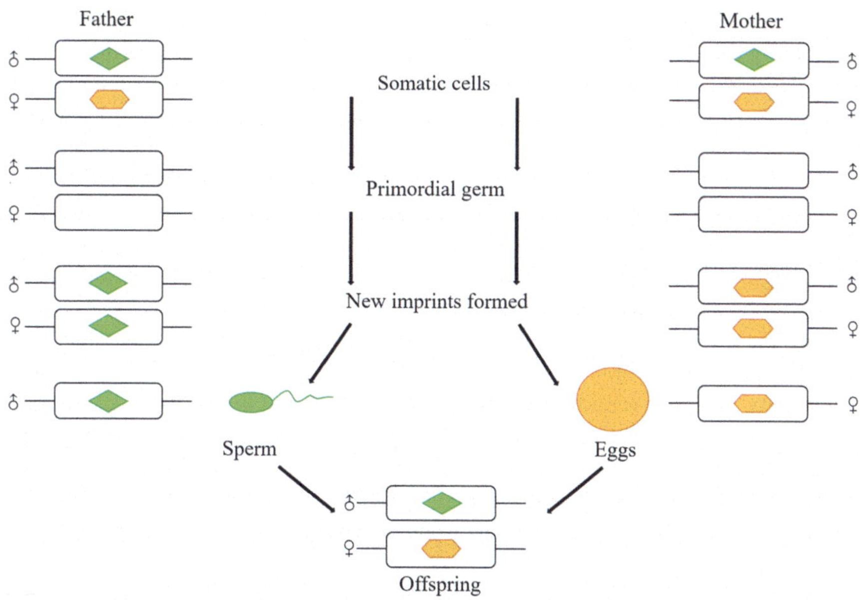

Fig. 2 The inheritable process of imprinted genes. The figure shows the reprogramming during germ cell development. A large number of imprinted genes controlled by epigenetics can resist reprogramming of fertilized eggs, but cannot resist reprogramming during germ cell development

4.5 Other Mechanisms

These three mechanisms are the most widely studied. Besides, researchers continue to seek breakthroughs from other perspectives. Maternal effects, dormant transposon activation, and some other mechanisms [57, 58] are not the points of this review. Last but not least, many diseases are not caused unilaterally by one mechanism, but by the abnormal occurrence of multiple mechanisms.

5 Development Prospects and Clinical Significance

In the past 50 years, modern medicine has developed by leaps and bounds. However, some non-communicable chronic diseases are still a thorny problem. As a result, the DOHaD theory has appealed to many people's eyes. Researchers in the field of public health around the world are trying to curb the development of diseases from the source. Many cases have confirmed that malnutrition during pregnancy can lead to a series of metabolic disorders such as diabetes and abdominal obesity in offspring [59]. In most countries that are developing or hard to develop themselves, the general level of economic development is not high, accompanied by material shortage and other adverse conditions, which has caused indelible harm to pregnant children, even through epigenetic mechanisms to the next generation [60]. Due to global resources distributing unevenly, the environmental exposure of young children during embryonic and early development varies from region to region [61]. Pertinent departments try their best to adapt to local conditions and analyze specific problems to improve the living standards of local inhabitants, the youth accounting for a large proportion particularly along with women in pregnancy. At the same time, children around the world should be educated about the DOHaD theory and improve their understanding of some important concepts. Only by understanding the role of early experience in promoting adult diseases can children improve their awareness of prevention and do a good job in preventing some chronic diseases [62, 63].

We should monitor these diseases with the help of large clinical data to facilitate further research [64]. Embryonic and early childhood development are "windows of opportunity" for intervention from the source of disease. On one hand, continuous intervention in the living environment of pregnant women and children during this period can help to prevent diseases [65]; on the other hand, by analyzing the environmental exposure of fetuses and young children in early stage, we can predict the risk of related diseases and be able to timely prevent and control them [66].

Acknowledgments This work was supported by National Natural Science Foundation of China (No. 81673217, 8197140).

References

1. Barker DJ, Winter PD, Osmond C, Margetts B, Simmonds SJ (1989) Weight in infancy and death from ischeamic heart disease. Lancet 2(8663):577–580
2. Sharp GC, Lawlor DA, Richardson SS (2018) It's the mother!: how assumptions about the casual primacy of maternal effects influence research on the developmental origins of health and disease. Soc Sci Med 213:20–27
3. Soubry A (2018) Epigenetics as a driver of developmental origins of health and disease:did we forget the fathers? BioEssays 40(1). https://doi.org/10.1002/bies.201700113
4. Soubry A (2018) POHaD: why we should study future fathers. Environ Epigenet 4(2):dvy007
5. Soubry A, Hoyo C, Jirle RL, Murphy SK (2014) A paternal environmental legacy: evidence for epigenetic inheritance through the male germ line. BioEssays 36(4):359–371
6. Wei Y, Schatten H, Sun QY (2015) Environmental epigenetic inheritance through gametes and implications for human reproduction. Hum Reprod Update 21(2):194–208
7. Wei Y, Yang CR, Wei YP, Zhao ZA, Hou Y, Schatten H, Sun QY (2014) Paternally induced transgenerational inheritance of susceptibility to diabetes in mammals. Proc Natl Acad Sci U S A 111(5):1873–1878
8. Duffle R, Ajjan S, Greenberg MV, Zamudio N, Escamilla del Arenal M, Iranzo J, Barbaux S, Fauque P, Bourc'his D (2014) The Gpr1/Zdbf2 locus provides new paradigms for transient and dynamic genomic imprinting in mammals. Genes Dev 28(5):463–478
9. Roseboom TJ (2019) Epidemiological evidence for the developmental origins of health and disease: effects of prenatal undernutrition in humans. J Endocrinol 242(1):T135–T144
10. Kim BJ, Kim Y, Hong EP, Jeon JP, Yang JS, Choi HJ, Kang SH, Cho YJ (2019) Correlation between altered DNA methylation of intergenic regions of ITPR3 and development of delayed cerebral ischemia in patients with subarachnoid Hemorrhage. World Neurosurg 130:e449–e456

11. Heard E, Martienssen RA (2014) Transgenerational epigenetic inheritance: myths and mechanisms. Cell 157(1):95–109
12. Wang L, Zhang J, Duan J, Gao X, Zhu W, Lu X, Yang L, Zhang J, Li W, Zhou Q, Aluru N, Tang F, He C, Huang X, Liu J (2014) Programming and inheritance of parental DNA methylomes in mammals. Cell 157(4):979–991
13. Remy JJ (2010) Stable inheritance of an acquired behavior in Caenorhabditis elegans. Curr Biol 20(20):R877–R878
14. Leitch HG, Tang WW, Surani MA (2013) Primordial germ-cell development and epigenetic reprogramming in mammals. Curr Top Dev Biol 104:149–187
15. Hanson MA, Skinner MK (2016) Developmental origins of epigenetic transgenerational inheritance. Environ Epigenet 2(1). pii: dvw002
16. Morrison JL, Botting KJ, Darby JRT, David AL, Dyson RM, Gatford KL, Gray C, Herrera EA, Hirst JJ, Kim B, Kind KL, Krause BJ, Matthews SG, Palliser HK, Regnault TRH, Richardson BS, Sasaki A, Thompson LP, Berry MJ (2018) Guinea pig models for translation of the developmental origins of health and disease hypothesis into the clinic. J Physiol 596 (23):5535–5569
17. King SE, McBirney M, Beck D, Sadler-Riggleman I, Nilsson E, Skinner MK (2019) Sperm epimutation biomarkers of obesity and pathologies following DDT induced epigenetic transgenerational inheritance of disease. Environ Epigenet 5(2):dvz008
18. Anway MD, Cupp AS, Uzumcu M, Skinner MK (2005) Epigenetic transgenerational actions of endocrine disruptors and male fertility. Science 308(5727):1466–1469
19. Skinner MK, Nilsson E, Sadler-Riggleman I, Beck D, Ben Maamar M, McCarrey JR (2019) Transgenerational sperm DNA methylation epimutation developmental origins following ancestral vinclozolin exposure. Epigenetics 14(7):721–739
20. Sarkies P (2019) Molecular mechanisms of epigenetic inheritance: Possible evolutionary implications. Semin Cell Dev Biol S1084-9521(18):30148–30144
21. Deichmann U (2016) Epigenetics: the origins and evolution of a fashionable topic. Dev Biol 416(1):249–254
22. Gayon J (2016) From Mendel to epigenetics: history of genetics. C R Biol 339:225–230
23. Milavetz BI, Balakrishnan L (2015) Viral epigenetics. Methods Mol Biol 1238:569–596
24. Ladd-Acosta C, Fallin MD (2016) The role of epigenetics in genetic and environmental epidemiology. Epigenomics 8(2):271–283
25. Moore DS (2017) Behavioral epigenetics. WIREs Syst Biol Med 9(1). https://doi.org/10.1002/wsbm.1333
26. Lester BM, Conradt E, Marsit C (2016) Introduction to the special section on epigenetics. Child Dev 87(1):29–37
27. Nicoglou A, Merlin F (2017) Epigenetics: a way to bridge the gap between biological fields. Stud Hist Phil Biol Biomed Sci 66:73–82
28. Kim S, Cho YH, Won S, Ku JL, Moon HB, Park J, Choi G, Kim S, Choi K (2019) Maternal exposures to persistent organic pollutants are associated with DNA methylation of thyroid hormone-related genes in placenta differently by infant sex. Environ Int 130:104956
29. Schacherer J (2016) Beyond the simplicity of Mendelian inheritance. C R Biol 339 (7–8):284–288
30. Aref-Eshghi E, Bourque DK, Kerkhof J, Carere DA, Ainsworth P, Sadikovic B, Armour CM, Lin H (2019) Genome-wide DNA methylation and RNA analyses enable reclassification of two variants of uncertain significance in a patient with clinical kabuki syndrome. Hum Mutat 40 (10):1684–1689
31. Brunet A, Berger SL (2014) Epigenetics of aging and aging-related disease. J Gerontol A Biol Sci Med Sci 69:S17–S20
32. Hata A, Nakajima T, Matsusaka K, Fukuyo M, Morimoto J, Yamamoto T, Sakairi Y, Rahmutulla B, Ota S, Wada H, Suzuki H, Matsubara H, Yoshino I, Kaneda A (2019) A low DNA methylation epigenotype in lung squamous cell carcinoma and its association with

idiopathic pulmonary fibrosis and poorer prognosis. Int J Cancer. https://doi.org/10.1002/ijc.32532
33. Potaczek DP, Harb H, Michel S, Alhamwe BA, Renz H, Tost J (2017) Epigenetics and allergy: from basic mechanisms to clinical applications. Epigenomics 9(4):539–571
34. Werner RJ, Kelly AD, Issa JJ (2017) Epigenetics and precision oncology. Cancer J 23 (5):262–269
35. Klein K, Gay S (2015) Epigenetics in rheumatoid arthritis. Curr Opin Rheumatol 27(1):76–82
36. van der Harst P, de Windt LJ, Chambers JC (2017) Translational perspective on epigenetics in cardiovascular disease. J Am Coll Cardiol 70(5):590–606
37. Barrertt JR (2017) Programming the future epigenetics in the context of DOHaD. Environ Health Perspect 125(4):A72
38. Goyal D, Limesand SW, Goyal R (2019) Epigenetic responses and the developmental origins of health and disease. J Endocrinol 242(1):T105–T119
39. Oblette A, Rondeaux J, Dumont L, Delessard M, Saulnier J, Rives A, Rives N, Rondanino C (2019) DNA methylation and histone post-translational modifications in the mouse germline following in- vitro maturation of fresh or cryopreserved prepubertal testicular tissue. Repord Biomed Online 39(3):383–401
40. Wang K, Tian Y, Zhang Y, Li X, Wei X, Hu H, Xu S (2019) Toxicity mechanism of sevoflurane in neural stem cells of rats through DNA methylation. Exp Ther Med 18(1):237–241
41. Wiklund P, Karhunen V, Richmond RC, Parmar P, Rodriguez A, De Silva M, Wielscher M, Rezwan FI, Richardson TG, Veijola J, Herzig KH, Holloway JW, Relton CL, Sebert S, Järvelin MR (2019) DNA methylation links prenatal smoking exposure to later life health outcomes in offspring. Clin Epigenet 11(1):97
42. Moody L, Wang H, Jung PM, Chen H, Pan YX (2019) Maternal and post-weaning high-fat diets produce distinct metabolic pathways within specific genomic contexts. Int J Mol Sci 20 (13):e3229
43. Yen RW, Vertino PM, Nelkin BD, Yu JJ, el-Deiry W, Cumaraswamy A, Lennon GG, Trask BJ, Celano P, Baylin SB (1992) Isolation and characterization of the cDNA encoding human DNA methyltransferase. Nucleic Acids Res 20(9):2287–2291
44. Leonhardt H, Page AW, Weier HU, Bestor TH (1992) A targeting sequence directs DNA methyltransferase to sites of DNA replication in mammalian nuclei. Cell 71(5):865–873
45. Mortusewicz O, Schermelleh L, Walter J, Cardoso MC, Leonhardt H (2005) Recruitment of DNA methyltransferase I to DNA repair sites. Proc Natl Acad Sci U S A 102(25):8905–8909
46. Hermann A, Goyal R, Jeltsch A (2004) The Dnmt1 DNA-(cytosine-C5)-methyltransferase to sites of DNA processively with high prefence for hemimethylated target sites. J Biol Chem 279 (46):48300–48359
47. Hendrich B, Bird A (1998) Identification and characterization of a family of mammalian methyl-CpG binding proteins. Mol Cell Biol 18(11):6538–6547
48. Taverna SD, Li H, Ruthenburg AJ, Allis CD, Patel DJ (2007) How chromatin-binding modules interpret histone modifications: lessons from professional pocket pickers. Nat Struct Mol Biol 14(11):1025–1040
49. Huang H, Sabari BR, Garcia BA, Allis CD, Zhao Y (2014) SnapShot: histone modifications. Cell 159(2):458–458
50. Lucca I, Hofbauer SL, Haitel A, Susani M, Shariat SF, Klatte T, De Martino M (2019) Urinary expression of genes involved in DNA methylation and histone modification for diagnosis of bladder cancer in patients with asymptomatic microscopic haematuria. Oncol Lett 18(1):57–62
51. Li D, Zhang Y, Zhang Y, Wang Q, Miao Q, Xu Y, Soares JC, Zhang X, Zhang R (2019) Correlation between the epigenetic modification of histone H3K9 acetylation of NR2B gene promoter in rat hippocampus and ethanol withdrawal syndrome. Mol Biol Rep 46 (3):2867–2875
52. Bergmann JH, Spector DL (2014) Long non-coding RNAs: modulators of nuclear structure and function. Curr Opin Cell Biol 26:10–18

53. Li YP, Wang Y (2015) Large noncoding RNAs are promising regulators in embryonic stem cells. J Genet Genomics 42(3):99–105
54. Henikoff S, Greally JM (2016) Epigenetics, cellular memory and gene regulation. Curr Biol 26 (14):R641–R666
55. Wang KC, Chang HY (2011) Molecular mechanisms of long noncoding RNAs. Mol Cell 43 (6):904–914
56. Panaud O (2016) Horizontal transfers of transposable events in eukaryotes: the flying genes. C R Biol 339(7–8):296–299
57. Harvey ZH, Chen Y, Jarosz DF (2018) Protein-based inheritance: epigenetics beyond 1 the chromosome. Mol Cell 69(2):195–202
58. Bianco-Miotto T, Craig JM, Gasser YP, van Dijk SJ, Ozanne SE (2017) Epigenetics and DOHaD: from basics to birth and beyond. J Dev Health Dis 8(5):513–519
59. Tu'akoi S, Vickers MH, Tairea K, Aung YYM, Tamarua-Herman N, 'Ofanoa M, Bay JL (2018) The significance of DOHaD for small island developing states. J Dev Orig Health Dis 9 (5):487–491
60. Haas SA, Oi K (2018) The developmental origins of health and disease in international perspective. Soc Sci Med 213:123–133
61. Macnab AJ, Mukisa R (2018) Priorities for Africa youth for engaging in DOHaD. J Dev Orig Health Dis 9(1):15–19
62. Oyamada M, Lim A, Dixon R, Wall C, Bay J (2018) Development of understanding of DOHaD concepts in students during undergraduate health professional programs in Japan and New Zealand. J Dev Orig Health Dis 9(3):253–259
63. Jaddoe VWV (2019) Translational challenges for the developmental origins of health and disease: time to fulfill the promises for innovative prevention strategies. J Dev Orig Health Dis 10(3):260–262
64. Holder LB, Haque MM, Skinner MK (2017) Machine learning for epigenetics and future medical medical applications. Epigenetics 12(7):505–514
65. Giordano C, Benyshek DC (2015) DOHaD research with populations in transition: a case study of prenatal diet remote recall with Yup'ik Alaskan women. J Dev Orig Health Dis 6(2):79–87
66. Connor KL, Bourque SL, Weaver ICG (2019) A Canadian perspective on the developmental origins of health and disease: understanding the past as a way forward. J Dev Orig Health Dis 10 (1):1–4

The manufacturer's authorised representative in the EU is Springer
Nature Customer Service Centre GmbH, Europaplatz 3, 69115 Heidelberg,
Germany. If you have any concerns regarding our products, please
contact ProductSafety@springernature.com

Printed and bound by CPI Group (UK) Ltd, Croydon, CR0 4YY
30/09/2026
02225557-0002